Orthopedic Massage

T0195418

To Elise

Your support for this project has been essential and my work would not be what it is without you.

For Elsevier

Publisher: Sarena Wolfaard
Development Editor: Helen Leng
Project Manager: Elouise Ball
Design Direction: George Ajayi
Illustration Manager: Gillian Richards
Photographer: Ross Chandler

Orthopedic Massage

Theory and Technique

Whitney Lowe, LMT

Director, Orthopedic Massage Education and Research Institute (OMERI), Sisters, Oregon, USA

Foreword by

Leon Chaitow ND DO

Osteopathic Practitioner and Honorary Fellow, School of Integrated Health, University of Westminster, London, UK

SECOND EDITION

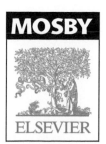

MOSBY

ELSEVIER

EDINBURGH   LONDON   NEW YORK   OXFORD   PHILADELPHIA   ST LOUIS   SYDNEY   TORONTO 2009

First edition 2003
Second edition 2009

ISBN 9780443068126

British Library Cataloguing in Publication Data
A catalogue record for this book is available from the British Library

Library of Congress Cataloging in Publication Data
A catalog record for this book is available from the Library of Congress

Notice
Knowledge and best practice in this field are constantly changing. As new research and experience broaden our knowledge, changes in practice, treatment and drug therapy may become necessary or appropriate. Readers are advised to check the most current information provided (i) on procedures featured or (ii) by the manufacturer of each product to be administered, to verify the recommended dose or formula, the method and duration of administration, and contraindications. It is the responsibility of the practitioner, relying on their own experience and knowledge of the patient, to make diagnoses, to determine dosages and the best treatment for each individual patient, and to take all appropriate safety precautions. To the fullest extent of the law, neither the publisher nor the author assumes any liability for any injury and/or damage to persons or property arising out of or related to any use of the material contained in this book.

The Publisher

Working together to grow
libraries in developing countries

www.elsevier.com | www.bookaid.org | www.sabre.org

ELSEVIER   BOOK AID International   Sabre Foundation

ELSEVIER
your source for books,
journals and multimedia
in the health sciences
www.elsevierhealth.com

The
Publisher's
policy is to use
**paper manufactured
from sustainable forests**

Printed in Great Britain
Last digit is the print number: 22

Contents

Foreword for Orthopedic Massage: Theory & Technique

Leon Chaitow, ND DO

What is Orthopedic Massage? At its simplest it can be said to be that form of massage that addresses orthopedic conditions, whether from the perspective of treatment, rehabilitation or, most importantly, prevention. Before considering the range and potential value of orthopedic massage it would be useful to acknowledge the foundations on which it has been built.

Abundant research shows that massage – in its most generic form, where its aim is to achieve relaxation, or wellness promotion – is non-invasive, almost totally safe, and with very few absolute contraindications. And when applied non-specifically, in this way, massage appears to produce consistently beneficial outcomes – involving individuals with a wide range of health problems – including autoimmune, pain and psychiatric conditions (Field 2006).

However, when massage adopts therapeutic intervention strategies, by incorporating physical medicine modalities (such as the use of heat and cold – via hydrotherapy for example), as well as a variety of active and passive soft tissue manipulation methods (such as myofascial release, muscle energy technique), or when it undertakes specific therapeutic goals, for example deactivation of trigger points, reduction of fibrosis, enhancement of lymphatic and venous drainage, etc., caution is required – particularly in cases involving pathology, active inflammation, and/or severe pain.

When massage is involved in active treatment, or rehabilitation settings associated with trauma, overuse, chronic or acute pain, post-surgical care – as examples – a requirement emerges for a comprehensive, validated (as far as this is possible in manual therapy) and above all systematic approach to therapeutic intervention. This needs to cover both assessment and treatment – and needs to include as a primary feature – contraindications and cautions. Safety becomes paramount, over and above efficacy.

Orthopedic massage – including as it does a wide range of adjunctive soft tissue modalities – as comprehensively described by Whitney Lowe in this admirable book, achieves these requirements, thoroughly.

Within the enormous range of techniques, methods, procedures and options used by the health care professions, a general rule can be seen to apply to the objectives inherent in almost all therapeutic endeavors, whether these involve brain surgery, spinal manipulation, medication, acupuncture, massage – or anything else.

Apart from the obvious desire to ease symptoms, without adding to the distress already being experienced by the individual, this 'rule' can be stated simply as an aim to reduce the adaptive load (biochemical, biomechanical, psychosocial) that the body is coping with, and/or to enhance the self-regulatory mechanisms of the body, so that they can better handle current adaptive demands.

The wide range of variations of manual techniques, as used in orthopedic massage and described in this book, comprises a number of basic generic elements, each of which carries inherent potentials for physiological change (Lederman 1997). Combinations of modes of manually applied loading – varied by the degree of force employed, the directions of force and whether this is applied constantly or intermittently; as well as the amount of time involved (brief, lengthy, pulsating) and the rate at which loads are applied (rapidly, slowly, variably, harmonically); whether the method is passive or active, or involves a combination of patient and practitioner effort, as well as which tissues are involved (muscle, fascia, scar tissue, joint, etc.), and their properties and stage of dysfunction (acute, chronic, subacute etc.), along with the practitioner's intent – create a huge range of variables that make up the potentially confusing variety of therapeutic options open to the practitioner, whether in active treatment or rehabilitation settings.

Orchestrating these variables into a systematic focus on named conditions, organised into the regions of the body, within a framework of orthopedic massage and associated modalities, in a logical and systematic manner, is one of the major achievements of this book.

Another is to place orthopedic massage, as described in the text, alongside established professional approaches to biomechanical problems, such as are used in physical medicine, osteopathy and chiropractic. The book should certainly form a resource for use in massage training, and should become an asset, from which to draw, for therapists and practitioners of all manual therapy professions.

Orthopedic Massage can be seen to be an evolving health care system, complementary to both mainstream medical, and CAM, approaches.

Reference

Field T 2006 Massage Therapy Research, Churchill Livingstone/Elsevier, Edinburgh.

Lederman E 1997 Fundamentals of Manual Therapy. Churchill Livingstone, Edinburgh.

Preface
to the First Edition

Massage as a health care treatment has been a part of medical practice in many cultures for hundreds – if not thousands – of years. However, with the rise of the pharmaceutical industry and the development of numerous technological treatments, it virtually disappeared from Western medical practice in the early twentieth century. Now we are in the middle of a resurgence – a time in which we see a renewed interest in the use of manual therapies for treatment of soft-tissue injuries and the use of massage as a therapeutic treatment.

Since Western society is notoriously plagued by stress-induced illnesses, massage has evolved into a popular remedy for helping many people reduce this stress and enhance wellness in their life. In addition, however, attention is now being focused on ways in which massage may be used to address specific pathological problems.

Soft-tissue injuries that impair function of the locomotor structures in the body are primarily addressed within the field of orthopedics. While there are numerous treatment methods for these soft-tissue problems, it is only recently that massage has come to be viewed as a beneficial treatment for specific complaints in more than a very general way.

Unfortunately, many of the individuals who have had the opportunity to learn proper application of massage techniques, especially massage therapists, have not had the background education in the field of orthopedics that leads to a comprehensive understanding of orthopedic disorders. At the same time, many of the individuals who have developed specialized knowledge and skills in the treatment of orthopedic disorders have not had the exposure to the highly specialized skills of massage therapy technique and application.

As a clinician, I have seen many individuals benefit from the effective application of massage as a therapeutic intervention for orthopedic problems. But I have also seen instances where improper application of massage treatment can be detrimental.

As an educator, I have noticed places where there are gaps in the knowledge and training of many practitioners who are using massage. Many of these individuals have good intentions, but don't understand all of the factors which must be considered in formulating an effective plan of care that includes massage.

Clinical experience has indicated that massage can be a very helpful treatment for many soft-tissue pain and injury conditions. However, in order for it to be most effective, it needs to be firmly rooted in clinical science, and applied with careful reasoning and skillful manual techniques.

While this text does not purport to be a comprehensive reference on the field of orthopedics, I have included certain fundamental principles with which a practitioner of orthopedic massage should be familiar. These principles are presented in the first several chapters. This text should also not be considered a comprehensive reference on basic massage techniques for those who have not had prior training in massage. However, I felt it important to include information on basic applications of massage in order for the reader to understand many of the treatment suggestions that are presented. Chapters 4 and 5 are designed to give a good background understanding of the use of massage as a therapeutic intervention.

The chapters that focus on a specific region of the body address commonly occurring soft-tissue pain and injury conditions. I feel that it is important for the practitioner of orthopedic massage to understand the treatments traditionally used for each problem. Therefore, I have included a description of how each condition is commonly treated, prior to a discussion of the ways in which massage may or may not be appropriate as a treatment for that particular pathology.

While knowledge of pathological conditions is valuable, that knowledge alone is not enough to ensure that an individual will be an effective practitioner of orthopedic massage. Personal interaction skills are important for any health care provider, but especially for any practitioner of massage, because the nature of the treatment brings the practitioner and patient into a very close relationship with one another. Therefore, while exploring the detailed facets of kinesiology, anatomy, mechanics, and pathology that go along with the field of orthopedics, it is essential that we never lose sight of the fact that we must work with each person as a unique individual.

It is my hope that this text will serve as a bridge to complement the skills and abilities of all those who may choose to incorporate massage as an intervention for orthopedic disorders. I have written this book with that in mind, intending that it should appeal not only to massage therapists, but physical (physio-) therapists, chiropractors, athletic trainers, nurses, physicians and any other interested professionals.

I would be delighted if this book were to become a starting point for a much larger inquiry into the use of massage for orthopedic problems. We are badly in need of research to validate the clinical experiences that form the basis for the theories presented in this book.

Finally, I hope this book will promote a fuller understanding of both pain and injury conditions, and the subsequent benefits of massage as a therapeutic intervention. Such an understanding might then bring together health care providers from these diverse professions – all of whom share a mutual interest in the healing power of touch.

Bend, Oregon, 2003
Whitney Lowe

Preface
to the Second Edition

More than six years have passed since the first edition of this book. In that short span of time there has been an increasing awareness of the valuable benefits of massage for treating soft-tissue pain and injury conditions. With musculoskeletal disorders being so prevalent worldwide, there is no shortage of need for knowledgeable and skilled massage practitioners to serve the public.

The shifting curricula in many massage education programs reflect this awareness that more people are seeking the help of massage therapists for a wide array of orthopedic disorders. Consequently, massage practitioners are looking for resource material that gives them sound guidance in developing appropriate treatment strategies to best assist those seeking their care. The changes in this second edition are a result of extensive feedback from students, educators and practicing professionals describing what would make an even better resource for them.

A great deal of advanced education in the massage field focuses on the acquisition of new techniques. Acquiring new skills is clearly a central component on the path to developing expertise. Yet, too often the emphasis on technique alone causes the practitioner to oversimplify each individual's condition and look for a simplistic recipe or routine to apply in a standard fashion. A skilled clinician must also incorporate sound clinical reasoning to determine if, and when, modification of any treatment approach is needed to fit the unique needs of each individual.

The most significant change in this second edition is in the section describing massage techniques for the various orthopedic conditions listed in the book. Many readers requested more thorough guidelines for massage treatments that were presented. In this new edition the description of specific massage techniques is greatly expanded. There is also a new section included under each condition called *Rehabilitation Protocol Considerations*. These considerations describe factors the practitioner should consider for modifications of any of the treatment techniques to make them appropriate to the stage or severity of each client's condition. This new edition has also been enhanced with color and improved photos of treatment procedures to make them more understandable. It is my sincere hope that this text becomes a guide that helps expand each practitioner's clinical skills to help the plethora of people who need care for soft-tissue pain.

Sisters, Oregon, 2008
Whitney Lowe

Acknowledgments

This book has been a continual work in progress for many years. It would not have been possible without the experiences I have had through teaching and clinical practice throughout that entire time. For that reason I am greatly indebted to the thousands of people who have contributed in that manner without realizing they were an essential part of this project.

Several people and organizations were instrumental in the early stages of supporting my interest in bringing together the field of orthopedics and massage. In particular I would like to thank the faculty, staff and students at the Atlanta School of Massage as well as the clinical staff I worked with at the Emory Clinic Sports Medicine Center in Atlanta, GA and at Timberhill Physical Therapy in Corvallis, OR. I would also like to offer special thanks to Benny Vaughn, who has been a wonderful teacher, colleague and friend all along the way.

A great deal of the material in this book has come out of my work in teaching massage. I have had the great fortune to share teaching responsibilities with some highly talented individuals and their input

and feedback has made this book far better. In particular I would like to thank Howard Weingarten, Lauren Felice, Bruce Lloyd and Lee Stang who have been working with me for years and helping refine this material. As a writer, I would also like to acknowledge the invaluable editorial assistance I have received from Elise Wolf. Her assistance in this project made it a far greater final product than I could ever have produced without her.

Thanks to Ross Chandler, David Eveland and Chelsie Hatch who all worked very hard in the preparation of the photo images in the book. I have also had great support, patience and encouragement from Sarena Wolfaard, Helen Leng, Elouise Ball and the staff at Elsevier.

Finally I would like to thank you, the readers of this book, because you will be the ones that fully bring it to life. Those of you who are practitioners are the ones out there 'in the trenches'. You will have a unique opportunity to test the concepts put forth in this text and identify new ways that this material can grow and expand in order to reduce the pain and discomfort in people's lives.

SECTION 1

General principles

For any discussion of orthopedic massage to be complete, it is essential to address some fundamental concepts. Section one addresses the basic principles necessary for the practitioner to have a proper context in which to understand the use of massage in treating orthopedic problems. The field of orthopedics is expansive, since it is the branch of medical science that deals with the movement systems of the body. To accurately address pathological problems in locomotor structures, the practitioner must understand how they work in a healthy system as well as when they are injured. A comprehensive discussion of how each of the primary locomotor tissues works in the healthy body is beyond the scope of this text. However, the most common pathological problems with the major locomotor tissues are discussed. Understanding these processes will be essential for the practitioner to identify the nature of most soft-tissue problems, and to determine the appropriateness and application of massage treatment.

This first section also discusses the fundamental principles of massage as a therapeutic intervention. While this text is not meant as an instructional manual in basic massage therapy applications, it is important to include general guidelines about the methods of massage for those who have not had much exposure to it. There are numerous books, videos and educational programs that cover the basics of massage in more detail. The reader is strongly encouraged to get adequate training in basic massage skills before attempting the advanced treatment methods suggested in this text.

Chapter 1

Introduction to orthopedic massage

Orthopedic massage is a relative newcomer to the many current massage modalities. As a broader category, orthopedic massage applies to treatment of conditions resulting from any number of activities, such as work, sports, or accidents. Current studies show increasing use and acceptance of massage.[1,2] One of the primary reasons for massage's popularity is the success massage has had in therapeutic applications. In the last 50 years massage has developed from a primarily relaxation and stress release solution to a therapeutic modality applied to complicated musculoskeletal disorders.

Orthopedic massage offers practitioners working in this setting an organized and effective approach to handling the greater needs of today's clients. Orthopedic massage practitioners are found working with professional sports and dance teams, in occupational therapy settings, and with physical therapists, chiropractors, and osteopaths. In many cases, massage is proving to be more effective than other modalities for treating certain conditions. In fact, millions of people have sought complementary care for musculoskeletal problems.

Similar to sports massage, there are different systems of orthopedic massage and it has yet to be standardized as one system or approach. Consequently, those educators using the term orthopedic massage to refer to a particular system may or may not be talking about the same thing. While there are distinct differences in these systems, there are also fundamental similarities, particularly assessment, treatment variability, and knowledge of common pain and injuries.

In this text, orthopedic massage is presented as a comprehensive system for the treatment of soft-tissue orthopedic disorders. By system, it is meant that to effectively treat pain and injuries a systematic approach should be employed. As in other orthopedic massage approaches, assessment and technique variety are key components. What sets this system apart perhaps is its emphasis on establishing a physiological rationale for a particular treatment approach or technique. Thus, matching the condition to the treatment is argued to be essential for effective therapeutic solutions. This system also promotes the idea that a full therapeutic treatment must understand and integrate standard rehabilitation protocols for the various soft-tissue dysfunctions. The orthopedic massage system presented in this text is increasingly emerging as a generally accepted model of orthopedic massage as evidenced in trade journal publications and courses taught in schools.

MUSCULOSKELETAL DISORDERS AND MASSAGE

Musculoskeletal disorders (MSDs) are one of the primary reasons people seek medical care worldwide. In the United States MSDs are rampant and are the second most common reason for visits to the doctor, infectious diseases being the first.[3–5] Many of these disorders result from the repetitive demands of work-related activities. These repetitive stress injuries (RSIs), also called cumulative trauma disorders (CTDs), are a pressing burden on our health care system. Estimates suggest RSIs may account for as much as 56% of all occupational injuries in the United States.[6]

Recreational and daily activities place additional strains on the body's soft tissues. Sports, gardening, hobbies, exercise (or lack of), and general household tasks are prime scenarios for developing pain or injuries. Of course, accidents also motivate individuals to seek treatment for musculoskeletal dysfunction. Common conditions include a wide array of soft-tissue problems including strains, sprains, tendinosis, myofascial trigger points, nerve entrapment, and the ever-present host of biomechanical problems resulting from chronic muscle tightness.

Because MSDs primarily affect tissues of the locomotor (movement) system, they are properly classified as orthopedic conditions. Orthopedics is the "branch of medical science that deals with prevention or correction of disorders involving locomotor structures of the body especially the skeleton, joints, muscles, fascia, and other supporting structures such as ligaments and cartilage."[7] With the locomotor soft tissues making up the majority of our body structure, it is no wonder that MSDs are so pervasive.

Physicians, physiotherapists (physical therapists in the USA), occupational therapists, chiropractors, massage therapists, acupuncturists, athletic trainers, nurses, and other movement system specialists treat MSDs. Individuals seeking care for MSDs are increasingly turning to various complementary and alternative medicine (CAM) approaches; particularly massage.[2,8–11,18] In the United States data suggest that individuals visit massage therapists over 114 million times per year.[2]

A 2005 study on the practice patterns of massage therapists found that about 60% of visits to massage therapists each year were for musculoskeletal symptoms.[10] Extrapolating those figures one could estimate over 68 million office visits to massage therapists each year to address MSDs. This number is likely to increase significantly with the aging of the baby-boomer population. Part of the reason for this movement away from mainstream treatment for these conditions is that historically the treatment options offered in that setting focused on drugs and surgery. Critiques of mainstream MSD treatment point to a deficiency in training to address minor musculoskeletal dysfunction.[3,12–14] A result is a gap in effective treatment options.

People are choosing massage treatment because soft-tissue therapy for MSDs is proving to be an effective and comparably affordable option. Massage therapists are the primary group offering massage treatment for MSDs and their hands-on, palpatory skills set them apart from other health care practitioners. Physical therapists help fill the treatment gap and are increasingly adding more manual soft-tissue therapy to their treatment protocols. Practitioners in other fields use massage for soft-tissue treatment as well. In this text we consider massage therapy a practice performed by professionals in a number of fields. In this text, references to practitioner and client designate the individual performing the treatment and the individual receiving the treatment, respectively, regardless of the practitioner's profession.

Unfortunately and for a variety of reasons, appropriate entry-level training for treating MSDs is lacking in massage therapy education. As a result, massage practitioners generally use continuing education seminars and workshops to improve their skills and knowledge in this area. However, the education gained in continuing education courses often does not go past simply amassing an arsenal of new treatment techniques. Clinical reasoning and analysis, in addition to sound knowledge of anatomy, physiology, and MSDs, are essential for effective treatment.[15,16]

Given the new popularity of massage as a pain and injury treatment, the goal of massage education today should be proper training at the entry and advanced levels. It is important to remember that while massage is generally a safe treatment, it is not benign. Massage produces effects; these effects can be beneficial or adverse. The first test of a qualified practitioner is the ability to determine the appropriateness of massage as a treatment for a condition. The better a practitioner understands anatomy, physiology, kinesiology, and massage treatment, the more likely that person is going to be capable of creating an effective treatment plan. For both practitioners and massage educators, this text provides a solid foundation in knowledge, skills, and abilities in using massage therapy for relieving the pain and suffering of common musculoskeletal disorders.

WHAT IS ORTHOPEDIC MASSAGE?

The orthopedic massage system presented here offers practitioners a systematic and effective approach to treating pain and injuries. *Orthopedics* is the "branch of medical science that deals with prevention or correction of disorders involving locomotor structures of the body especially the skeleton, joints, muscles, fascia, and other supporting structures such as ligaments and cartilage."[7] Thus, orthopedic massage is a modality that seeks to address *orthopedic conditions* – those pain and injuries affecting the locomotor soft tissues.

Orthopedic massage is often referred to as a comprehensive system. What this means is that an orthopedic massage approach moves beyond a focus on a particular technique to include a more comprehensive approach to rehabilitation. The orthopedic massage system presented here includes several key components: assessment, treatment technique variety, knowledge of conditions and physiology, understanding of the physiological effects of techniques, and rehabilitation protocols.

Similar to the learning of any skill, orthopedic massage takes practice and continual learning. Yet, becoming a superior clinician working with orthopedic disorders is a far greater challenge. One constantly faces unique clinical decisions that require creative thought and analysis. The ability to mentally step away from routine and assumptions, and apply analytical thought processes is the mark of an advanced clinical massage practitioner. Combining foundational knowledge with clinical decision processes allows the practitioner to adapt to the unique presentations of the client. This over-arching skill is a critical component of competent soft-tissue therapy.

THE FOUR PRIMARY COMPONENTS OF ORTHOPEDIC MASSAGE

Four components characterize the system of orthopedic massage: (1) orthopedic assessment; (2) matching the physiology of the tissue injury with the physiological effects of treatment; (3) treatment adaptability; and (4) appropriate use of the rehabilitation protocol.

Orthopedic assessment

A critical component to any orthopedic massage system is *assessment* and evaluation. Assessment is more than an abbreviated interview. Client expectations of massage therapists today demand more thorough evaluation skills. Massage practitioners who treat clients with either mild or more severe pain or injuries must develop the skills necessary to assess the nature of the client's condition and continue to evaluate it through the progression of treatment. A practitioner should never assume that a client's pain or discomfort is a matter of simple tension or stress. Initial assessment evaluates the appropriateness of massage in addition to the nature of the complaint.

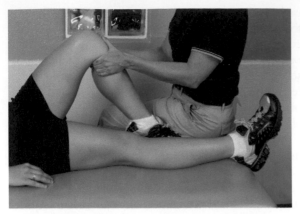

Figure 1.1 Assessment is a crucial component of orthopedic massage.

Assessment does not need to be a drawn out activity. Indeed, sometimes evaluations are quick and simple. However, having the capability to pursue the suspicion of something more involved requires assessment knowledge and skill. Without knowing more about a client's condition, treatment becomes guesswork based on assumptions, not critical reasoning and thinking. Even with a physician's diagnosis, the skilled practitioner should be able to perform their own evaluation in order to gain the information needed for treatment.

While there can be basic treatment protocols for most conditions, treatment approaches should not be condensed into simplistic recipes. Orthopedic massage promotes the use of scientific and research-based knowledge in its treatment protocols. Sufficient and valid knowledge and understanding of the locomotor system, its tissues, and common pain and injury conditions is a prerequisite for orthopedic massage. Without adequate understanding of soft-tissue function, treatment may be at minimum futile and at worse complicate the condition. The goal of treatment is to reduce symptoms and improve tissue function in the involved tissues. This requires the practitioner should have some inclination as to the nature of the tissue pathology. Assessment also allows the practitioner to determine if massage is in fact appropriate for the condition and to refer the client to another health care provider if massage is contraindicated.

Assessment is *the systematic process of gathering information to make informed decisions about treatment*. Treating pain and injuries requires the

practitioner be able to assess the nature of the condition and understand its physiological characteristics. Fundamental questions about a condition are often answered in assessment; this allows the practitioner to make educated treatment decisions. What tissues are involved, and how, and the status of those tissues can be revealed through a proper evaluation. In the simplest terms, the practitioner should know whether the tissues involved are muscle, fascia, tendon, ligament, joint capsule, nerve, cartilage, or bursa.

A practitioner can also evaluate the potential type of dysfunction in the tissue (tear, hypertonicity, myofascial trigger point, strains, sprains, nerve conduction impairment, etc.). Evaluating the biomechanical forces that produce these tissue effects will also help the practitioner understand the status of the tissues. Assessment provides the practitioner with important information about the client's tissues in order to create a clinically sound treatment plan.[17]

Box 1.1   Basic Assessment Tools

History
Observation
Palpation
Range-of-Motion and Resistance Testing
Special Tests

There is a distinct difference between assessment and diagnosis. A physician uses assessment and the information gathered to determine a diagnosis. Diagnosis is the identification and labeling of a disease, illness or condition made by a licensed medical professional. Diagnosis is not within the scope of practice for the massage therapist; however, it is for other health care practitioners who may be using soft-tissue treatment in their practice. For the massage therapist, the point of assessment is not to come up with a hard and fast name for the client's problem. A massage practitioner should never tell a client they have a specific condition, as that is giving a diagnosis. A practitioner can discuss with the client the tissues they believe to be involved and how. Further identification of the condition should be referred to another health care practitioner.

Assessment used by the massage practitioner is an ongoing process that begins with the initial visit and continues throughout the duration of treatment(s). Gauging the client's pain levels and symptoms is integral to assessment. Noting these symptoms in an initial evaluation provides a baseline against which progress is measured. It allows the practitioner to keep track of their client's progress and make educated decisions about continued therapy approaches. In addition, both the initial and ongoing evaluations can supply information to other health care professionals working with the client. Skilled assessment also builds the client/practitioner relationship, further enhancing treatment.

Assessment, however, is not an exact science. It relies heavily on the skilled clinical reasoning of the practitioner. There are no specific evaluation techniques that can provide a 100% positive result in establishing the tissues and dysfunction involved. In some cases, the nature of the client's pain is straightforward. In other cases, the condition can be far more complicated. An immediate assumption about the nature of a client's pain or problem is best avoided. It is not uncommon for conditions to have similar or identical symptoms. In many cases, finding the source of a client's complaint is not possible, regardless of practitioner's experience or knowledge. In this case, continual exploration, monitoring, and referral to another professional are the best approaches.

Proper application of assessment strategies decreases the practitioner's guesswork and helps make accurate, knowledge-based decisions about treatment or referral. Those involved in finding solutions for musculoskeletal problems with soft-tissue therapy know that massage is not benign. Massage produces significant tissue changes and effects; thus its effectiveness in treating such conditions. While massage's effects are often beneficial, they can also be ineffective or contraindicated. It is advisable to refer clients with more severe pain or injuries to a more qualified health care professional.

Matching treatment to injury

A second integral component of this orthopedic massage approach is to *match the physiology of the injury with the physiological effects of the treatment technique*. A host of therapeutic techniques are available to the massage practitioner.

Yet, no single massage modality effectively treats all of the diverse pain and injury conditions. A practitioner should have a solid foundation in the most common treatment approaches for conditions. Having a diversity of techniques to draw from to address a client's complaint is advisable. However, the practitioner must understand how their techniques interact with tissues involved in a pain or injury condition. The orthopedic massage practitioner needs to be familiar with the physiological effects of each treatment technique to make a decision about the most appropriate treatment strategy.

Understanding the physiological effects of a technique means knowing physiologically how and in what way a technique is helpful for a particular tissue dysfunction. For the most effective treatment, the physiological effects of the treatment should specifically address the nature of the pain or injury condition. An example is soft-tissue treatment for carpal tunnel syndrome. Massage is a highly effective treatment for this condition, often preventing the need for surgery or other invasive techniques if the appropriate techniques are chosen. However, carpal tunnel syndrome involves entrapment of the median nerve underneath the flexor retinaculum. Any soft-tissue technique that exacerbates the nerve compression is contraindicated, for example transverse friction massage. A massage technique that would more effectively match the physiology of the condition would be deep longitudinal stripping to the wrist flexor muscle group, thus leading to a decrease in cumulative tension in the muscle-tendon units and subsequent reduction in the tenosynovitis that aggravates the median nerve.

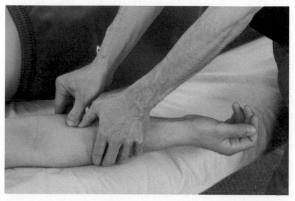

Figure 1.2   Deep stripping to the wrist flexor muscles.

Adaptability is key, however, when applying a technique to a tissue dysfunction. Variations in injury or condition may result in a treatment working in one instance and not in another. Informed treatment decisions come not from the simple amassing of techniques, but more from being able to apply knowledge and critical thinking skills to the unique presentations of their clients. In addition, symptoms can mimic those of other conditions. For example, what may seem like an obvious case of carpal tunnel syndrome, using the example above, may not be. If the condition is due to nerve compression in the thoracic outlet longitudinal stripping on the wrist flexors, while perhaps resolving local wrist symptoms, would not lead to complete resolution of the problem. Without further exploration of the unique physiology of the condition, the client's symptoms would likely continue and could worsen. In this example, resolving tension and compression on the nerves in the thoracic outlet region is a crucial part of treatment.

Treatment adaptability

The third component of orthopedic massage is treatment adaptability. The practitioner should be skilled in the basic treatment techniques most frequently used for pain and injury massage. The techniques discussed in this text will provide soft-tissue practitioners with a solid foundation from which to build their skill base. The more techniques the practitioner masters, the more potential treatment tools they have at their disposal. Mastering the treatment techniques presented in this text is a wise goal for those working with orthopedic conditions. The best treatment plan for a condition is not based on highly specialized techniques but on the best technique for that particular tissue injury and client. Effective clinical reasoning plays a critical role in choosing which of those techniques are most effective in a particular clinical case.

Clearly, considering the diversity of problems with which clients may present, the practitioner should not rigidly adhere to any one particular technique. There is no single technique or method that works for all soft-tissue pathology. However, the practitioner should also be careful

about simply amassing an encyclopedic array of different techniques. As the practitioner's practice develops and the basic therapeutic techniques are mastered, expanding one's technique options is an advisable goal. Further study of the techniques presented here will advance the practitioner's understanding of the techniques and their skills. The practitioner can then choose from a wide variety of treatment methods to find the approach that is most appropriate for each client's unique rehabilitation needs.

This text provides suggested treatment protocols for the conditions discussed, but these are a basic framework. These treatments should not be interpreted as prescribed treatment routines. The practitioner must be prepared to adapt to a particular presentation and/or alter a treatment course. Ignoring the uniqueness of the client's particular presentation will blind a practitioner to essential information needed for addressing the client's complaint. The practitioner must use their assessment and critical thinking skills to choose and adapt treatment methods or techniques to address the unique situation of each individual client.

Appropriate use of the rehabilitation protocol

The rehabilitation protocol is the final component in this system of orthopedic massage. The rehabilitation protocol is the course of injury management used to support recovery. Following this protocol is important for recovery. Rushing the soft-tissue injury repair process is a leading cause of treatment failure for musculoskeletal disorders. Massage can play an integral role at various stages of this process, particularly in normalizing tissues and regaining flexibility. How involved the soft-tissue practitioner is in managing a client's rehabilitation will depend on their skills and qualifications. However, the orthopedic massage practitioner can play an important part in the rehabilitative process with a wide-range of pain and injury conditions.

The rehabilitation protocol is a four-step process; although the steps often overlap. Each step is important and necessary for complete recovery from soft-tissue dysfunction or injury. These steps are especially important if the client will be subjected to the offending activity that created the problem initially. For example, the athlete who must return to training or the carpenter who must go back to work will benefit from following through on the process. At the same time, elements such as motivation, time pressures, and psychological factors must be considered when determining an effective rehabilitation plan.

The four steps of the rehabilitation protocol are to normalize soft-tissue dysfunction, improve flexibility, restore proper movement patterns, and strengthen and condition the tissues. An easy way to remember the four steps is with the acronym, NIRS. For proper rehabilitation from soft-tissue injury, the client should generally progress through these stages in the order presented. However, it is common for the steps to overlap and one step need not be fully complete before moving on to the next. However, following the general outline and order of the steps is important.

Box 1.2 Rehabilitation Protocol

Normalize soft-tissue dysfunction
Improve flexibility
Restore proper movement patterns
Strengthening and conditioning

The first step is to normalize the soft-tissue dysfunction. The practitioner should understand what the healthy function of the involved tissues is in order to return the tissues to as near that state as possible. For example, if chronic muscle tightness and myofascial trigger points are the complaint, then therapy that normalizes muscular tone and neutralizes myofascial trigger points would be used. Massage is a valuable treatment option in this stage of rehabilitation. Other modalities are also used at this stage including thermal modalities and therapies used by other health care providers.

The use of multiple modalities to normalize soft-tissue dysfunction is of great advantage. Interdisciplinary treatment encourages practitioners of different methods to work together for the most effective outcomes. Combining different treatment modalities can offer distinct advantages for certain conditions. For example, chiropractic treatment performed in conjunction with massage therapy can prove more beneficial because proper alignment of bony structure is easier to achieve if the muscles pulling on the bones are in a more relaxed state.

The second stage of the rehabilitation protocol is to improve flexibility. When this rehabilitation step should be introduced depends on the client's condition and other factors. Improving flexibility is sometimes integrated into initial therapies that seek to normalize the tissues. However, stretching may or may not be beneficial in the early stages of recovery. In some cases, stretching is not recommended. For example, if a client has severe carpal tunnel syndrome, any attempts to stretch the flexor muscles of the wrist may cause severe pain and aggravate the condition by stretching the median nerve. In this instance, flexibility training is not appropriate until a later stage in the treatment. Knowledge of the condition, client history, and the stage of rehabilitation are critical (see assessment above).

Dysfunctional compensating neuromuscular patterns can develop as a result of injury. Along with regaining normal function and flexibility, rehabilitation should include re-integrating proper movement patterns. Protective muscle spasm or biomechanical imbalance result from compensation as the body

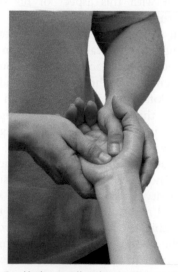

Figure 1.3 Understanding how massage fits in with other aspects of any soft-tissue rehabilitation process is essential for effective outcomes.

attempts to compensate for the injury. Acquiring new neuromuscular patterns will be more successful when the patterns are repeated regularly and frequently.[18] Rehabilitation protocols generally incorporate methods to encourage the client to return to proper movement patterns. Biomechanical corrections such as postural change are an example. Massage can play a role in this aspect of rehabilitation as well. In an ideal situation, the tissue dysfunction is normalized and flexibility is restored prior to this step; however, this is not always possible and this step becomes interspersed with steps 1 and 2.

Strength training and conditioning for specific activities is the last stage of the rehabilitation protocol. Once flexibility and proper movement patterns are initiated, strengthening and conditioning help the body prepare for future movement demands. Rehabilitative exercises and stretching should only be performed when the tissues are able to accomplish these activities without being further injured or impaired. With greater conditioning, the likelihood of re-injury is reduced. Conditioning activities are routinely performed while the client is still establishing proper movement patterns (which can be a long process). Engaging increased muscular demand while focusing on correct mechanics facilitates proper movement coordination.

The average client is not always inclined to follow through with this aspect of his or her recovery, but this step remains important. Those in professional sports understand the critical role of conditioning. The physical demands from many occupations and weekend activities are enough to warrant the client follow through on a conditioning regimen. Soft-tissue practitioners can assist their clients in this process by explaining why rehabilitation is important and encouraging their clients to follow through.

For the average person strengthening and conditioning does not have to be a time consuming or difficult activity. Often it is a matter of simply using household items already available or simple exercises. Rehabilitation protocols are provided for each of the conditions discussed in this text (see the Section 2 chapters). Certain aspects of the rehabilitation protocol, such as supervised exercise programs, may be out of the scope of practice for some soft-tissue practitioners. In this case, the massage practitioner can work alongside other health care professionals for the most effective results. The practitioner who understands the rehabilitation process and can follow the different stages of their client's progress is much more effective in treating their client's complaint.

PRACTITIONER CARE

Orthopedic massage can be a particularly successful style of massage to incorporate in a practitioner's practice. Today's clients are increasingly seeking this type of therapy and meeting these demands can stimulate one's career. At the same time, orthopedic massage can be a physically demanding practice as are many other styles of more engaged massage. The soft-tissue practitioner who chooses to treat pain and injury conditions often uses techniques that require a high degree of force or effort; for example, the deep longitudinal stripping methods performed with active engagement. Longevity in today's massage career requires practitioners take as much care of their own physical needs as they do their clients.

Massage practitioners benefit from strength training and flexibility programs, not just for the wrist and hands, but for the forearms, shoulders, and back. General and regular conditioning is a good policy for massage therapists. Employing proper postural form is critical not only for correct technique application, but for reducing

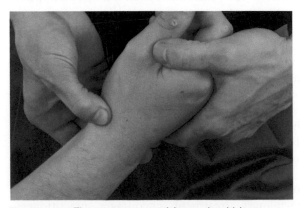

Figure 1.4 The massage practitioner should be conscious about self-care in order to encourage the greatest career longevity. Massage is a physically demanding occupation and should be conditioned for accordingly.

practitioner discomfort and dysfunction. Following the standard body mechanics entry-level therapists learn is a great starting point. Many therapists also find tai chi practice to be particularly useful training, as the basic posture of tai chi is quite similar to that used in massage practice. A simple conditioning activity of drawing the letters of the alphabet in the air with a broom, while holding it in one hand is a great way to condition many of the muscles subjected to overuse in the daily practice of massage. Finally, massage therapists are vulnerable to cumulative trauma injuries. Utilizing the massage techniques for these types of conditions will prevent long-term dysfunction for the soft-tissue practitioner. Massage is always recommended for the massage practitioner!

References

1. Cherkin DC, Sherman KJ, Deyo RA, Shekelle PG. A review of the evidence for the effectiveness, safety, and cost of acupuncture, massage therapy, and spinal manipulation for back pain. Ann Intern Med. 2003;138(11):898–906.
2. Eisenberg DM, Davis RB, Ettner SL, et al. Trends in alternative medicine use in the United States, 1990–1997: results of a follow-up national survey. JAMA. 1998;280(18):1569–1575.
3. Craton N, Matheson GO. Training and clinical competency in musculoskeletal medicine. Identifying the problem. Sports Med. 1993;15(5):328–337.
4. McCaig LF, Burt CW. National Hospital Ambulatory Medical Care Survey: 2001 emergency department summary. Adv Data. 2003(335):1–29.
5. Praemer A, Furner S, Rice DP. Musculoskeletal Conditions in the United States. Rosemont, IL: American Academy of Orthopedic Surgeons; 1999.
6. Melhorn JM. Cumulative trauma disorders and repetitive strain injuries. The future. Clin Orthop. 1998(351):107–126.
7. Thomas C. Taber's Cyclopedic Medical Dictionary. 15th ed. Philadelphia: F.A. Davis Company; 1987.
8. Barnes PM, Powell-Griner E, McFann K, Nahin RL. Complementary and alternative medicine use among adults: United States, 2002. Adv Data. 2004(343):1–19.
9. Tindle HA, Davis RB, Phillips RS, Eisenberg DM. Trends in use of complementary and alternative medicine by US adults: 1997–2002. Altern Ther Health Med. 2005;11(1):42–49.
10. Sherman KJ, Cherkin DC, Kahn J, et al. A survey of training and practice patterns of massage therapists in two US states. BMC Complement Altern Med. 2005;5:13.
11. Sherman KJ, Dixon MW, Thompson D, Cherkin DC. Development of a taxonomy to describe massage treatments for musculoskeletal pain. BMC Complement Altern Med. 2006;6:24.
12. Callahan DJ. The adequacy of medical school education in musculoskeletal medicine. J Bone Joint Surg Am. 1999;81(10):1501–1502.
13. Matzkin E, Smith EL, Freccero D, Richardson AB. Adequacy of education in musculoskeletal medicine. J Bone Joint Surg Am. 2005;87-A(2):310–314.
14. DiCaprio MR, Covey A, Bernstein J. Curricular requirements for musculoskeletal medicine in American medical schools. J Bone Joint Surg Am. 2003;85-A(3):565–567.
15. Butler D. Mobilisation of the Nervous System. London: Churchill Livingstone; 1991.
16. Epstein RM, Hundert EM. Defining and assessing professional competence. JAMA. 2002;287(2):226–235.
17. Lowe W. Orthopedic Assessment in Massage Therapy. Sisters, OR: Daviau-Scott; 2006.
18. Fritz S. Mosby's Fundamentals of Therapeutic Massage. 2nd ed. St. Louis: Mosby; 2000.

Chapter 2

Understanding soft–tissue injuries

Treating orthopedic disorders effectively requires that the practitioner have a working knowledge of the soft tissues in health as well as in pathology. This chapter focuses on the basic function of the human body's major soft tissues and the most common ways in which they are injured or dysfunctional. The reader is encouraged to review their favorite anatomy and physiology texts for a more comprehensive discussion of healthy physiological function for these tissues.

The following will prepare the practitioner with a basic understanding of the common disorders that affect the soft tissues. There are a few basic injuries that can occur to the various soft tissues, for example hypertonicity, strains, sprains, and tears. The emphasis here is placed on the most commonly occurring problems as they appear in the particular tissue, for example hypertonicity in muscle or sprains in ligaments. Orthopedic disorders do not always have a special name, but are simply these common dysfunctions. Knowing how each tissue can be injured prepares the practitioner with information for evaluating a treatment protocol.

Section 2 (starting with Chapter 6) discusses the specific conditions that have unique clinical characteristics; again, the discussion is limited to those disorders most seen in the massage therapy clinic. This chapter provides the reader with information not presented in the later chapters on specific conditions. Understanding the basic framework of conditions discussed below will facilitate the reader's understanding of the conditions discussed in later chapters.

MUSCLE

Skeletal muscle is the most abundant tissue in the body, and makes up about 40–45% of the body's total weight.[1] With such a large amount of muscle tissue in the body it is not surprising there are so many muscle-related complaints. Despite their ubiquitous presence, muscles are often overlooked as a cause of soft-tissue pain and disability.[2,3]

The primary function of muscles is to contract in order to produce the acceleration, deceleration or static position of skeletal structures. Muscles must have a high degree of pliability and elasticity in order to function properly. They also have neurological connections for the transmission of sensory and motor signals to and from the central nervous system.

There are three types of muscle contraction. A concentric contraction is one in which the muscle shortens. Shortening occurs because the tension developed within the muscle overcomes the external resistance. For example, when the biceps brachii receives a contraction stimulus, and its contraction force is greater than any resistance, the forearm flexes at the elbow in a concentric contraction (Fig. 2.1).

When forces on the muscle are equal, i.e. when the tension developed within the muscle matches the external resistance, an isometric contraction occurs. No movement is produced at the joint with isometric contraction. In an eccentric contraction the external resistance is greater than the tension developed

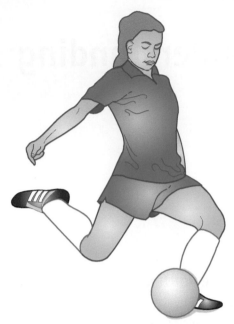

Figure 2.2   Muscle injury in quadriceps from eccentric contraction.

within the muscle. As a result, the muscle must lengthen while still receiving a contraction stimulus from the nervous system. Essentially the muscle is slowly letting go of its contraction. Eccentric contractions occur during the deceleration of movement. Eccentric contractions are the most common cause of muscular injury (Fig. 2.2).[4–7]

Numerous factors cause muscle injuries. Overuse, lack of proper conditioning, metabolic stress, or fatigue are some of the most common causes.[8,9] These factors can lead to a number of specific pathological processes in the muscle tissue. The most common types of muscle pathology include hypertonicity, atrophy, strain and contusion. Each of these problems is explored in greater detail to develop a comprehensive understanding of muscular dysfunctions.

Hypertonicity

One of the most commonly occurring soft-tissue pathologies is muscular hypertonicity, or more simply, tight muscles.[10] Yet this problem rarely receives the level of attention it deserves based on its frequency of occurrence. It is almost as if the idea of tight muscles is too simple to be considered an orthopedic 'condition' in its own right. However, biomechanical disturbances are routinely attributed to muscle imbalance and tightness.

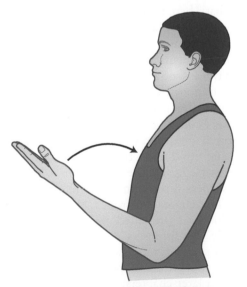

Figure 2.1   Concentric contraction of the biceps brachii.

Muscle tightness appears for several reasons. It frequently develops due to an increased rate of contraction stimulus, causing the muscle to hold a higher degree of resting tonus than it normally would. Some form of stress causes the increased muscular tone. Possible stresses include: mechanical, such as a postural distortion; chemical, such as excessive intake of caffeine; or psychological.

Hypertonic muscles may appear shortened during postural evaluation or range-of-motion testing. They will feel tight when investigated with palpation compared to other unaffected tissues. Hypertonic muscles are also more resistant to stretching, and may therefore have limitations in range of motion. The client usually reports some degree of pain and/or discomfort with palpation or stretching of the muscle.

Trigger points

Another dysfunctional process that is related to muscular tightness is the myofascial trigger point. Trigger points have begun to receive attention as a serious cause of soft-tissue pain. It is through the monumental work of Janet Travell, MD and her colleagues that these issues first received widespread attention. Travell defined a myofascial trigger point as 'A hyperirritable spot in skeletal muscle that is associated with a hypersensitive palpable nodule in a taut band. The spot is painful on compression and can give rise to characteristic referred pain, referred tenderness, motor dysfunction, and autonomic phenomena'.[11]

Medical researchers still don't fully understand trigger points, but current theories are evolving as to their cause. McPartland states that trigger points result from dysfunctional activity at the motor end plates in the muscle.[12] Trigger points result from lack of exercise, muscle overload, postural distress, metabolic problems, sleep disturbances, or various other causes.[10,12,13]

Identification of myofascial trigger points and their characteristic referral patterns is a crucial skill for any practitioner using orthopedic massage. There are numerous charts and maps of myofascial trigger point pain referral patterns that are useful references. However, the practitioner is encouraged to use these diagrams as a reference point, not as an infallible map because trigger point pain referral patterns can differ between individuals.

Atrophy

Muscular atrophy impairs function due to disuse and denervation (loss or impairment of nerve supply to the muscle). Denervation may be the result of nerve compression syndromes, systemic disease, or traumatic damage to the nerve or neuromuscular interface. Lack of proper neurological stimulation quickly leads to a loss in the size and contractile strength of the muscle. This size and strength loss can have significant detrimental effects on normal biomechanics.

Disuse atrophy is a frequent problem in muscles because it usually accompanies another injury where a limb is partially or fully immobilized during the healing process. There is greater atrophy if the muscle is immobilized in a shortened position. The primary anti-gravity muscles – such as the quadriceps, gluteals, and erector spinae – are most affected by disuse atrophy. The anti-gravity muscles are those that resist the downward pull of gravity when one is engaged in normal locomotion.

For example, muscle disuse atrophy that occurs with knee injuries is more common in the quadriceps than in the hamstring muscles. The quadriceps muscles are anti-gravity muscles, whereas the hamstrings are not. In addition, most injuries that require knee immobilization maintain the knee in an extended position, which puts the quadriceps in a shortened position while the hamstrings are lengthened.[8] Pain avoidance from an injury also leads to disuse atrophy. It is remarkable how quickly disuse atrophy may develop, and muscles affected by it will rapidly lose significant strength.[14]

Strain

Excessive tensile stress on a muscle can produce tearing of the muscle fibers; this injury is defined as a strain. The common name for a muscle strain is a pulled muscle. However, it is not an excess of stretch alone that produces the greatest number of strains on a muscle. Muscle strains occur most often from some degree of stretch tension on a contracted muscle, usually an eccentric contraction.[5,15] The forces are greater on a muscle in an eccentric contraction than during isometric or concentric contractions. It is this increased load on the fibers that causes more strain injury from eccentric contractions.[16]

The muscles that are most susceptible to strain injury are those which cross more than one joint (multi-articulate muscles), such as the hamstrings. Multi-articulate muscles are not designed to allow full lengthening over all joints at the same time.[5] Thus they are more vulnerable and their capacity to extend can be reached with abnormal stress, and injury can result. Strains can occur in any region of the muscle, but they are most prevalent at the musculotendinous junction.[17,18] The musculotendinous junction is a region where one tissue that has a great deal of pliability (muscle) is meeting another tissue that has very limited pliability (tendon). The point of interface between these two tissues is a site of mechanical weakness.

Muscle strains are graded at three levels – first degree or mild, second degree or moderate, and third degree or severe.[19] In a first-degree strain only a few muscle fibers are torn. There is likely to be some level of post-injury soreness, but the individual will be back to normal levels of activity rather quickly. In a second-degree strain there are more fibers involved in the injury. There is likely to be a greater level of pain with this injury, and a clear region of maximum tenderness in the muscle tissue. A third-degree strain involves a severe tear or a complete rupture of the muscle tendon unit. In a complete rupture there is likely to be significant pain at the time of the injury. Notably, pain may be minimal if the muscle ends are completely separated because moving the limbs will not put additional tensile stress on the separated ends of the muscle.

Third-degree strains usually require surgery to repair the ruptured muscle. However, in some instances the muscle may not have a crucial role, and the potential dangers of surgery do not outweigh the loss of partial muscle action. In this situation the physician may recommend leaving the injury alone. Ruptures to the rectus femoris, for example, are commonly left as is since the other three quadriceps muscles can usually make up for the strength deficit.

Contusion

A contusion is an injury – usually caused by a direct blow – to the muscle that causes a disruption in the

---

> **Box 2.1** Signs of Muscle Strains
>
> - First degree:
>   - Minor weakness evident
>   - Minor muscle spasm
>   - Swelling possible, minor
>   - Minor loss of function
>   - Minor pain on stretch
>   - Minor pain in resisted isometric contraction
> - Second degree:
>   - Weakness more pronounced
>   - Weakness due to reflex inhibition
>   - Moderate to major spasm in injured muscles
>   - Moderate to major spasm in nearby muscles
>   - Moderate to major swelling
>   - Moderate to major impaired function
>   - Pain likely strong during stretch
>   - Pain likely strong with resisted isometric contraction.
> - Third degree:
>   - Pronounced muscle weakness
>   - Muscle may not function
>   - Spasm if muscle is intact
>   - Surrounding muscles in spasm
>   - Moderate to major swelling
>   - Loss of function due to reflex inhibition
>   - Pain severe at injury, but may recede

---

fibers and/or their neurovascular supply. Ecchymosis (bruising) usually follows a contusion as the blood from damaged capillaries leaks out into the muscle tissue. The period of healing for a muscle contusion depends on how severe the impact trauma was, and how much disruption of muscle fibers and neurovascular structures has occurred.

In some cases, a contusion can develop bone tissue (ossification) within the muscle during the healing process; this is called myositis ossificans. Massage practitioners should be watchful for this condition after a contusion injury. Deep pressure of an area that has developed myositis ossificans could be detrimental to the healing process and can cause further injury.[20] It is most common in some of the anterior muscles of the body that are vulnerable to direct blows, such as the quadriceps group, biceps brachii, brachialis, and deltoid muscles.

TENDON

The primary function of tendon is to transmit the contraction force of the skeletal muscles to the bones in order to generate movement. Therefore, it is necessary for the tendon to have a great deal of tensile strength. Within the tendon, collagen fibers are oriented in a parallel direction to give the greatest amount of tensile strength in a longitudinal direction.

The tendons are a fundamental part of the contractile unit, but unlike muscles they are rarely injured with significant fiber tearing like a muscle is with a strain. The tensile strength in a tendon is often more than twice that of the associated muscle.[1] As a result, a severe tear or rupture will likely be in the muscular fibers near the musculotendinous junction rather than the tendon.

Tendinosis

The most common pathological problem involving tendons is caused by repetitive mechanical load placed on the tendon. It was previously thought that the tendon fibers tore and subsequently led to an inflammatory reaction in the tendon, thus the name tendinitis (-itis meaning inflammation). However, research into the cellular pathology of tendinitis has repeatedly demonstrated that this is not the case. This conclusion is supported by numerous studies of the condition. Research shows the pathology in the tendon to be devoid of inflammatory cells in this type of injury.[21–24]

The term tendinosis is proposed as a more appropriate referent to indicate a degenerative condition; this text uses this term. Note that many clinicians continue to define the condition as inflammatory. There is such a thing as tendon fiber tearing with inflammation (true tendinitis), but it is not the common tendon pathology that is associated with so many repetitive stress injuries.[25]

The primary problem in tendinosis appears not to be the tearing of tendon fibers, but a collagen breakdown in the tissue. Collagen breakdown leads to chronic pain and a significant loss of tensile strength in the tendon. This explains the greater time it takes to heal from tendinosis problems; if tissue tearing were the primary problem then the tissue would heal more quickly. Rebuilding damaged collagen is a much slower process.

While the collagen breakdown of tendinosis seems mostly caused by repetitive mechanical load, other factors play a role as well. Studies indicate that an increase in vascularity (blood flow) can be a significant part of tendinosis pathology.[25,26] Other studies show that decreased vascularity may also contribute to chronic tendon pathology.[27,28]

Tenosynovitis

Another chronic overuse problem affecting certain tendons is tenosynovitis. This condition does not affect all tendons only those enclosed within a synovial sheath. The synovial sheath, also called the epitenon, surrounds tendons in the distal extremities and a few other locations where excessive friction may irritate the tendon (Fig. 2.3). For example, a synovial sheath surrounds the tendon of the long head of the biceps brachii as it passes through the bicipital groove. The purpose of the sheath is to reduce friction between the tendon and the retinaculum that binds the tendon close to the joint. The tendon must be able to glide freely within the synovial sheath.

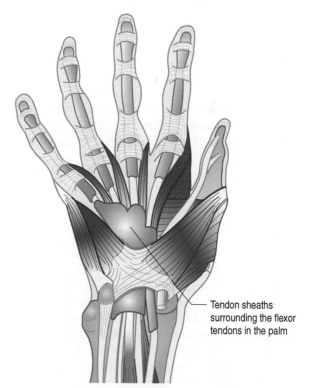

Tendon sheaths surrounding the flexor tendons in the palm

Figure 2.3 Tendon sheaths and their surrounding retinacula.

In tenosynovitis, chronic overloading or excess friction causes an inflammatory reaction between the tendon and the enclosing synovial sheath. The inflammatory reaction creates a roughening of the surface of the tendon and fibrous adhesion develops between the tendon and the sheath. The roughening of the tendon surface may cause crepitus when the joint is moved through a range of motion. The symptoms of tendinosis and tenosynovitis are very similar, but massage treatment of these conditions is virtually identical.

LIGAMENT

The primary function of ligament tissue is to connect adjacent bones to each other to establish stability in the skeletal structure. Ligament fibers are oriented primarily in a longitudinal plane to give the ligament fiber the greatest amount of resistance to tensile stress. Within the ligament there are also fibers that are oriented in other planes, to give the ligament some pliability and strength against forces in other directions.[1] Strength in multiple directions is important because joints are subjected to forces in multiple directions.

Sprains, plastic deformation

Ligament injuries usually occur from sudden high tensile loads on the fibers. For example, a blow from the lateral side of the knee puts excess tensile stress on the medial collateral ligament on the medial side of the knee. The severity of the injury is dependent on how much force the ligament must withstand. Ligament fibers have some degree of pliability and resistance to stretch. If the tensile stress is minor, the ligament can usually absorb the force with minor stretching of the fibers.

If the force is greater, the ligament fibers may stretch slightly. Stretching the ligament past the initial level of pliability in the tissue causes permanent lengthening called plastic deformation.[1] In plastic deformation the tissue stretches, but does not recoil to its original length. Plastic deformation of ligaments leads to joint instability and hypermobility, and may be the source of other disorders as well. Tensile forces that exceed plastic deformation produce tearing of the ligament fibers.

Ligament fiber stretching or tearing is referred to as a sprain. Magee describes the range of sprain injury as mild or grade 1, moderate or grade 2, and severe or grade 3.[19] In a mild sprain only a few ligament fibers are torn and the ligament has likely undergone stretching that is not permanent. The client is likely to feel pain with stretching the ligament, the joint may be swollen, and the muscles around the joint may be in spasm.

In moderate or grade 2 sprains a more significant number of ligament fibers are torn. The ligament has likely undergone some degree of overstretching, and will remain somewhat overstretched, with the result being some degree of joint laxity. Pain will usually be moderate to severe when the ligament is stretched, local spasm is likely in surrounding muscles, and there will likely be moderate swelling.

When the ligament is severely torn or ruptured the sprain is a grade 3 or severe sprain. Most if not all ligament fibers will no longer be intact, and will need to be reattached. Permanent changes in joint stability are likely. Pain will usually be severe at the time of injury, but may not be present later on with joint movement if the ends of the ligament are no longer connected. There will be a moderate level of swelling around the affected joint and local muscle spasm is likely.

Box 2.2 Signs of Ligament Sprains

- Mild or grade 1:
  - Few ligament fibers torn.
  - Temporary ligament stretching possible
  - Mild to moderate pain with stretch
  - Minor swelling
  - Local muscle spasm likely
- Moderate or grade 2:
  - More ligament fibers torn
  - Ligament overstretching likely
  - Joint laxity likely
  - Moderate to severe pain with stretch
  - Moderate swelling likely
  - Local muscle spasm likely
- Severe or grade 3:
  - Severe tear or rupture
  - Fibers likely need repair
  - Permanent changes in joint stability likely
  - Pain severe at injury
  - Pain may recede if ends detached
  - Moderate swelling likely
  - Muscle spasm likely

JOINT CAPSULE

There are two layers to the joint capsule, the outermost layer called the fibrous capsule, and the inner layer called the synovial membrane (Fig. 2.4). The fibrous capsule is primarily ligamentous in most joints as ligament tissue makes up a significant portion of the capsule around synovial joints. The joint capsule acts like a ligament to help maintain stability and support, but also houses synovial fluid and provides a protective covering for the synovial membrane. The synovial membrane secretes synovial fluid, which helps to lubricate the joint, supply nutrients, and remove metabolic waste products from the area. The fibrous capsule is richly innervated, so even minor levels of damage cause significant pain and discomfort.

Tears, adhesions, fibrosis

Damage to the capsule is often an acute injury. Examples include joint dislocation or injuries in which the joint is exposed to significant stress that tears the supporting ligamentous structure. The capsule is also susceptible to fibrotic changes that

may occur for a number of reasons. Fibrous adhesion within the capsule may cause it to adhere to itself, such as occurs in adhesive capsulitis. Pain from osteoarthritis is also commonly ascribed to pathological changes that occur in the joint capsule.[29]

Tears to the joint capsule that occur from acute trauma are evaluated in the same manner as ligament sprains. Other pathological problems in the capsule, such as fibrosis, are evident with a specific pattern of movement restriction that is unique to each joint called a capsular pattern. Not all joints have capsular patterns; joints not directly controlled by muscles do not have capsular patterns, such as the sacroiliac joint.[19] If the joint's pattern of motion restriction is not the characteristic capsular pattern for that joint, the restriction is referred to as a non-capsular pattern. Testing for capsular patterns is performed in an assessment.

FASCIA

Fascia is an abundant connective tissue in the body and is intricately woven around organs as well as wrapped around every individual muscular fiber. It is the ultimate connective tissue, as one of its

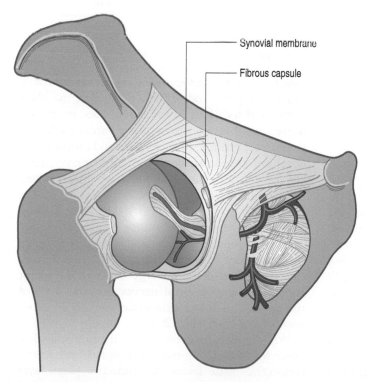

Figure 2.4 The components of a typical joint capsule.

— Synovial membrane

— Fibrous capsule

primary functions is connecting different bones, organs, and other soft tissues together. Fascia is primarily composed of elastic collagen fibers. Its consistency ranges from thin and pliable to very dense and resistant. It has multiple functions, including providing support, shape, and suspension for most of the soft tissues of the body, aiding in force transmission, and providing extensive proprioceptive feedback.[30,31]

Fascia is found throughout the body and there is a special interdependent relationship between muscle tissue and fascia, both structurally and functionally. This relationship is so extensive that the two are described as *myofascial* tissues. From a structural standpoint, fascia is crucial in transmitting muscle contraction force to the bones (though some anatomy texts attribute all force to muscle–tendon attachments). Without the fascia that envelopes muscles and their individual fibers, the muscles would not be able to generate anywhere near the amount of force necessary for proper movement and function.[32–34] Notably, the force from muscles can be still be delivered to distal bones after cutting the muscle's primary tendon because of fascial connections with adjacent muscles.[30]

Fascia also plays a crucial role in neuromuscular function. Numerous receptor cells in myofascial tissues generate extensive sensory information that is necessary for regulation of movement and posture. This supply of sensory input is so extensive that it produces the greatest amount of afferent (sensory) information coming in to our central nervous system.[31] Consequently, the myofascial system is our largest sensory organ – greater than the eyes, nose, ears, and skin.

The importance of fascia in soft-tissue pain and injury conditions has gained increasing visibility with new research on fascial tissues. Previously fascia was considered an inert tissue, although one that was stretched by prolonged tensile force to the tissue. Fascia was previously described as a colloidal substance that responded to mechanical force or thermal applications by changing from a more gelatinous (*gel*) state to a more fluid (*sol*) state.[35,36] Recent investigations into the anatomical and physiological function of fascia provide an alternative explanation.

Current cellular physiology research has found active contractile cells within fascial tissue itself.[31,37–40] The presence of active contractile cells indicates that fascia is able to contract and elongate with some degree of neurological control. Changes in tissue consistency appear to result from neurological activity in these contractile cells and not from a conversion from gel to fluid.

Fascia also contains an abundance of specialized sensory receptors called Ruffini endings which respond to forces applied to tissues connected to or adjacent to them.[39] Activation of the Ruffini endings with tangential force techniques appears to cause a neurological response that decreases contractile activity in the fascia itself. Consequently the 'fascial release' felt by many practitioners is likely a neurological response of relaxation in the fascia just as it is in muscle tissue.

Fascia is injured in a variety of ways. Fascia has a great deal of elasticity, but extreme tensile stress on the fascia can cause it to tear or perforate. Many injuries involve damage to fascia as well as to the tissues it envelops, such as muscle. When fascia remains in a shortened position for prolonged periods it will have a tendency to adopt that shortened position.[41] Tension in associated muscle fibers activates contractile fibers within the fascia to maintain the shortened position. Long periods in a shortened position can also lead to fibrous cross-linking within the fascial tissue, which can result in motion limitation.

NERVE

Injuries to nerve tissue are an important source of soft-tissue pain and dysfunction. Due to their anatomical locations in the extremities, numerous nerve trunks are particularly susceptible to mechanical trauma. Both sensory and motor nerve fibers are at risk, so symptoms from nerve injury can involve both motor and sensory disturbances.

The nerves that leave the spinal cord have a dorsal root that carries sensory information and a ventral root that carries motor signals; these are called the spinal nerve roots. The two sections of the nerve root blend together shortly after leaving the spinal cord, and converge to make the major trunks of the peripheral nerves that travel down the upper and lower extremities and to all other areas of the body (Fig. 2.5).

Within the major nerve trunks there are individual nerve fibers that transmit nerve signals and several connective tissue layers. A connective tissue layer called the endoneurium surrounds each individual

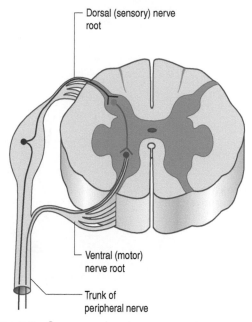

Figure 2.5   Sensory and motor nerve roots.

nerve fiber. The nerve fibers are collected into bundles called fascicles, and another connective tissue layer called the perineurium surrounds the fascicles. The fascicles are collected in bundles, which are all enclosed within another connective tissue layer called the epineurium (Fig. 2.6). It is the numerous bundles of fascicles that make up an entire peripheral nerve.

The different layers of connective tissue within a nerve play an important role in nerve tissue pathologies. Peripheral nerves are provided more support and protection from the connective tissue layers than the spinal nerve roots. The epineurium surrounding the spinal nerve fibers are poorly

developed or non-existent.[42] This lack of protection makes the spinal nerves more susceptible to injury, particularly compression trauma.

The nerve needs adequate blood circulation to function properly so there is an intricate vascular supply to each nerve. There is a complex web of tiny blood vessels within the nerve. Neural ischemia due to compression is a known cause of neurological symptoms.[43] Most people are familiar with the experience of pins and needles that comes with neural ischemia from holding a limb or sitting in a static position for a length of time. Once circulation returns the sensations recede. Nerve tissue is generally pliable and resilient to mechanical injury, but excessive force can produce tissue damage.

In addition to carrying sensory and motor impulses, the nerve fiber serves another important function. The nerve carries its own nutrient proteins necessary for proper function. These substances are carried through the nerve by a slow flowing cytoplasm within the nerve cell called axoplasm. This two-way flow of axoplasm inside the nerve is called the axoplasmic flow. Disturbances to the axoplasmic flow affect the nerve in the local area as well as throughout the entire length of the nerve.

Most major nerve trunks carry sensory and motor fibers so pathology can produce both sensory and motor symptoms. Some nerve pathologies are more likely to produce sensory symptoms while others produce motor dysfunction due to the number of sensory and motor fibers in their associated nerve trunks. In the upper extremity, for example, the median nerve has a greater percentage of sensory fibers than motor fibers, so symptoms of carpal tunnel syndrome tend to be sensory before there is motor impairment. In contrast, compression of posterior interosseous nerve, which has mostly motor fibers, creates weakness before there is sensory impairment.[43]

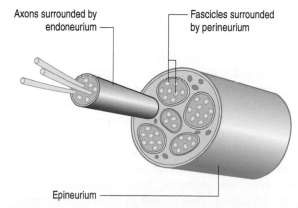

Figure 2.6   Connective tissue layers in the nerve.

Box 2.3   Nerve Compression/Tension Signs/ Symptoms

- Reduced sensory input
- Reduced motor impulses
- Pain in a specific dermatome
- Motor weakness in a specific myotome
- Hyperesthesia or paresthesia sensations

Dermatomes, cutaneous innervation, myotomes

Becoming familiar with dermatomes, cutaneous innervation, and myotomes will help practitioners better understand nerve injury symptoms. A dermatome is an area of skin supplied by fibers from a single nerve root. The fibers from that one nerve root make up several peripheral nerves and innervate specific areas of the body. For example, the C8 nerve root has branches that make up portions of several upper extremity nerves, such as the median and ulnar nerves. Sensory symptoms from C8 nerve root irritation are felt in the ulnar side of the hand and medial side of the forearm and arm (Fig. 2.7).

Each peripheral nerve is made up of fibers deriving from the different nerve roots. A skin region supplied by a peripheral nerve is called the cutaneous innervation of that nerve (Fig. 2.8). There can be some overlap between the dermatome and the area of cutaneous innervation. For example, the ulnar nerve in the arm has fibers from C7, C8, and T1, yet its sensory fibers only supply the ulnar aspect of the hand and the last two fingers, whereas the C8 dermatome covers the ulnar aspect of the hand, as well as the entire medial forearm and arm.

Information about dermatomes and regions of cutaneous innervation is valuable in the clinical evaluation process. Using the example above, if

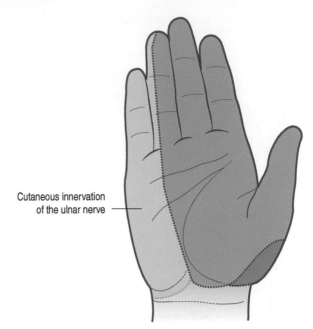

Cutaneous innervation of the ulnar nerve

Figure 2.8 Cutaneous innervation for a peripheral nerve.

sensory symptoms are felt throughout the C8 dermatome, one would suspect nerve root involvement rather than a problem with the ulnar nerve. This is because the symptoms extend outside the ulnar nerve's cutaneous innervation area on the ulnar side of the hand. If symptoms are only in the ulnar side of the hand, ulnar nerve pathology is more likely. Keep in mind that symptoms may appear in only a part of the dermatome. Whenever sensory symptoms are reported in an extremity one should consider the possibility of the nerve root being the source of the problem.

Myotomes are somewhat similar to dermatomes. A myotome is a group of muscles that are innervated by the same nerve root. A single muscle can have fibers that come from several different nerve roots. Each peripheral nerve also has a number of muscles that it innervates. If there is weakness apparent in a group of muscles innervated by the same nerve root, i.e. the same myotome, then the problem is most likely at the nerve root level. Muscle weakness in a myotome is not always easy to detect because the muscle may only have a small number of fibers that come from the affected nerve root. For more on these conditions see the text, Orthopedic Assessment in Massage Therapy.

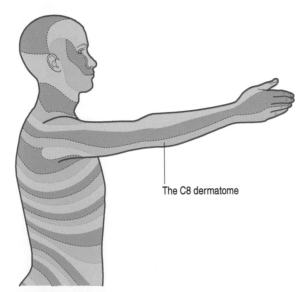

The C8 dermatome

Figure 2.7 Dermatomes of the upper extremity. Each dermatome is associated with a specific nerve root.

Nerve injuries

Nerve injuries generally develop from compressive loads, such as a direct blow to the nerve or a chronic low level of compression. With excess tensile stress the overall diameter of the nerve decreases compressing the fibers within the nerve; this condition is called adverse neural tension.[44–46] The symptoms of compression or tension pathology are similar because both cause degeneration of the nerve. Compressive and tensile forces can occur in numerous locations along the nerve, but several sites are most vulnerable for nerve damage.[46]

Radiculopathy, neuropathy

There are two terms that describe nerve injuries and which indicate the location of the pathology in the nerve. A *radiculopathy* is a nerve pathology that occurs at the nerve root. A common radiculopathy is the herniated nucleus pulposus (HNP) or herniated disc, in which the disc presses on a nerve root. Pathology farther along the length of the nerve is a *neuropathy*. It is also called a peripheral neuropathy indicating that the injury is in the peripheral nerves, distant from the nerve roots and spinal cord. Many nerve compression syndromes, such as thoracic outlet and carpal tunnel syndrome, are examples of peripheral neuropathies.

Nerve degeneration

Nerve degeneration results from mechanical forces or from systemic disorders that attack the nerve, such as multiple sclerosis. Nerve injuries are classified by severity into three levels: neurapraxia, axonotmesis, and neurotmesis.[47,48] Either compression or tension injuries can produce these levels of nerve injury.

When there is impairment of the axoplasmic flow in one part of a nerve, the remainder of the nerve becomes nutritionally deficient and thus more susceptible to pathological changes. With additional regions of the nerve more susceptible to degenerative changes, a client may have symptoms of more than one nerve pathology. The presence of multiple sites of neurological pathology is called the double or multiple crush phenomenon.[49–51]

The nerves of the upper extremity provide a good illustration of double crush pathology. Brachial plexus compression near the thoracic outlet impairs axoplasmic flow and subsequent function of the distal regions of the upper extremity nerves. As a result simultaneous symptoms of thoracic outlet syndrome and carpal tunnel syndrome can develop.

Neurapraxia, axonotmesis, neurotmesis

Neurapraxia is the least severe nerve injury and involves the blocking of axon conduction. The nerve continues to conduct some signals above and below the primary area of compression or injury, but conduction velocity slows. Common symptoms include

---

Box 2.4 Areas Where Nerves Are Most Vulnerable

Tunnels – soft or bony tissues may create tunnels the nerve must travel through, compression is the risk. Ex: carpal tunnel in the wrist, the cubital tunnel in the elbow or the tarsal tunnel in the foot.

Nerve branches – anywhere nerve tissue branches out to other areas there is the potential for increased neural tension. Ex: where the posterior interosseous nerve branches from the main radial nerve near the elbow.

Nerve is fixed – anywhere the nerve is tethered to an adjacent structure for stability is a region for potential compressive or tensile stress on the nerve. Ex: deep peroneal nerve where it is attached to the upper region of the fibula in the lower extremity.

Nerve passes by unyielding surface – passing close to unyielding surfaces like bone there is a greater chance of compression or tension. Ex: brachial plexus as it goes over the first rib in the upper thoracic region.

Tension points – the mid-point of a stretched nerve fiber, called the tension point of the nerve, is more susceptible to pathology.

Box 2.5 Nerve Injury Levels

Neurapraxia – mild sensory and motor deficits

Axonotmesis – sensory and motor dysfunction, significant pain

Neurotmesis – altered sensation or function, or no recovery

mild sensory and motor deficits, which usually decrease when the nerve is no longer compressed.

The next level of nerve damage is called axonotmesis. There is a loss in continuity of the axon, but the surrounding endoneurium may still be intact. The outer layers of connective tissue are still intact as well. Typical symptoms include sensory and motor dysfunction, as well as significant pain. If the connective tissue layers are intact the nerve axon is likely to regenerate, although slowly. The rate of regeneration of nerve axons is estimated to be 1 mm per day or 1 inch per month, but in certain cases slower.[46]

A severe nerve injury is neurotmesis. At this level, damage affects not only the axons, but also their connective tissue layers. Because these layers are damaged, recovery from neurotmesis may not be possible. Neurotmesis occurs in severe crush injuries or situations where the nerve is severed. Axons can regenerate once severed, but because the connective tissue template is disrupted the axons may not grow back in their original locations. This is one reason some surgical repairs produce altered sensation or function in the region when the individual regains use.

CARTILAGE

There are three different types of cartilage. The first two, hyaline and fibrocartilage, are those which are relevant for orthopedic disorders. A third type, elastic cartilage, is the type that is found in areas such as the external portion of the ear or the epiglottis. Hyaline cartilage is located on the ends of long bones. It is also called articular cartilage. It provides a smooth gliding surface for movement at the joints, and aids in joint flexibility and support. The most common pathology affecting hyaline cartilage is compressive stress that causes a breakdown in the integrity of the cartilage matrix, and will eventually cause degenerative changes in the joint.

At the ends of the long bones cartilage performs as an important protective cushion. The cartilage is mostly devoid of nerve fibers, so there is very little, if any, sensation from the cartilage when degeneration occurs. Most pain sensations come from the subchondral bone (the layer of bone just below the cartilage) because it is richly innervated. Friction develops between the long bones as the hyaline cartilage degenerates, causing pain.[52]

Fibrocartilage is the other type of cartilage involved in orthopedic disorders. This is the strongest type of cartilage, and it is designed to provide rigidity and support. Fibrocartilage is located in areas of high compressive force between bones such as the intervertebral discs and the menisci of the knee. As with hyaline cartilage, the most common type of injury to fibrocartilage is with high levels of compressive stress that cause it to break down. The compressive forces causing the greatest problems are those involving heavy loads over a long period of time. Poor posture that increases the compressive load on the intervertebral discs in the lumbar spine is a good example.

While compressive loads routinely injure the menisci in the knee, fibrocartilage in the knee can also be injured from tensile forces. The tearing of the medial meniscus is an example. The medial meniscus of the knee has a fibrous connection to the medial collateral ligament. When there is excessive valgus force on the knee, the medial collateral ligament may stretch or tear. Since there is a fibrous connection of the medial meniscus with the medial collateral ligament, pulling the ligament fibers pulls on the cartilage as well. The cartilage may tear, especially near its edge, from these high tensile forces.

References

1. Nordin MA, Frankel V. Basic Biomechanics of the Musculoskeletal System. 3rd ed. Baltimore: Lippincott Williams & Wilkins; 2001.
2. Craton N, Matheson GO. Training and clinical competency in musculoskeletal medicine. Identifying the problem. Sports Med. 1993;15(5):328–337.
3. Travell J, Simons D. Myofascial Pain and Dysfunction: The Trigger Point Manual. Vol 2. Baltimore: Williams & Wilkins; 1992.
4. AAOS. Athletic Training and Sports Medicine. 2nd ed. Park Ridge: American Academy of Orthopaedic Surgeons; 1991.
5. Garrett WE. Muscle strain injuries. Am J Sports Med. 1996;24(6 Suppl):S2–S8.
6. Paddon-Jones D, Muthalib M, Jenkins D. The effects of a repeated bout of eccentric exercise on indices of muscle damage and delayed onset muscle soreness. J Sci Med Sport. 2000;3(1):35–43.
7. Lieber RL, Friden J. Mechanisms of muscle injury after eccentric contraction. J Sci Med Sport. 1999;2(3):253–265.
8. McComas A. Skeletal Muscle: Form and Function. Champaign: Human Kinetics; 1996.

9. Croisier JL. Factors associated with recurrent hamstring injuries. Sports Med. 2004;34(10):681–695.

10. Mense S, Simons DG. Muscle Pain: Understanding Its Nature, Diagnosis, & Treatment. Baltimore: Lippincott Williams & Wilkins; 2001.

11. Travell JS, D. Myofascial Pain and Dysfunction: The Trigger Point Manual. Vol 1. 1st ed. Baltimore: Williams & Wilkins; 1983.

12. McPartland JM. Travell trigger points – molecular and osteopathic perspectives. J Am Osteopath Assoc. 2004; 104(6):244–249.

13. Simons DG. Review of enigmatic MTrPs as a common cause of enigmatic musculoskeletal pain and dysfunction. J Electromyogr Kinesiol. 2004;14(1):95–107.

14. Lindboe CF, Platou CS. Effect of immobilization of short duration on the muscle fibre size. Clin Physiol. 1984; 4(2):183–188.

15. McCully KK, Faulkner JA. Characteristics of lengthening contractions associated with injury to skeletal muscle fibers. J Appl Physiol. 1986;61(1):293–299.

16. Faulkner JA, Brooks SV, Opiteck JA. Injury to skeletal muscle fibers during contractions: conditions of occurrence and prevention. Phys Ther. 1993;73(12):911–921.

17. Connell DA, Schneider-Kolsky ME, Hoving JL, et al. Longitudinal study comparing sonographic and MRI assessments of acute and healing hamstring injuries. AJR Am J Roentgenol. 2004;183(4):975–984.

18. Garrett WE, Jr., Safran MR, Seaber AV, Glisson RR, Ribbeck BM. Biomechanical comparison of stimulated and nonstimulated skeletal muscle pulled to failure. Am J Sports Med. 1987;15(5):448–454.

19. Magee D. Orthopedic Physical Assessment. 3rd ed. Philadelphia: W.B. Saunders; 1997.

20. Ryan JM. Myositis ossificans: a serious complication of a minor injury. CJEM. 1999;1(3):198.

21. Almekinders LC, Temple JD. Etiology, Diagnosis, and Treatment of Tendinitis – An Analysis of the Literature. Med Sci Sport Exercise. 1998;30(8):1183–1190.

22. Cook JL, Khan KM. What is the most appropriate treatment for patellar tendinopathy? Br J Sports Med. 2001;35(5):291–294.

23. Kraushaar BS, Nirschl RP. Tendinosis of the elbow (tennis elbow). Clinical features and findings of histological, immunohistochemical, and electron microscopy studies. J Bone Joint Surg Am. 1999;81(2):259–278.

24. Whiteside JA, Andrews JR, Conner JA. Tendinopathies of the Elbow. Sport Med Arthroscopy. 1995;3(3):195–203.

25. Khan KM, Cook JL, Taunton JE, Bonar F. Overuse tendinosis, not tendinitis – Part 1: A new paradigm for a difficult clinical problem. Physician Sportsmed. 2000;28(5):38.

26. Astrom M, Westlin N. Blood flow in chronic Achilles tendinopathy. Clin Orthop. 1994(308):166–172.

27. Ahmed IM, Lagopoulos M, McConnell P, Soames RW, Sefton GK. Blood supply of the Achilles tendon. J Orthop Res. 1998;16(5):591–596.

28. Carr AJ, Norris SH. The blood supply of the calcaneal tendon. J Bone Joint Surg Br. 1989;71(1):100–101.

29. Cyriax J. Textbook of Orthopaedic Medicine Volume One: Diagnosis of Soft Tissue Lesions. Vol 1. 8th ed. London: Baillière Tindall; 1982.

30. Huijing PA. Muscle as a collagen fiber reinforced composite: a review of force transmission in muscle and whole limb. J Biomech. 1999;32(4):329–345.

31. Schleip R. Fascial plasticity – a new neurobiological explanation. Journal of Bodywork and Movement Therapies. 2003;7(1):11–19.

32. Fourie W. Fascia lata: Merely a thigh stocking, or a coordinator of complex thigh muscular activity. Paper presented at: Fascia Research Congress, 2007; Harvard Medical School, Boston, MA.

33. Vleeming A. A clinical anatomical look at the human thoracolumbar fascia. Paper presented at: Fascia Research Congress, 2007; Harvard Medical School, Boston, MA.

34. Gracovetsky S. Is the lumbodorsal fascia necessary. Paper presented at: Fascia Research Congress, 2007; Harvard Medical School, Boston, MA.

35. Rolf I. Rolfing. Rochester, VT: Healing Arts Press; 1977.

36. Juhan D. Job's Body. Barrytown, NY: Station Hill Press; 1987.

37. Tomasek J, Haaksma C. Mechanoregulation of myofibroblast formation and function. Paper presented at: Fascia Research Congress, 2007; Harvard Medical School, Boston, MA.

38. Hinz B, Gabbiani G. Mechanisms of force generation and transmission by myofibroblasts. Curr Opin Biotechnol. 2003;14(5):538–546.

39. Schleip R. Fascial plasticity – a new neurobiological explanation Part 2. Journal of Bodywork and Movement Therapies. 2003;7(2):104–116.

40. Schleip R. Fascia is able to contract in a smooth muscle-like manner and thereby influence musculoskeletal mechanics. Paper presented at: Fascia Research Congress, 2007; Harvard Medical School, Boston, MA.

41. Schultz RL, Feitis R. The Endless Web. Berkeley: North Atlantic Books; 1996.

42. Rydevik B, Brown MD, Lundborg G. Pathoanatomy and pathophysiology of nerve root compression. Spine. 1984;9(1):7–15.

43. Dawson D, Hallett M, Wilbourn A. Entrapment Neuropathies. 3rd ed. Philadelphia: Lippincott-Raven; 1999.

44. Gallant S. Assessing adverse neural tension in athletes. J Sport Rehabil. 1998;7(2):128–139.

45. Turl SE, George KP. Adverse neural tension – a factor in repetitive hamstring strain. J Orthop Sport Phys Therapy. 1998;27(1):16–21.

46. Butler D. Mobilisation of the Nervous System. London: Churchill Livingstone; 1991.

47. Seddon HJ. Three types of nerve injury. Brain. 1943;66:237.

48. Sunderland S. Nerves and Nerve Injuries. 2nd ed. Edinburgh: Churchill Livingstone; 1978.

49. Upton AR, McComas AJ. The double crush in nerve entrapment syndromes. Lancet. 18 1973;2(7825):359–362.

50. Golovchinsky V. Double crush syndrome in lower extremities. Electromyogr Clin Neurophysiol. 1998; 38(2):115–120.

51. Mackinnon SE. Double and multiple "crush" syndromes. Double and multiple entrapment neuropathies. Hand Clin. 1992;8(2):369–390.

52. Moore K, Dalley A. Clinically Oriented Anatomy. 4th ed. Philadelphia: Lippincott Williams & Wilkins; 1999.

Chapter **3**

Thermal modalities as treatment aids

Applied appropriately, thermal modalities can be helpful adjuncts to soft-tissue manipulation. To use thermal modalities effectively, however, requires the practitioner understand a few fundamental principles of physics and physiology in the body, such as the nature of pain, methods of heat transfer, and physiological responses to temperature change. Thermal agents such as ice bags, hot packs, or ultrasound units are used to increase circulation and soft-tissue extensibility, increase or decrease the local tissue metabolic rate, and to decrease inflammation. In addition, a primary purpose for using thermal modalities in the rehabilitation environment is pain management.

UNDERSTANDING PAIN

Pain is generally defined as an unpleasant sensory and emotional experience due to actual or possible damage to tissues.[1] Because of the soft-tissues' extensive innervations they are a primary source of pain when injured or dysfunctional. Musculoskeletal dysfunction, inflammation or neurological excitation caused by injury, trauma and or degenerative disease are the primary causes of most soft tissue pain.[2,3] The effectiveness of thermal modalities at interrupting pain signals becomes clear when the nature of pain transmission is understood.

Nociceptors, also called free nerve endings, are the key sensory cells (neurons) that report pain to the central nervous system (CNS). They are present in varying quantities in most types of soft tissues, including skin, joints, muscle, and organs. As a response to mechanical, chemical, or thermal stress that could cause the body damage the nociceptors send signals to the CNS that are interpreted by the brain as pain. The number of nociceptors influences the level of pain. For example, due to the high number of nociceptors in muscles and joint capsules considerable pain can result when these tissues are injured. In contrast, the intervertebral discs can withstand high levels of compression and significant damage without the individual feeling pain due to the discs having few nociceptors.[4,5]

Signals are sent from nociceptors to the central nervous system by two types of small diameter afferent fibers called C and A-delta fibers.[6] Due to the small diameter of these fibers they do not transmit signals as fast as the other non-pain receptors, the mechanoreceptors and proprioceptors. The difference in signal transmission rate between nociceptors and the mechanoreceptors or proprioceptors plays an important role in pain management and is explained more thoroughly further in the chapter.

A-delta fibers have a myelin sheath which functions to speed up the transmission rate of signals. A-delta fibers are most sensitive to high levels of mechanical stress and produce sensations generally described as sharp, pricking, or stabbing.[2,7,8] C fibers are slower than A-delta fibers because they are unmyelinated (Fig. 3.1). Pain from C fibers has a slower onset but lasts longer and produces dull, throbbing, aching, or burning sensations.[7,8]

The A-delta and C fibers work in conjunction with each other in reporting pain sensations, but have different timing. For instance, imagine what happens when one stumbles and falls, hitting the knee on a rock. There is an immediate sharp pain sensation in the knee which is then transmitted primarily by A-delta fibers. A day later a more pervasive dull and throbbing pain, transmitted by the C fibers, replaces the initial sharp pain. Interestingly, a person's immediate reaction with such an accident is to rub the stricken area and to move the knee. The stimulation of mechanoreceptors and proprioceptors (associated with movement and touch) sends signals to the CNS that outpace the nociceptors, thus overriding some of the pain signals.

There are three primary categories of pain – acute, chronic and referred. Acute pain occurs as an immediate result of a causative event (ex: injury) and resolves within a relatively short period of time. Pain that lasts less than 6 months and where an identifiable pathology is found is called acute by some.[9] Chronic pain continues past what would be considered the normal time period for healing of a particular condition. Some references put a time frame on chronic pain and say it is any pain that has persisted for longer than 3–6 months.[2] When pain is referred, the sensations are experienced elsewhere from the location of dysfunction.[10] A site of referred pain can be either nearby the dysfunction or remote from it.

Minimizing a client's pain sensations with thermal modalities is an important rehabilitative goal. Not only is continual pain uncomfortable and indicative of tissue dysfunction, but it slows down the healing process as well. Chronic pain produces increased muscle hypertonicity which causes further pain and biomechanical dysfunction.[10] While attempting to correct a soft-tissue disorder, the more the pain can be reduced the better chance there is to make positive changes.

There are several theories that work to explain the means by which thermal modalities address pain. The most prominent is the gate control theory, originally proposed by Melzack and Wall in the 1960s.[11] According to the gate theory, only a limited amount of sensory information can make it through to the central nervous system. This limitation keeps the body from being totally overwhelmed with the massive amount of sensory information that it processes. Thermal modalities produce strong sensory impulses that shut off, or at least reduce the pain signals that reach the CNS. Signals from the C and A-delta fibers are

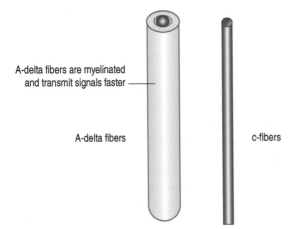

A-delta fibers are myelinated and transmit signals faster

A-delta fibers

c-fibers

Figure 3.1   Myelinated and unmyelinated nerve fibers.

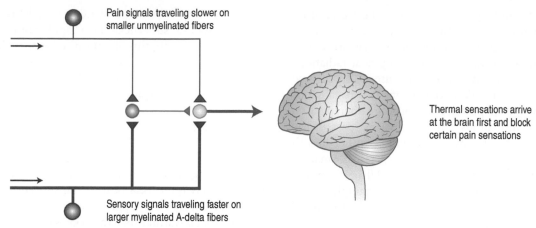

Figure 3.2 Schematic representation of the gate control theory.

slower than many of the other non-nociceptive afferent fibers. Thermal applications produce additional signals from afferent fibers which arrive at the central nervous system first and essentially override some of the pain signals from the injury or condition (Fig. 3.2).

The gate theory of pain has been dominant in pain research for decades. However, one of its founders has expanded the theory to be more inclusive of phenomena that were not adequately explained in the original theory. Ronald Melzack now suggests pain perception is a more complex process than initially envisioned. Melzack's current *neuromatrix theory* argues that pain "is a multidimensional experience produced by characteristic neurosignature patterns of nerve impulses generated by a widely distributed neural network – the 'body-self neuromatrix' – in the brain. These neurosignature patterns may be triggered by sensory inputs, but they may also be generated independently of them."[12,13] The neuromatrix concept includes aspects of cognitive and emotional experience that were not originally part of the gate theory. There is still validity to the gate control concepts, and there is much to learn about how various therapeutic interventions interact with Melzack's neuromatrix model.

HEAT TRANSFER

Thermal modalities work by taking advantage of temperature variances between the body and a physical agent. The laws of thermodynamics instruct that the production of heat or cold occurs as a result of the movement of heat from a warmer to a colder object. Heat is transferred in an attempt to reach equilibrium. There are four methods of heat transfer: conduction, convection, radiation, and conversion. Heat applications can employ any of the four methods of heat transfer, while cold applications require either conduction or convection to produce their results.

Conduction is a common method of heat transfer in thermal modalities. In conduction there are two objects in contact with each other. Heat is transferred from the object with the higher temperature to the object with the lower temperature. In hot applications, heat moves from the warmer modality to the cooler body part. Cold is produced in the same way but instead of the heat moving toward the body it moves away and toward the cooler modality (such as an ice bag). In essence, cold is created by the removal of heat. Conduction modalities include heat packs and ice bags.

Some thermal modalities employ convection. Conduction still occurs in convection but the medium of transfer – air or water – is moving. The constant movement of the heated medium, for example water, allows heat transfer to occur quicker and more efficiently than if the heated medium was static. Movement allows new areas of the warm medium to come into contact with the body part, thus allowing the body part to remain in contact with the warmest part of the heated medium. Thermal modalities employing convection include Jacuzzi tubs or foot baths of moving water.

Radiation is a third method of heat transfer. Radiation is the movement of electromagnetic energy through space. This type of heat is emitted as thermal radiation (there are other types of radiation). Infrared heat lamps and saunas are examples of thermal modalities utilizing heat radiation.

Some therapeutic modalities use a fourth type of heat transfer called conversion. It is usually out of the scope of practice for massage therapists to use these modalities but they may be part of the client's treatment protocol with another health care practitioner. Conversion is a transformation of non-thermal energy into heat. Ultrasound and pulsed short-wave diathermy are examples. Diathermy is not used much anymore. With pulsed ultrasound, high-frequency sound waves convert into heat as different tissues in the body selectively absorb them. Devices which use conversion do not get hot themselves generally; heat is not produced until the tissues absorb the ultrasonic energy.

HEAT APPLICATIONS

Integrating thermal modalities effectively into the clinical practice requires understanding how they function and of their benefits and disadvantages. In general, heat therapies are soothing and the soft-tissue practitioner can take advantage of their effects to enhance relaxation and decrease excessive sensory activity in the nervous system. However, there are situations where the effects of heat are not desired, and even contraindicated.

The following are the most commonly used types of heat modalities in the massage therapy clinic. There may be other forms of heat applications the client may have available to them if the therapist works alongside other health care practitioners, such as physical therapists and chiropractors. Understanding the nature of the client's complaint is paramount to knowing how and when heat modalities are beneficial and appropriate. Assessment should always be performed prior to treatment in order for the therapy to be most effective and not further complicate a condition.

An important factor to consider when selecting a heat modality is the depth of penetration. Most thermal applications are superficial as they are placed directly on the skin. A superficial application of either heat or cold can have a number of beneficial effects. Yet the depth of penetration of superficial thermal modalities is only about 1 cm below the skin.[14–16] Therefore, if the intention is

to heat a deep soft-tissue structure such as the joint capsule, a superficial heat application will not be effective. In this situation a form of heat application that has the capability to produce heat in the deeper tissues, such as ultrasound or diathermy, would be required.

Heat modalities

Localized applications

The following are heat modalities that work by conduction. Increasing local heat in the superficial tissues is accomplished by applying a source of heat to the body that is warmer than the body's temperature. For example, if a hot pack is placed on the body and the hot pack is above 98°F, there will be a transfer of heat from the hot pack to the body. This type of heat will not penetrate deeper tissues, such as the muscles lying underneath layers of other muscles.

It is important to monitor the client's response because all the applications below can cause burns. Additional towels may be needed to protect the client with the hot pads or wet packs, which may be removed once the pack is tolerable level. Always test the heat of the item before applying to confirm it is not too hot. No heat source should be left on the body for long periods (15–20 minutes is standard) and they should be frequently monitored. Stones have caused burns because it is harder to control their heat. Always check in with the client as to heat tolerance, some people cannot stand heat well.

Box 3.1 Heat Modalities

- Local applications:
  ○ Moist heat pack
  ○ Dry heating pads
  ○ 'Moist heat' heating pads
  ○ Chemical gel packs
  ○ Heated gel packs
  ○ Rice/buckwheat pillows
  ○ Hot stones
  ○ Melted paraffin wax
  ○ Whirlpool tubs
- Whole-body applications:
  ○ Whirlpool tubs
  ○ Steam room
  ○ Sauna

The moist heat pack is one of the most effective superficial heat applications. Wet packs are cloth packs of silica gel in various shapes and sizes that are submerged in hot water. After removing from the water they are wrapped in a fitting terry cloth cover and placed on the body. Moisture in these heat packs improves the conduction of heat from the hot pack to the body. Additional towels are sometimes needed, and removed as the pack cools. A moist heat pack is usually applied for about 20 minutes. Dry heat should never be left on the body for extended periods; frequently check in with the client on temperature and location.

Dry heating pads are probably the most commonly used commercial form of heat application. The conduction of heat is not as good as with moist heat because the water molecules in a moist heat application aid the heat transfer. Dry heating pads are usually electric and have a switch that allows different heat settings from low to high. There are several forms of 'moist heat' electric heating pads that aren't a true moist heat application. A special cloth covering over the heating pad draws moisture out of the air and creates more moisture than the dry heating pad alone. These units are a convenient alternative to full moist heat packs, and usually more effective than the traditional dry heating pad.

There are a host of heat bags and pillows designed for heating in a microwave. These usually contain buckwheat, rice or some other fill that heats up without cooking. These are handy to have in the clinic for specific local applications and for keeping the client warm. These can be used, as can the dry heating pad, with moist washcloths for a moist heat effect.

Certain types of chemical gel packs may be heated for use as a heat pack. These packs contain a chemical compound that gets either hot or cold. Some gel packs may be heated in the microwave. They are usually designed to fit a certain region of the body, and may have Velcro fasteners or straps that hold them in place. Chemical gel packs are commercially popular and convenient.

Hot stones are primarily used in the spa environment. The stones are heated in water-filled tubs and then placed directly on the body. The density of rock allows it to retain heat for a longer time than some other heat modalities. Some practitioners use the heated stone as a soft-tissue manipulation tool with effective results. It can be challenging to monitor and control the temperature of the stone.

To prevent burns, the practitioner must closely monitor the client, frequently checking in for comfort levels.

Melted paraffin is applied, usually to the hands or feet, as a local heat treatment. The hand or foot is dipped into melted paraffin and then remains covered as the paraffin solidifies and cools. The paraffin acts as an insulator that keeps heat applied to the application area. Wrapping the paraffin-covered body part in a towel or plastic wrap helps prolong the heat application. The paraffin bath is helpful to apply heat to areas, such as the hands or feet, that are harder to reach with other topical heat applications due to their shape. Monitoring the heat of the wax is important to prevent burns; practitioners should always test the heat of the wax on their own skin before applying to client.

The whirlpool is an effective method of applying localized moist heat to a particular area. In a rehabilitation environment, such as a physical therapy clinic or athletic training facility, the smaller whirlpools, which treat distal limb injuries, are more common.

Whole-body applications

These modalities work through either conduction if the water or air is non-moving or convection if the water or air is moving. In a whirlpool, movement allows the water molecules that have transferred their heat to the cooler body to be moved away, while warmer molecules of water move in to replace them. Thus, there is a continual renewal of the warmer elements as they come in contact with the body.[?] The medium's movement allows a more efficient transfer of heat. The steam room works by convection as steam moves across the body. A sauna works by radiation as there is a static heat source (wood fire or electrical element) that is radiating heat toward the body. Whole-body applications are effective at enhancing circulation throughout the body as opposed to just a small area as in local heat applications.

However, the benefits of heat come from the neurological reactions not an increase in temperature in the deep tissues. Although some whole-body applications do raise the temperature in the deeper tissues, this increase is not considered therapeutic.

The whirlpool uses jets of air that continuously circulate to move the water, stimulate circulation and provide an analgesic (pain relieving) response. Hot tubs with moving water accomplish the same effects as smaller whirlpool baths.

A steam room is a form of moist heat. The contact of steam with the body surface produces a whole-body moist heat application. The moist heat of the steam room prevents the evaporation of moisture from the skin, so it is easy to become overheated. Client time in a steam room should be monitored to make sure the body is not overheating.

A sauna is a form of dry heat. Sauna treatments are in a small enclosed room or cabinet that the person sits in for the length of the treatment. The sauna's heat source is usually electric in a clinic environment. The sauna is desirable in situations where flushing of the body's toxins through sweating is desired. Some people will prefer the sauna over a steam room or whirlpool as well.

The rehabilitation clinic

In a clinic with other health care practitioners such as physical therapists, chiropractors, or sports medicine doctors, clients may have access to other modalities. Ultrasound is the most frequently used conversion heat modality. Although its use is usually out of the scope of practice for massage therapists, therapists should be familiar with how ultrasound works.

Ultrasound is the most effective method to heat the deep tissues. With continuous wave ultrasound, high frequency sound waves are transmitted into the body through the head of the ultrasound device. Various tissues in the body absorb the ultrasonic energy at different rates. The denser is the tissue, the faster it absorbs ultrasound energy. Consequently, the denser tissues, such as bone, absorb ultrasonic energy at the greatest rate while thinner tissues are harder to heat. Therefore, heating dense and deep tissues that connect to bone, such as ligament or joint capsule, is most effective with ultrasound.

Heat benefits and contraindications

Heat applications have a number of physiological effects. Heat can be an effective compliment to the soft-tissue therapist's efforts to promote tissue healing and pain relief. Heat has general overall effects as well as those that are localized to a treated body part or region. Heat's effects also depend on the type of heat and its depth of penetration (the more adipose a client has the less penetration in those areas; and the reverse for those particularly thin).

As with all modalities, thermal and non, there are instances in which the therapy can produce effects opposite or even harmful to the goal of recovery. There are instances where there are both positive and potentially negative results with the use of heat, such as using heat on acute injuries which may increase lymphatic fluid movement but also swelling. The practitioner must evaluate the situation and make an educated decision. Consulting with a client's other health care practitioners may be beneficial. Knowing the effects of heat will help with these therapeutic choices.

Box 3.2   Benefits of Heat

- Increases local tissue metabolism
- Increases local circulation bringing nutrition and removing waste
- Viscosity of blood is reduced improving blood flow
- Increases lymphatic fluid movement, removing damaged cellular debris
- Increases the extensibility and elasticity of various connective tissues
- Relaxes neurological cells within fascia that govern fascial contractility
- Increases elasticity in superficial connective tissues and reduces fascial tension
- Relaxes deeper muscles through neurological effects
- Assists therapeutic stretching procedures
- Decreases excess neurological activity and hypertonicity
- Improves motor nerve conduction so reduces biomechanical dysfunction
- Increases nerve conduction velocity so reduces muscle tightness
- Breaks the pain–spasm–pain cycle and reduces pain

Benefits

Metabolism   Heat increases local tissue metabolism as it speeds up various chemical and metabolic processes. In many cases, such as hypertonic muscle that is ischemic, this effect is desirable. In other situations, an increase in local tissue metabolism could cause problems (see precautions below).

Circulation   Some of the most beneficial effects of thermotherapy involve increases to local circulation.

Superficial heat applications cause a reflex vasodilation of the blood vessels and a corresponding increase in local tissue circulation. Circulation is also increased because the viscosity of blood is reduced which allows for easier movement of blood through the vessels.[2] Increased circulation is of vital importance in the healing of most injuries. Increasing circulation helps injuries and other conditions because the blood brings in nutrients and oxygen, while removing waste products.

Increased lymphatic fluid movement Lymphatic fluids remove damaged cellular tissue debris. There is an increase in the movement of lymphatic fluid with heat applications and stimulating this effect with heat modalities is important for injuries.[17] Acute injuries can sometimes benefit from this treatment (see precautions below).

Increased connective tissue pliability Heat applications increase the extensibility and elasticity of various connective tissues. In muscles and tissues closest to the skin, using superficial heat modalities works to raise the tissue temperature and thus increase tissue pliability. Current research in fascial physiology shows that there are neurological cells within fascia that govern fascial contractility.[18,19]

While significant thermal change from a heat application does not penetrate to the depth of many muscle tissues, topical thermal applications can still reduce tension in deeper muscles. The reason for this is that heat increases elasticity in superficial connective tissues and reduces fascial tension. There is a neurological integration of superficial fascia with that which permeates deeper muscles. Consequently a reduction in superficial fascial tension from the heat application produces neurological responses that are followed in the deeper fascia producing a similar muscular relaxation response.

Because muscles have such a large percentage of connective tissue in them, it is helpful to use a heat modality before performing therapeutic stretching procedures. Stretching the connective tissues is more effective when they are warmer and the neurological response of the heat is transmitted to deeper muscles, making them easier to stretch as well.

A superficial heating modality provides little increase in connective tissue pliability for connective tissues around deep joints such as the joint capsule of the shoulder or ligaments of the hip. These joints

are too deep for any significant thermal effects to reach. Heating these tissues requires a thermal modality other than topical applications. To cause a temperature change in these deeper muscle tissues, a qualified practitioner would have to use a deep heating modality such as ultrasound or diathermy.

Decreased muscle tightness Heat has a soothing effect which decreases excess neurological activity and reduces muscular hypertonicity. Heat is thought to reduce the firing rate of muscle spindle cells and decrease activity in the gamma efferent system of the spindles. The reduction in muscle spindle activity reduces muscle tightness. Heat may also increase the firing rate of Golgi tendon organs, also a factor that will lead to the reduction in muscle tension.[20]

Increase in nerve conduction velocity Reductions in muscle tightness that result from increased heat sensations are likely related to the increase in nerve conduction velocity of various sensory impulses.[21] Increased tissue temperature may also improve coordination in muscular activities and reduce biomechanical dysfunction because of improved conduction of motor nerve impulses.

Increased pain threshold A reduction in pain sensations helps break the pain–spasm–pain cycle, so a reduction in pain has lasting effects for many soft-tissue disorders. Thermal applications produce additional signals from afferent fibers which arrive at the central nervous system first and essentially override some of pain signals. Nerve conduction can also be reduced by raising the skin temperature and thus change the perception of pain. Any reduction in hypertonicity or spasm would also reduce pain.

Precautions and contraindications for heat

Heat, whilst usually and generally a positive modality for treating pain and injury, can cause further injury or delay healing in some situations. Taking precautions in using heat modalities overall and knowing when not to use them is important for the soft-tissue therapists. A proper assessment is necessary to ascertain the appropriateness of heat.

Acute injury or inflammation Heat applications can aggravate an acute injury or inflammatory condition. Heating the tissues speeds up metabolic processes and increases the inflammatory response. The acute inflammatory phase of most acute injuries is mostly complete after about 72 hours. After

Box 3.3 Precautions and Contraindications for Heat

- Acute injury or inflammation
- Recent or potential hemorrhage
- Increased formation of edema
- Impaired sensation
- Modalities that are too hot
- Impaired mental ability
- Thrombophlebitis
- Malignancy
- Pregnancy
- Broken or irritated skin
- Topical analgesics

this time, heat modalities are safer to use; however, one should use caution. In systemic inflammation, such as rheumatoid arthritis, heat can be contraindicated as it furthers damage.

Recent or potential hemorrhage Because heat applications stimulate circulation heat modalities should not be used if there is any suspicion of uncontrolled bleeding in the area. By decreasing the viscosity of the blood, the heat could aggravate this type of problem.

Increased formation of edema Edema (swelling) develops in response to traumatic tissue damage in the region of the injury. Heat applications increase the movement of fluids to the area. The clinician should be judicious in the use of heat modalities when swelling is present.

Impaired sensation If an individual has some form of sensory nerve impairment and is not able to feel sensations on the skin, heat applications should be used with great caution. Individuals can receive burns from heat applications because they do not perceive the pain sensations from the excess heat. Local nerve damage or systemic neurological disorders could also cause nerve damage severe enough to impair the perception of excess heat.

Modalities that are too hot Certain modalities, such as moist heat packs or hot stones that are heated in hot water, can be very hot. The client can be burned if the heat modality is placed directly on the skin without proper insulation. A general guideline is that if you can't comfortably leave your hand in the hot water that the modality was heated in, you need some level of insulation before placing it on the client's body. Always test the temperature of the modality prior to placing it upon the client.

Impaired mental ability An individual with impaired sensation or cognitive function is not able to determine if there is an excess of temperature applied to the body. Impaired mental abilities may result from genetic disorders, trauma, disease, medications, or other substances the client may have taken.

Thrombophlebitis An increase in circulation and/or reduction in viscosity of the blood from the heat application can dislodge the clot and cause a cerebro-vascular accident (stroke) or even death. Local swelling, particularly in the lower extremity, could involve clotting. Always ask the client if they have a blood clot.

Malignancy If the individual has malignant tumors, thermotherapy in the region is contraindicated. There is a possibility that growth of the tumor could be encouraged through an increase in circulation or an increase in local cellular metabolic activity.

Pregnancy Local applications of heat are generally not a problem for pregnant women. What is of concern is any form of heat that could increase the temperature which the fetus is exposed to. For example, therapeutic ultrasound that produces heat effects could be detrimental if aimed in the direction of the fetus. The density of the bones in the fetus could selectively absorb the ultrasonic injury and cause injury. The frequency level of diagnostic ultrasound (which is used frequently during pregnancy) is much different, and does not produce heat changes in the tissue. Full body immersions in hot water, especially for longer than 15 minutes, could cause adverse effects because the body temperature could be raised to a level that is harmful to the fetus.

Broken or irritated skin When the skin is broken there is an increased chance of infections being started. Any broken skin should be kept clear of thermotherapy to prevent risk of infection or transmission of infection to another individual. In most instances, the client is going to be aware of any broken or irritated skin and their pain is most likely to discourage the application of any thermal modality on the broken skin.

Topical analgesics Some advise against applying heat over topical analgesics that cause the skin to vasodilate, such as menthol or capsaicin due to a concern over burns possibly resulting.

COLD APPLICATIONS

Cold applications, or cryotherapy, have effects that are, for the most part, opposite to those of heat. Cryotherapy is the ideal treatment modality for acute injuries because of its effect on arresting inflammation and slowing local tissue metabolism. They are used extensively in the athletic environment as cold helps injured athletes to return to activity sooner.[22]

There are no deep, penetrating cold modalities as there are with heat; all cold modalities are superficial applications. In order for a cold application to be effective, the target tissue must cool by transferring heat out of itself. There is little significant temperature change at depths greater than about 1 cm below the skin.[14,16,23] Consequently, cryotherapy is impractical for deep anatomical structures. Practitioners must also consider the insulating capabilities of adipose tissue as its presence reduces the impact of cold applications on deeper tissues.[24] Monitoring cold applications is just as important as with heat. Frequently check in with the client for comfort and tolerance levels.

Box 3.4 Cold Modalities

- Ice bag
- Chemical gel packs
- Ice massage
- Cold immersion
- Whirlpool tub
- Vapo-coolant sprays

Cold modalities

An ice bag is applied to the body using a plastic or rubber bag that holds the ice and helps it mold to the shape of the body. The plastic bag acts as a partial insulator and keeps the ice from causing tissue damage from prolonged direct exposure to cold. Since the ice bag treatment uses conduction as a means of heat transfer, the bag (plastic) will never get as cold as ice placed directly on the skin. Therefore, the plastic provides a degree of insulation to keep the ice application from causing damage.

Although suggestions for treatment times vary, a generally accepted period of application is about 10–20 minutes.[25–27] One study found that repeated applications of 10 minutes was the most effective cryotherapy application for generating beneficial tissue temperature changes and avoiding adverse affects.[28]

In many situations, an ice bag is the preferred treatment because it can effectively mold to a body part that has an odd shape. Bags of frozen vegetables like peas or corn are used for this purpose as well, and make a great home treatment. The benefit of frozen vegetables, peas for example, is that they are much smaller than ice cubes, and will often provide a more effective contour to the body part. However, they are not as effective as crushed ice. Bags of crushed ice or ice water immersion appear to be the most effective cryotherapy methods.[29,30]

Chemical gel packs contain a chemical compound that gets very cold when frozen. Gel packs are frozen in a freezer and can be reused. They are usually designed to fit a certain region of the body, and may have Velcro fasteners or straps that hold them in place. The approximate length of time for a chemical ice pack application is 20 minutes. However, the client should be monitored when using a chemical cold pack (or tell them to pay close attention to signs and symptoms if using them alone). Some of chemical cold packs freeze at a lower temperature than water, and may be colder than initially apparent.

Chemical gel packs are commercially popular and convenient. Ice that melts in a plastic bag when you apply it can sometimes be messy. There is no similar mess with the chemical gel packs. However, comparative studies of different cryotherapeutic modalities have found gel packs to be some of the least effective at achieving beneficial therapeutic results.[29,30] Gel packs are not as effective as ice applications.

Ice massage allows the beneficial effects of cold to be combined with tissue manipulation. Ice massage is also an effective way to produce a cryotherapy treatment in a short duration of time.[31] This cold application begins with forming ice in a shape that is easy to handle. The most common method is freezing a paper cup filled with water. Once the water in the cup is frozen, the top of the cup is peeled away to reveal the ice. The cup provides an insulated handle for the practitioner to use when applying the ice treatment. The ice is rubbed over the area until the client experiences the four stages of cryotherapy treatment (see below). Ice application times vary, but they are usually no longer than 5 minutes in any one area because the ice is directly touching the skin. Ice massage is effective when performed in conjunction with massage treatments such as deep transverse friction.

Cold immersion is an effective cryotherapy treatment for regions such as the distal extremities. In this application the extremity is submerged in ice water. Because cold is applied directly to the skin, this treatment should not last longer than 5 minutes. Closely monitor the client in ice immersion treatments because the area being treated (such as an ankle) will cool faster than connected areas left out of the water (like the toes). Extensive ice immersion treatments can cause tissue damage to distal extremities where circulation is poor, and should therefore be used with caution.

Cold immersion is also done in whirlpools where the cold water is continuously circulated around the affected area. The water temperature in any of these ice immersion treatments can be adjusted so it is not too cold for the length of treatment. Ice water immersion is one of the most effective methods of cryotherapy application.[25]

Vapo-coolant sprays, such as fluori-methane, are another superficial cold application.[32] Fluori-methane and other vapo-coolants are substances kept in a pressurized bottle and then sprayed onto the skin surface. When exposed to air, these liquids evaporate rapidly, causing the underlying tissue to be chilled. Vapo-coolant sprays have become less popular in recent years because their use is linked to environmental damage such as ozone depletion.[33,34]

Cold benefits and contraindications

As with heat applications, selection of the proper cryotherapy method is dependent on the physiological goals of treatment. These goals arise from an understanding of the physiological effects of cold applications. The length of time for a cryotherapy treatment is dependent on a number of variables. For most cryotherapy treatments there are four distinct stages of cryotherapy treatment, which indicate stages of the body's response to the cold. These stages generally occur in the following order:

- Appreciation or strong sensation of the cold
- Burning sensations in the skin
- Deep aching sensations
- Numbness (lack of sensation).

When the stage of numbness is achieved, the cryotherapy application can be terminated. Decrease of sensory input (numbness) is the end goal of most cryotherapy treatment. Continued use of a cryotherapy treatment past the point of numbness can be dangerous, especially if the source of the cold, such as ice, is put directly on the skin without any insulating barrier. Prolonged application of cryotherapy can lead to frostbite or nerve damage. It is important to closely monitor the client during cryotherapy treatment.

While there are general guidelines for cryotherapy application, several factors can alter those guidelines and should be considered. The effect of

---

Box 3.5   Benefits of Cold

- Cellular metabolism is slowed, shortening healing time
- Swelling from acute injuries is reduced
- Blood flow is inhibited, also reducing inflammation
- Heat from inflammation is reduced
- Sensory signals are slowed, reducing pain
- Pain tolerance is heightened
- Acute spasm may be inhibited
- Reduces muscle soreness
- Decreases muscle tightness
- Helps break the pain–spasm–pain cycle

any thermal application can vary among individuals so the length of treatment for one person may be different than for another. The subcutaneous body fat is a highly effective insulating layer so the discrepancy in body fat percentage makes a difference in how two different people respond to any thermal modality.[24] Differences in adipose tissue in different body regions in one person also affect how long cryotherapy applications should be applied.

Benefits

Metabolism   Cold applications slow down the cellular metabolic activity in the region where the cold is applied. Reduced metabolism is a primary benefit of cold applications, especially in acute injuries. The excess cellular metabolic activity in acute injuries is one factor that prolongs the healing process. Using cryotherapy immediately after the injury brings this metabolic activity under control and shortens the recovery period from the injury. Compression is usually applied to an acute injury along with ice applications. Reducing metabolic activity at the injury site is more effectively done when using ice in combination with compression.[35]

Circulation   In response to cold sensations, the smooth muscle cells in the walls of the superficial blood vessels contract and produce vasoconstriction. Vasoconstriction is more pronounced with cold applications in some regions of the body, the distal extremities in particular. Blood flow is reduced with cold application in order to keep the overall body from becoming too cold. Circulation is usually decreased initially with cold applications, but a reaction called 'the hunting response' can occur after about 15 minutes, especially in the distal extremities. This response may repeat as a cycle of vasoconstriction and vasodilation during the entire application of the cryotherapy.[36] Attempting to incite vasodilation with cold is not recommended as a therapy. (The physiological effects on circulation can be either a benefit or a contraindication depending on the circumstances.)

Decreased edema   Swelling and inflammation from an acute injury can be reduced with cryotherapy. Accumulation of excess fluids in the tissues around an injury is a primary cause of pain with injuries in the acute stage. By reducing the temperature in the tissues, heat is reduced. Cold also reduces blood viscosity and capillary permeability, which along with vasoconstriction inhibits blood flow and thus, the movement of fluids to the inflamed area.

The use of cryotherapy for the reduction of edema should be limited to acute injuries. Chronic edema due to poor circulation or immobility benefits more from heat applications that increase connective tissue pliability and encourage greater tissue fluid movement.

Decreased nerve conduction velocity and pain   Cryotherapy slows the rate at which nerve impulses are propagated along a peripheral nerve. The slowing of this impulse affects both sensory and motor signals in the nerve. Slowing of motor signal transmission is evident by the lack of muscular coordination in an area that has had cryotherapy application. Sensory signals are slowed as well. The reduction of sensory signals is beneficial in reducing pain sensations following an injury. Pain reduction helps break the pain–spasm–pain cycle and contributes to a decrease in muscular hypertonicity.

If the cold application is of short duration (about 15 minutes), nerve conduction velocity returns to normal relatively soon. In cold applications that are 20 minutes or longer, it may take close to 30 minutes for nerve conduction velocity to return to baseline levels.[2] With a decrease in nerve conduction velocity, there is a decrease in the reporting of pain sensations. This nerve signal reduction gives the individual a heightened level of pain tolerance. However, the higher pain tolerance is limited to the tissues that are chilled with the cryotherapy application.

Decreased stretch reflex   A corresponding part of the reduction in nerve conduction velocity is a reduction in the myotatic or stretch reflex. This reflex is activated by the muscle spindles when they are stretched either too far or too fast (as in whiplash). Overstretching a hypertonic muscle can also activate the muscle spindles, causing increased muscle tension. Cryotherapy is one avenue to decrease the activation of the muscle spindles so that stretching procedures can be more effective. This physiological effect will be most useful in acute muscle spasm where there is significant muscle tension that is difficult to reduce. However, cold applications decrease the pliability of connective tissues so attempting to aid stretching with cryotherapy may be limited. The practitioner will need to weigh the benefits of decreased neurological activity vs decreased connective tissue pliability.

Reduction in muscle soreness   Cryotherapy helps reduce certain types of muscle soreness, especially the delayed onset muscle soreness (DOMS) associated with increased levels of unaccustomed exercise.[37,38] In addition, cryotherapy is used to reduce post-treatment soreness after certain methods of soft-tissue manipulation.

Decreased muscle tightness   A reduction in muscle tightness occurs as a result of the reduction in motor nerve conduction velocity. By reducing motor signals and concurrently reducing pain sensations, cold application helps break the pain–spasm–pain cycle.

Contrast treatments   In some instances, the beneficial effects of both heat and cold are desired. Alternating heat and cold modalities is called a contrast treatment. The use of heat and cold in quick succession is theorized to produce a flushing of the blood and tissue fluids. While contrast treatments are used routinely in rehabilitation settings, the research does not support many of the ideas behind contrast treatments. There are claims that contrast therapy enhances circulation though cyclical temperature fluctuations. However, in several studies contrast therapy did not appear to produce many of these purported temperature fluctuations.[16,39]

While contrast therapy may not produce the significant tissue temperature changes once thought, it still has benefits. There are valuable neurological responses to the alternating heat and cold, which are the most likely reason for clinical successes with contrast therapy. Recommendations for how long heat is used compared to how long the cold is used are variable. Time constraints of the two treatments often depend upon the situation and the individual. A general guideline is a 3:1 ratio of heat to cold. For every 3 minutes of heat there will be 1 minute of cold.[14] Consider the physiological effects of both the heat and cold applications when designing a contrast treatment.

Precautions and contraindications to cold

Many of the precautions for heat applications are the same as for cold. The following list of contraindications is relative – meaning a modality may be contraindicated in some cases, but not in all. Apply thoughtful clinical reasoning to determine if the physiology of the condition and treatment goals warrant one of the different cold applications mentioned. In some cases certain physiological effects of cold are desirable, but not others. If that is the case, then it is best to estimate if the benefits of using the cold application outweigh the drawbacks. Evaluation should always assess the client for the conditions listed below.

Box 3.6   Precautions for Cold

- Broken or irritated skin
- Cold intolerance or cold allergy
- Raynaud's disease
- Conditions of circulatory compromise
- Decreased connective tissue pliability
- Areas of superficial nerves
- Sensory nerve impairment
- Impaired mental ability

Broken or irritated skin   Keep cryotherapy applications clear of broken skin to prevent the risk of infection or transmission of infection to another individual.

Cold intolerance or cold allergy   Some individuals are not able to tolerate cryotherapy, and may have allergic reactions that are visible on the skin. They may break out in hives or rashes immediately or within a few minutes of placing a cold application on them. In many cases, the person does not know they have a cold allergy, so it is important to monitor the client when the cold application is first applied.

Raynaud's disease   This is a condition involving arterial spasm that most commonly affects females between the ages of 18 and 30. The condition involves abnormal vasoconstriction in the extremities when they are exposed to cold. Emotional stress can also play a role in setting off the reaction.[40] The individual does not need to be exposed to extremes of cold for symptoms of Raynaud's to be evident. Most people who have this problem are aware of it because they have experienced the symptoms before.

Conditions of circulatory compromise Cryotherapy could further aggravate any condition that involves an undesirable reduction in circulation.

Decreased connective tissue pliability Heat increases the pliability in connective tissues and cold does just the opposite. In most instances, the goal of therapeutic procedures is to increase connective tissue pliability, so this physiological effect is usually undesirable. The practitioner should weigh the benefits of using cold application if an increase in connective tissue pliability is a primary goal of the treatment procedure.

Over regions where nerves are superficial Nerve damage can occur from cryotherapy if the nerve is close to the skin, and does not have adequate insulating protection from the cold. Two common examples where nerves can be injured from superficial cold applications are the ulnar nerve on the posterior aspect of the elbow and the peroneal nerve on the lateral aspect of the knee near the fibular head.

Impaired sensation If an individual has sensory nerve impairment and is not able to feel sensations on the skin, use caution or don't use cryotherapy at all. Always ask the client whether the client has a condition that impairs their sensations. Frostbite or nerve damage could occur because an individual does not feel the skin go through the various stages of cold application.[38]

Impaired mental ability As with impaired sensation if an individual does not have full and normally functioning cognitive powers, they might not be able to determine if there is an excess of temperature applied to the body. Impaired mental abilities can result from genetic disorders, trauma, disease, medications, or other substances they might have taken.

TOPICAL ANALGESICS AS THERMAL AGENTS

Analgesics are substances or agents that relieve pain without causing a loss of consciousness.[41] Most of us are familiar with oral analgesics such as aspirin or ibuprofen. Topical analgesics (TAs) are pain-relieving substances placed or rubbed directly on the skin in order to relieve pain and are popular forms of pain relief. A 1987 survey indicated that 34% of adults in the United States use TAs for some form of pain relief.[42]

Advertisements for topical analgesics sometimes tout their benefits in producing heat or cooling effects on the body. However, these claims can be misleading because topical analgesics are not true thermal modalities. Yet, there are therapeutic benefits to their use in certain conditions. The practitioner should understand how topical analgesics work in order to evaluate their physiological effects and if they are appropriate for specific clients.

Categories of topical analgesics

There are several categories of topical analgesics, depending upon their active ingredients. Some analgesics contain medications that are not legally dispensed in over-the-counter preparations, so they are not used by most massage practitioners.[43] The more common TAs that massage practitioners use fall into a category sometimes called rubefacients. A rubefacient is an agent that reddens the skin by producing active or passive hyperemia.[41] The majority of rubefacient TAs fall into one of three categories: counterirritants, salicylates, and capsaicin. The physiological properties of each category are described below. Several brand names are mentioned so it is clear which category various products fall into. All brand names listed are considered trademarked names.

Counterirritants

The majority of TAs used by massage practitioners is counterirritant. A counterirritant is an agent that produces a superficial irritation in one part of the body that is intended to relieve irritation in another part. The irritation produced by these substances is most commonly a chemical stimulation of thermal receptors in the skin, which produce a sensation of heat or cold. Popular brand names for counterirritants include: ArthriCare, Eucalyptamint, Atomic Balm, Icy Hot, Prossage Heat, Tiger Balm, Nature's Chemist, Biofreeze, and Therapeutic Mineral Ice.

The brand names for these various products reflect the emphasis on the sensation of heat or cold experienced from their use. For example, you would probably expect to have a sensation of heat from Prossage Heat or Atomic Balm. Likewise you would expect to have a sensation of cold from Therapeutic Mineral Ice. But what about Icy Hot? Each person's physiology may respond a little differently to the formula of the analgesic. Therefore some people may have a sensation of heat from Tiger Balm while others have a sensation of cold.

Salicylates

The salicylates are a group of related compounds derived from salicylic acid. They contain similar pharmacological agents as aspirin. Salicylates have several beneficial physiological effects. They are known to inhibit prostaglandin synthesis, reduce inflammatory activity, and aid in fever reduction and pain management. A review of salicylates show that in some cases they are beneficial, while in others they are only moderately helpful and in some cases not helpful at all (as in chronic arthritic and rheumatic pain).[44] Popular brand names for salicylates include: Aspercreme, Ben Gay, Flexall, Mobisyl, and Sportscreme.

Capsaicin

Many people are familiar with a sensation of heat felt on the skin when it is exposed to cayenne pepper. In cold weather climates or winter sports activities, people put cayenne pepper in their socks to keep their toes warm. The active ingredient in cayenne pepper that produces this warming sensation is capsaicin. It is an alkaloid irritation to the skin and mucous membranes that produces pain-relieving sensations. Capsaicin binds to the nociceptors of the skin where it produces an initial excitation of neurons (often felt as burning, itching, or prickling). After the initial sensation (sometimes as long as 2 weeks) there is some desensitization that leads to the analgesic effects. There are adverse effects with some forms of topical capsaicin because it can produce a burning sensation at the site of application.[43] Therefore it is not as popular as other TAs, such as the counterirritants. Brand names for analgesics containing capsaicin include: Zostrix, Zoxtrix HP, and Capzasin-P. Some sources suggest

not using heat modalities over TAs such as capsaicin. Gloves should be worn for application in order to prevent it getting into sensitive skin areas.

Therapeutic effects of topical analgesics

Counterirritants are members of the primary group of TAs that is used in thermal application (correctly or incorrectly), so this discussion of physiological effects emphasizes that group. The effects of the counterirritants can be grouped into three primary categories: neurological, circulatory, and thermal.

Neurological

Interestingly, the neurological responses are the most significant benefits of TAs. Counterirritants work by chemically stimulating (irritating) sensory receptors in the skin, especially those associated with thermal sensations. The irritation of receptors in the skin may also inhibit pain signals reported from the nociceptors (pain receptors), thereby blocking pain sensations sent to the brain. This description is based on the gate theory of pain described earlier in the chapter.

While the receptors that are activated by the TA are located in the skin, the neurological effects are not limited to the skin. For example, a reduction of muscle tension often results from the chemical stimulation of sensory receptors in the skin.[45] Muscular pain reduction is a goal in most soft-tissue treatments so these substances can be helpful. Note, however, that the other physiological effects of true heat or cold applications, such as changes in connective tissue pliability or nerve conduction velocity, are not necessarily present with TA application.

Circulatory

The chemical stimulation of receptors in the skin produces a superficial vasodilation. Cutaneous vasodilation produces local hyperemia and accounts for the redness that can result from certain analgesics. The increase in circulation is local and only in the superficial tissues, so TAs shouldn't be considered a means of increasing circulation to damaged tissues at deeper levels. The increase in circulation can produce a slight temperature increase due to the increased circulation in the skin. However, this temperature increase is relatively small and it is questionable whether the small increase can produce any therapeutic benefits from the heat increase alone. The thermal results of TAs are discussed in greater detail below.

Thermal

There is a difference between a sensation of heat or cold and an actual temperature change within the tissues. The primary effects of counterirritants result from chemically stimulating the thermal receptors in the skin. The stimulation of these receptors causes the brain to perceive sensations of heat or cold. Yet there is no ingredient in TAs capable of producing a therapeutically relevant temperature change in the tissues. The therapeutic benefits of heat for soft tissues, especially the deeper tissues do not occur until the tissues reach a temperature of between 104°F and 113°F.[46]

As mentioned above under circulatory effects, local circulation increases from TAs may create a small temperature increase in the skin. One study that evaluated Eucalyptamint found the local circulation increase caused a skin temperature rise of approximately 1.5°F.[47] This slight temperature increase was limited to the skin and did not penetrate to deeper tissues.

When a TA is applied it is likely at room temperature (about 70°F). Of the four methods of heat transfer (conduction, convection, conversion, and radiation) the only one that is feasible for a topically applied cream to heat tissues is conduction. Therefore, to reach the temperature level considered necessary for therapeutic change in deeper tissues, the TA would have to be at least 30°F–40°F warmer than room temperature. Without being at this temperature there may be a sensation of heat but no significant thermal change in the tissues.

Precautions

As with heat or cold modalities, there are contraindications for the use of TAs. Practitioners should not assume the therapy will make deeper tissues more pliable, as that assumption could lead the practitioner to be overzealous in their soft-tissue treatment. Likewise, a person who applies a cold sensation TA to an acute injury with the idea of reducing inflammation may, in fact, use it inappropriately by increasing local circulation to the injury site in the acute phase. Finally, some argue that one should never use a TA with a heat application, as burns can result due to the skin possibly reaching the limit of vasodilation.[2]

References

1. Cailliet R. Pain: Mechanisms and Management. Philadelphia: F.A. Davis; 1993.
2. Cameron MH. Physical Agents in Rehabilitation. Philadelphia: W.B. Saunders; 1999.
3. Schlereth T, Birklein F. The sympathetic nervous system and pain. Neuromolecular Med. 2008;10(3):141–147.
4. White A, Panjabi M. Clinical Biomechanics of the Spine. 2nd ed. Philadelphia: Lippincott Williams & Wilkins; 1990.
5. Adams M, Bogduk N, Burton K, Dolan P. The Biomechanics of Back Pain. Edinburgh: Churchill Livingstone; 2002.
6. Warfield C, Bajwa Z. Principles & Practice of Pain Management. New York: McGraw-Hill; 2004.
7. Ochoa J, Torebjork E. Sensations evoked by intraneural microstimulation of C nociceptor fibres in human skin nerves. J Physiol. 1989;415:583–599.
8. Torebjork HE, Ochoa JL. New method to identify nociceptor units innervating glabrous skin of the human hand. Exp Brain Res. 1990;81(3):509–514.
9. Bonica JJ. The Management of Pain. 2nd ed. Philadelphia: Lea & Febiger; 1990.
10. Mense S, Simons DG. Muscle Pain: Understanding Its Nature, Diagnosis, & Treatment. Baltimore: Lippincott Williams & Wilkins; 2001.
11. Melzack R, Wall PD. The Challenge of Pain. New York: Basic Books, Inc.; 1983.
12. Melzack R. Pain and the neuromatrix in the brain. J Dent Educ. 2001;65(12):1378–1382.
13. Melzack R. Evolution of the neuromatrix theory of pain. The Prithvi Raj Lecture: presented at the third World Congress of World Institute of Pain, Barcelona 2004. Pain Pract. 2005;5(2):85–94.
14. Prentice W. Therapeutic Modalities in Sports Medicine. 2nd ed. St. Louis: Mosby; 1990.
15. Robertson VJ, Ward AR, Jung P. The effect of heat on tissue extensibility: a comparison of deep and superficial heating. Arch Phys Med Rehabil. 2005;86(4):819–825.
16. Myrer JW, Draper DO, Durrant E. Contrast therapy and intramuscular temperature in the human leg. J Athl Train. 1994;29(4):318–322.
17. Tortora G, Grabowski S. Principles of Anatomy and Physiology. 8th ed. New York: Harper Collins; 1996.

18. Schleip R. Fascial plasticity – a new neurobiological explanation. Journal of Bodywork and Movement Therapies. 2003;7(1):11–19.

19. Schleip R. Fascia is able to contract in a smooth muscle-like manner and thereby influence musculoskeletal mechanics. Paper presented at: Fascia Research Congress, 2007; Harvard Medical School, Boston, MA.

20. Lehmann JF, DeLateur BJ. Therapeutic heat. In: Lehman JF, ed. Therapeutic Heat and Cold. 4th ed. Baltimore: Williams & Wilkins; 1990.

21. Kramer JF. Ultrasound: evaluation of its mechanical and thermal effects. Arch Phys Med Rehabil. 1984;65(5):223–227.

22. Hubbard TJ, Aronson SL, Denegar CR. Does cryotherapy hasten return to participation? A systematic review. J Athl Train. 2004;39(1):88–94.

23. Merrick MA, Jutte LS, Smith ME. Cold modalities with different thermodynamic properties produce different surface and intramuscular temperatures. J Athl Train. 2003;38(1):28–33.

24. Myrer WJ, Myrer KA, Measom GJ, Fellingham GW, Evers SL. Muscle temperature is affected by overlying adipose when cryotherapy is administered. J Athl Train. 2001;36(1):32–36.

25. Myrer JW, Measom G, Fellingham GW. Temperature changes in the human leg during and after two methods of cryotherapy. J Athl Train. 1998;33(1):25–29.

26. Palmer JE, Knight KL. Ankle and thigh skin surface temperature changes with repeated ice pack application. J Athl Train. 1996;31(4):319–323.

27. AAOS. Athletic Training and Sports Medicine. 2nd ed. Park Ridge: American Academy of Orthopaedic Surgeons; 1991.

28. Mac Auley DC. Ice therapy: how good is the evidence? Int J Sports Med. 2001;22(5):379–384.

29. Kennet J, Hardaker N, Hobbs S, Selfe J. Cooling efficiency of 4 common cryotherapeutic agents. J Athl Train. 2007;42(3):343–348.

30. Kanlayanaphotporn R, Janwantanakul P. Comparison of skin surface temperature during the application of various cryotherapy modalities. Arch Phys Med Rehabil. 2005; 86(7):1411–1415.

31. Zemke JE, Andersen JC, Guion WK, McMillan J, Joyner AB. Intramuscular temperature responses in the human leg to two forms of cryotherapy: ice massage and ice bag. J Orthop Sports Phys Ther. 1998;27(4):301–307.

32. Travell JS, D. Myofascial Pain and Dysfunction: The Trigger Point Manual. Vol 1. 1st ed. Baltimore: Williams & Wilkins; 1983.

33. Vallentyne SW, Vallentyne JR. The case of the missing ozone: are physiatrists to blame? Arch Phys Med Rehabil. 1988;69(11):992–993.

34. Simons DG, Travell JG, Simons LS. Protecting the ozone layer. Arch Phys Med Rehabil. 1990;71(1):64.

35. Merrick MA, Knight KL, Ingersoll CD, Potteiger JA. The effects of ice and compression wraps on intramuscular temperatures at various depths. J Athl Train. 1993; 28(3):236–245.

36. Knight K. Cryotherapy: Theory, Technique and Physiology. 1st ed. Chattanooga: Chattanooga Corporation; 1985.

37. Meeusen R, Lievens P. The use of cryotherapy in sports injuries. Sports Med. 1986;3(6):398–414.

38. Swenson C, Sward L, Karlsson J. Cryotherapy in sports medicine. Scand J Med Sci Sports. 1996;6(4):193–200.

39. Higgins D, Kaminski TW. Contrast therapy does not cause fluctuations in human gastrocnemius intramuscular temperature. J Athl Train. 1998;33(4):336–340.

40. Werner R, Benjamin B. A Massage Therapist's Guide to Pathology. Baltimore: Williams & Wilkins; 1998.

41. Dorland's Illustrated Medical Dictionary. Philadelphia: Saunders; 2003.

42. Barone J. Topical analgesics: how effective are they? Physician Sportsmed. 1989;17(2).

43. Sawynok J. Topical and peripherally acting analgesics. Pharmacol Rev. 2003;55(1):1–20.

44. Mason L, Moore RA, Edwards JE, McQuay HJ, Derry S, Wiffen PJ. Systematic review of efficacy of topical rubefacients containing salicylates for the treatment of acute and chronic pain. BMJ. 24 2004;328(7446):995.

45. Ichiyama RM, Ragan BG, Bell GW, Iwamoto GA. Effects of topical analgesics on the pressor response evoked by muscle afferents. Med Sci Sports Exerc. 2002;34(9):1440–1445.

46. Myrer JW, Measom GJ, Fellingham GW. Intramuscular temperature rises with topical analgesics used as coupling agents during therapeutic ultrasound. J Athl Train. 2001;36(1):20–25.

47. Hong CZ, Shellock FG. Effects of a topically applied counterirritant (Eucalyptamint) on cutaneous blood flow and on skin and muscle temperatures. A placebo-controlled study. Am J Phys Med Rehabil. 1991;70(1):29–33.

Chapter 4

Introduction to specific massage techniques

Chapter 1 described orthopedic massage as a comprehensive rehabilitation system and not a particular technique. Consequently, an orthopedic massage treatment plan is capable of integrating a variety of massage techniques. Practitioner's who have a diversity of treatment techniques in their massage 'tool belt' are allowed a wider range of treatment options. Yet, the fundamental lesson of orthopedic massage is not 'how many', but how well one applies their knowledge and critical thinking skills. Thus, a really astute therapist with only the basic number of techniques in their tool belt is likely to be a more effective therapist than someone who has a host of techniques but is not yet skilled enough in evaluation and application.

This chapter presents the most common techniques that have been shown to be clinically effective in treating the soft-tissue pathologies described in Section 2. There is no single technique that is ideal for every condition. The hallmark of an excellent clinician is one who can determine the nature of each client's complaint and choose the most appropriate methods for each unique client. The techniques presented in this chapter should be viewed as a foundation upon which one builds a clinical treatment approach. The following provide practitioners with a basic set of tools that they may expand upon.

While there are innumerable treatment techniques available, the following basic set have defendable physiological rationales for their employment. The crucial factor is to match the physiological effects of the technique used (physiological effects are discussed in Chapter 5) with the physiology of the client's injury condition. Creative clinical thinking will allow the practitioner to use tried and tested techniques or consider new ways to apply familiar techniques with an innovative approach. No technique in and of itself is either good or bad; its effectiveness is directly related to the situation in which it is used by the clinician. Exceptional clinical results are a combination of effective manual techniques, correctly applied by the practitioner, and sound clinical judgment about the most effective treatment approach.

The discussion below begins with some of the traditional massage methods and progresses to several newer techniques that have evolved from the classical methods. I have found the following valuable in treating a wide array of soft-tissue disorders. Exclusion of any particular technique does not necessarily imply that the technique is not valuable or helpful; only, perhaps that it is not widely used in treating most soft-tissue disorders. These techniques may be applied to virtually any region of the body.

MASSAGE TECHNIQUES

Massage techniques go by a wide variety of names. What one practitioner calls trigger point therapy, another calls pressure point release, acupressure, or shiatsu. In describing these techniques, I have attempted to use simple and/or the most common names whenever possible to avoid confusion. In some cases treatment techniques are identified with the individual that made the technique popular, e.g. Rolfing, Graston technique, or Bowen Therapy. These 'named' techniques are often modifications or elaborations of the basic methods presented in this chapter.

Sound palpatory skills and an awareness of the client's response to a technique are prerequisites for effective massage. Most massage techniques have a range of pressure levels understood to be more or less effective. Understanding what the average pressure level is for a particular technique is only half of the equation. The other half is the knowledge of what the client's tolerance level is. Adequate pressure is usually defined as the point of the pain/pleasure threshold for that particular client. The importance of a quality

communicative environment for the client to express him/herself cannot be understated, particularly with pain and injury treatment.

In addition to the client's feedback, the practitioner must be skilled in reading the client's tissue response to gauge the appropriate pressure level. If the client is tightening up with reactive muscle splinting in the treatment area, then the pressure is too much. The practitioner must gauge how the client's tissues react and not rely solely on the client's feedback for pain or pressure levels. Developed palpation skills will provide the practitioner with much information about their client's responses and the effectiveness of the treatment.

Effleurage (gliding)

The most common massage technique is the gliding stroke and is commonly referred to within the Swedish system as effleurage. Many massage treatments begin with this stroke. It is beneficial for spreading lubricant, warming the tissues, reducing muscular tension, and enhancing tissue fluid movement. In this technique the hands mold to the body part being treated and a smooth gliding stroke is applied (Fig. 4.1). Effleurage is performed parallel to the primary fiber direction.

This technique significantly affects the circulatory system and produces mechanical pressure on the veins so it should always be performed toward the heart, especially in the lower extremities.[1,2,3] Performing effleurage toward the heart will reduce the likelihood of dislodging a thrombus.[4] Effleurage strokes can be performed with a variety of contact surfaces. The broad surface of the hand is

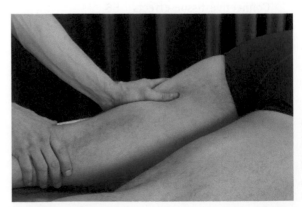

Figure 4.1   Effleurage applied to the hamstring muscles.

used most often. In less accessible or smaller body regions, the fingers or thumb can be used. In larger body regions, such as the back or posterior lower extremity, the gliding stroke can be applied with a broad contact surface such as the back of the hand or forearm.

Unfortunately, too many practitioners consider effleurage to be only a means of starting treatment and spreading lubricant. Effleurage is a versatile treatment method and one of the most effective massage strokes. You can alter the pressure level, speed of application, and angle of pressure to create many different variations of this simple technique. Several of the techniques described later in this chapter are based on effleurage strokes.

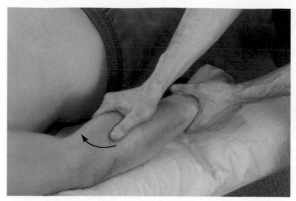

Figure 4.2 Sweeping cross fiber to the wrist extensor muscles.

Box 4.1   Foundational Techniques

- Effleurage (gliding)
- Sweeping cross fiber
- Compression broadening
- Friction massage
- Deep longitudinal stripping
- Static compression
- Massage with passive engagement
- Massage with active engagement
- Myofascial approaches
- Stretching methods

Sweeping cross fiber

Sweeping cross fiber is similar to effleurage in that it is primarily a gliding stroke, but there is a superficial cross fiber component. While the strokes of effleurage are parallel to the primary fiber direction, in the sweeping cross fiber technique the stroke moves diagonally across fibers of the muscle being treated. A common method of performing this movement is with a sweeping motion of the thumb and wrist. During the sweeping motion flex the thumb toward the palm and move the wrist in ulnar deviation (Fig. 4.2). These combined movements of the hand and thumb produce the stroke that diagonally sweeps across the fiber direction. The primary pressure of the stroke is underneath the moving thumb.

This technique is similar to the method called *Deep Muscle Therapy* developed by Therese Pfrimmer in Canada in the 1940s. The pressure level of the stroke is usually moderate, but could be more or less depending on the physiological effects desired and the client's pressure level tolerance. Sweeping cross fiber techniques encourage tissue fluid flow, warm the soft tissues, enhance pliability, and reduce tension in the muscular fibers. The sweeping motion that moves diagonally across the fiber direction is believed to enhance pliability through broadening and separating muscular fibers.

Compression broadening

To be healthy and fully functional a muscle must be able to fully contract and elongate. When a muscle contracts, it also broadens due to the overlapping sarcomeres within the fiber.[5] *Compression broadening techniques* are designed to mimic this natural broadening action of the whole muscle, although they do not actually broaden individual muscle fibers. The technique enhances elasticity and pliability in the muscle by using deep pressure perpendicular to the muscle fiber direction. Pliability is improved through the reduction of intramuscular adhesion among parallel fibers.[6] This stroke is particularly effective when used as part of the active engagement methods described later.

To perform compression broadening you must apply pressure to the target muscle whilst performing a broad cross fiber stroke (perpendicular to the muscle fiber direction) (Fig. 4.3). In areas of large muscle mass, apply the compression

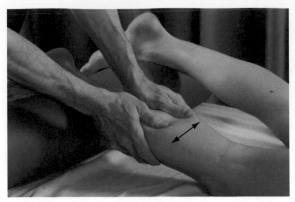

Figure 4.3 Compression broadening to the posterior calf muscles.

with a broad contact surface, such as the palm of the hand. On small muscle groups, such as the wrist flexors or extensors, the region to be treated is much smaller so use the thenar aspect of the hand or thumb.

Friction

Friction treatments move adjacent tissues in relation to each other (usually superficial over deeper tissues). There are several variations of friction but all emphasize moderate to deep pressure and mobilizing adjacent tissues. Circular friction is performed with a broad contact surface such as the heel of the hand for more general applications or a small contact surface, such as the fingertips for treating a specific area. The hand, fingers, or thumb do not glide over the skin but retain contact with the skin and move with it during treatment (Fig. 4.4).

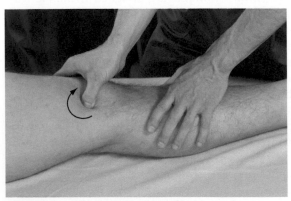

Figure 4.4 Circular friction around the patellar retinaculum.

Circular friction can start with light pressure to address the superficial tissues and then increase to more significant pressure to decrease tension in the deeper tissues.

Many soft-tissue injuries, especially those involving fibrous scar tissue, are treated with friction that is transverse (perpendicular) to the fiber direction, instead of circular.[7-10] Deep transverse friction (DTF), originally described by James Cyriax, is the primary technique used for this approach.[11] Transverse friction is used for separating adhesions between damaged fibers.[10,12-14]

Transverse movement is important for conditions where there is a disruption or tearing of the tissue fiber, such as in muscle strains or ligament sprains. In these conditions a back-and-forth friction movement is valuable because of its ability to break the cross linking bonds of fibrous scar tissue that have bound adjacent muscle, tendon or ligament fibers together.[6,10] Transverse friction is also helpful in tenosynovitis, in which the transverse movement helps break up the fibrous adhesions that have developed between the tendon and its surrounding synovial sheath.

Deep friction treatment is also used to treat tendinitis/tendinosis, with the idea that the transverse movement helps decrease fibrous adhesions between torn tendon fibers.[15] However, recent studies into the nature of tendinitis indicate that common overuse tendon disorders do not involve fiber tearing or an inflammatory reaction, but a degeneration of collagen fiber within the tendon instead. For this reason, the term tendinosis is preferred over tendonitis (see Tendinosis, Chapter 2).[16-18] Despite the lack of torn fibers and inflammatory activity in tendinosis, DTF is effective in treating these complaints.

The primary benefit of DTF in treating tendinosis appears to be stimulation of fibroblast activity in the degenerated tendon and not reducing adhesions between torn tendon fibers.[19] Thus, friction massage does not need to be transverse to the primary fibers to be effective when treating tendinosis. Longitudinal friction (applied parallel to the tendon fiber direction) can achieve the same results as transverse movement. The fibroblast mobilization in damaged tendon fibers that is stimulated by friction appears to result from the combination of pressure and movement and not from the direction in which pressure is applied.[20]

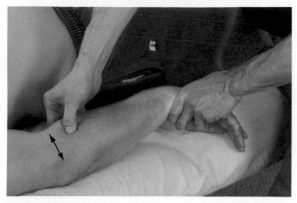

Figure 4.5 Deep transverse friction to the wrist extensor tendons.

The practitioner performs DTF by placing the fingers on the skin and then applying a back and forth motion that is perpendicular to the fiber direction (Fig. 4.5). The friction technique is applied directly to the site of the soft-tissue lesion. DTF applications use a significant amount of pressure. However, too much pressure can cause reactive muscle splinting or further tissue injury. Deep friction is most effective when the client reports the sensation as uncomfortable, even mildly painful, but bearable. If the pressure is within tolerable limits a sensation of analgesia can develop after a few minutes of treatment, decreasing the discomfort and making the treatment more tolerable.[10] The analgesia effect is likely due to stimulation of non-pain sensory receptors and nociceptor inhibition as described in the gate theory of pain.[21–23]

There are different views on how long DTF should be applied. Cyriax advocated treatments of 20-minutes' duration given every other day in an ideal treatment setting.[24] Some recommend shorter treatments, such as 10 minutes.[10] The author has found it effective to apply much shorter durations of friction treatment and to intersperse the friction with other techniques. For example, apply deep friction for 20–30 seconds and then follow with other techniques, such as compressive effleurage, sweeping cross fiber, or compression broadening. Active and passive range of motion and stretching procedures can then be performed to encourage proper tissue remodeling. This combination of techniques is repeated several times during the treatment session.

Incorporating a variety of techniques along with the friction treatment gives maximum opportunity to mobilize the affected tissues and prevents the client from having to withstand long durations of DTF that can be uncomfortable. More specific guidelines for how to incorporate DTF with other treatments are given in the specific treatment suggestions for each condition in Section 2.

Deep longitudinal stripping

Deep longitudinal stripping technique involves a slow longitudinal gliding stroke applied to muscle or other soft tissue with the intent of encouraging tissue elongation and elasticity. *Deep tissue massage* is another common name for this technique, although this term can be misleading because many different techniques access deep tissues of the body. It is an excellent method for reducing hypertonicity and increasing pliability in muscles and connective tissues. When deep longitudinal stripping technique is applied to muscle fibers, it helps encourage lengthening and elasticity in those fibers leading to a reduction in hypertonicity (muscle tightness) and increased flexibility.

The deep, long gliding strokes create tangential pulling forces on superficial and deep connective tissues. These tangential forces stimulate Ruffini endings (a specialized sensory receptor cell in the skin) in the connective tissue creating a neurological response that leads to increased tissue relaxation.[25] Deep longitudinal striping is also the most effective way to inactivate myofascial trigger points when using a direct manual approach.[26] Deep longitudinal stripping techniques are parallel to the direction of the muscle fibers being treated. The stroke usually extends from one tendinous attachment of the muscle to the other. In some cases short segments of muscle or other soft tissue are treated without covering the entire length of the tissue.

The technique can be applied with varying levels of pressure, although it is most effective when the pressure level is moderately deep. Adequate pressure is usually when the client perceives it as right on the pain/pleasure threshold. In addition to the client's feedback, the practitioner must be skilled in reading the client's tissue response to gauge the appropriate pressure level. If the client is tightening up with reactive muscle splinting in the treatment area, then the pressure is too much. The practitioner must gauge how the client's tissues react and not rely solely on the client's feedback for pain or pressure levels. A detailed knowledge of anatomy and muscle fiber direction is also required to perform this technique correctly.

Stripping techniques are performed slowly due to the depth of pressure. If the practitioner is moving too fast across the tissue while applying significant pressure, the sensation can be very abrupt and uncomfortable for the client. Moving too fast across tissues also causes the practitioner to miss valuable tissue consistency changes perceived with palpation. Deep stripping techniques are particularly valuable for their diagnostic as well as treatment capabilities.

Longitudinal stripping can be performed with a broad contact surface, such as the palm, fist, or forearm (Fig. 4.6). With a broad contact surface the pressure is spread over a larger surface area so the pressure is not as intense for the client. Applying stripping techniques with a broad contact surface first is helpful to reduce tension in superficial tissues before treating deeper tissues. Muscles or other soft tissues can be treated more precisely with longitudinal stripping using a small contact surface. In these techniques pressure is delivered over a smaller surface area, so pressure is more concentrated on those tissues directly under contact. Examples of small contact pressure surfaces include thumbs, fingertips, knuckles,

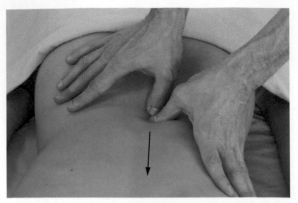

Figure 4.7 Small contact surface deep stripping on the intrinsic spinal muscles.

elbow, or pressure tools (Fig. 4.7). As with the broad contact surface treatments, the stroke should be slow, deep, and preferably close to the client's pain tolerance. All longitudinal stripping techniques should follow circulatory guidelines and move toward the heart when working on the extremities.

Static compression

Static compression is a technique of pressing directly on soft tissue in one location without moving the treatment hand. Numerous systems and techniques use static compression as a primary method of treatment. These systems differ mostly in their theoretical models and not in the way pressure is applied to the client's body. Examples of these systems include shiatsu, acupressure, myotherapy, and neuromuscular therapy. Static compression on pain points in the body can produce several physiological effects.[27] In this text attention focuses on static compression for its neuromuscular effects of reducing hypertonicity and deactivating myofascial trigger points in muscle tissue.

The amount of pressure used in static compression techniques varies depending on the practitioner's intended results. In their original discussions of myofascial trigger point treatment, Travell & Simons called their static compression technique ischemic compression, emphasizing a pressure level that would produce local tissue ischemia of the irritable trigger point.[28] However, later research developments led to a change in perspective for the most

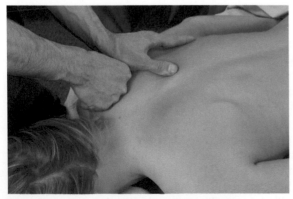

Figure 4.6 Broad pressure application of deep stripping with the back side of the right hand.

effective method to treat myofascial trigger points with static compression.

Myofascial trigger points appear to result from dysfunctional activity at the motor-end plate. In addition the hypertonic muscles compress local sensory nerves and lead to greater pain generation.[29] Pressure that is strong enough to produce local tissue ischemia could aggravate these sites in the muscle. Therefore, a gentler pressure on the trigger point appears to produce better treatment results, especially when combined with tissue stretching. This newer static compression technique for trigger points is called trigger point pressure release.[26,30]

As with deep stripping techniques, static compression is an important technique for identifying areas of hypertonicity or restriction in the tissues as well as the tissue's response to treatment. Palpation and static compression techniques have proven to be one of the most reliable methods of identifying myofascial trigger points in muscle tissue. However, the practitioner must have well-developed skills of palpation to identify these dysfunctional regions of muscle tissue.[31–33]

Another use of static compression is its integration with a technique called positional release. In positional release the practitioner uses static compression to identify a tender point in the target tissue. Pressure is maintained on the tender point while moving the body region in a variety of different positions. The client is asked to monitor the pain sensations in the tender point during the movement. Using these different positions, the practitioner attempts to find the position with the least discomfort and to hold the static compression along with the position.[34,35] After holding the compression and position for anywhere from a few seconds to more than a minute there is a reduction in local neurological activity that decreases muscle tightness.

Static compression can be performed with a broad base of pressure such as the palm, fist, or forearm (Fig. 4.8). Hold the pressure until you feel the tissues relax. If you have identified myofascial trigger points or regions of muscle tissue that appear hypertonic these regions can be treated with small contact applications of static compression, such as the thumbs, fingers, elbow, knuckles, or pressure tools (Fig. 4.9). Pressure is held for varying lengths of time, but you can usually achieve a therapeutic response in about 8–10 seconds. The

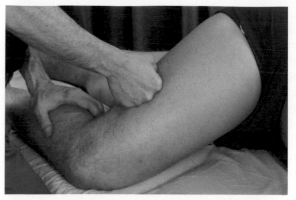

Figure 4.8 Broad contact surface static compression to the lateral thigh region.

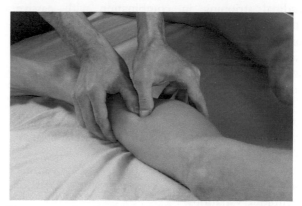

Figure 4.9 Small contact surface static compression to the tibialis posterior.

therapeutic response is a reduction in tissue tightness or the client's report of reduced local or referred pain from pressure applied to the region.

MASSAGE WITH ACTIVE AND PASSIVE MOVEMENT

This next section introduces a number of techniques that combine some of the methods described above along with either active or passive movement. Proper application of these techniques requires a sound knowledge of *kinesiology* (the study of human movement) due to the use of movements along with the soft-tissue manipulation. Different variations and positions can be used to access each muscle making a wide variety of treatment options.

Not every technique is appropriate for every client. For example, the techniques involving active engagement can be more uncomfortable than passive techniques for a client at the early stages of a soft-tissue injury because more muscle fibers are engaged in the active technique. In those cases it is best to keep the active techniques for the later stages of the rehabilitation process. More specific guidelines about active and passive engagement techniques are discussed with the injury treatment recommendations for each condition in Section 2.

Massage with passive engagement

Massage with passive engagement uses static compression, compression broadening, or deep longitudinal stripping in combination with passive joint movement. Joint movements are used that produce either shortening or lengthening of the target tissue being treated. Performing movement with specific soft-tissue manipulation magnifies some of the physiological effects of the technique.

Compression broadening, static compression, and deep longitudinal stripping techniques use a variety of contact surfaces both broad and small for different effects. The choice of contact surface and pressure level as well as the use of shortening or lengthening strokes creates a wide variety of technique variations.

Shortening strokes

In a shortening stroke the practitioner applies static compression to an area of the muscle that has a heightened neurological response, such as a myofascial trigger point, an area of restricted fascial movement, or muscle tightness. Once static pressure is applied over the area, the tissues underneath the pressure are shortened by moving the affected joint passively (Fig. 4.10). Most clients will feel a decrease in painful sensations as the tissue is brought into a shortened position.

The idea behind this technique is that decreasing the sensation of pain and restriction in the muscle tissue by moving it to a shortened position instead of forcibly trying to stretch it, may help decrease tension, trigger point activity, and neuromuscular dysfunction in that muscle. This procedure is particularly helpful in situations of severe muscle spasm, such as those which occur following an acute injury.

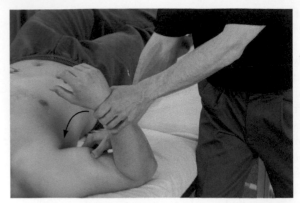

Figure 4.10 Passive engagement/shortening applied to the elbow flexors.

The final shortened position of the muscle may be held for longer periods to achieve a better neurological release. There are different theories about how long is a beneficial time to hold this position ranging from about 20 to 90 seconds.[35]

The primary effect of the shortening strokes is a reduction in neurological activity in the muscle. By applying pressure to a muscle and then decreasing the intensity of the pressure through passively shortening the muscle, there is less tension on the muscle fibers while they are being compressed. There may also be some myofascial effects of moving the muscle while pressure is maintained on it. This technique is very similar to procedures that go by the name of positional release or strain/counterstrain.[34,35]

Lengthening strokes

Lengthening strokes are most effective for mobilizing connective tissue, decreasing muscle tension, and increasing elongation in the myofascial tissues. Lengthening strokes are particularly effective for helping to encourage elongation and flexibility in tight muscles. The pressure applied to the tissue while it is being elongated helps in the stretching of both connective tissue and contractile elements within the muscle. There are two ways to perform lengthening strokes:

1. Static compression is applied to a particular area of the muscle while it is in the shortened position. The target muscle (the one being treated) is placed in a shortened position (for

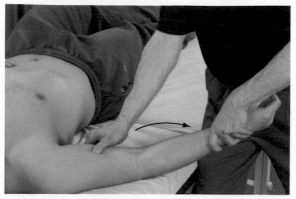

Figure 4.11   Passive engagement/lengthening with static compression applied to the elbow flexors.

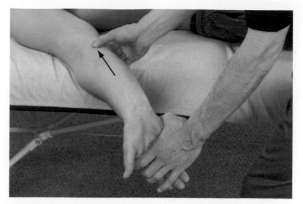

Figure 4.12   Passive engagement/lengthening with longitudinal stripping applied to the wrist flexors.

example, elbow flexion is a shortened position for the biceps brachii). With static compression continually applied, the client's related joint or limb is moved so the target tissues are elongated. This technique is also called *pin and stretch* (Fig. 4.11). The static compression can be applied with a broad base of contact, such as the palm or back side of the hand initially. Using a broad base of contact allows the technique to feel a little less intense for the client. A broader contact surface also allows a greater expanse of connective tissue to be pulled and stretched. If a more specific application is desired or the area being treated is not large, a small contact surface such as thumbs, finger tips, elbows, or pressure tools can be used.

2. Another lengthening stroke is to use deep longitudinal stripping on the target muscle while moving the related joint or limb passively to lengthen the muscle (Fig. 4.12). Place the target muscle in a shortened position. Perform the deep stripping technique with a broad contact surface for more general applications or a small contact surface for more specific ones. The stripping technique can be repeated several times, working in parallel strips on the muscle, until the entire area is treated.

Massage with active engagement

The following techniques use static compression, compression broadening, or deep longitudinal stripping in combination with active movements of a muscle. The primary effects of active engagement techniques are both neurological and mechanical. In both variations, shortening (broadening) and lengthening, the pressure applied while the muscle is under contraction helps to reduce excessive muscle spindle activity and decrease overall muscle tension, just as any static compression technique would do. These techniques also help increase connective tissue mobility. In the shortening techniques the cross fiber movement performed with pressure helps to spread and broaden muscle fibers thereby decreasing any intramuscular adhesions and enhancing pliability. In the lengthening techniques, pressure applied while the muscle is increasing in length helps to pull and stretch the myofascial tissues and decrease overall muscle tension.

Massage with active engagement is effective for magnifying the muscle's neurological and mechanical responses to the techniques. For example, with muscles that are tight and also deep, it is hard to apply effective pressure when doing a longitudinal stripping technique without using a great deal of force. By having the client actively engage the area, the cumulative effect of the pressure is magnified because the density of the tissue is increased when the muscle is engaged in active contraction. Pressure during active contraction also helps mobilize some of the deep fascia surrounding these muscles.

A benefit to this approach is that practitioners don't have to exert as much effort in treating large or deep muscles. With the deeper muscles it can be hard to apply effective pressure when doing a longitudinal stripping technique without using a great deal of force. Working deep or large muscles is advantageous with this technique, but it is just as effective in treating small or easily accessible tissues as well. Compression can be performed with the palm, knuckles, thumb, fingers, elbow, or a pressure tool.

Shortening strokes

The primary purpose of the shortening strokes is to enhance the broadening effect of the muscle during concentric contractions. Efforts to enhance muscle broadening with various cross-fiber techniques help reduce inter-fiber adhesions within muscle tissue.[15] The amount of muscle contraction can be varied with either of the following methods by adding additional resistance. The additional resistance will recruit a greater number of muscle fibers and make the pressure level more effective. The practitioner can increase muscular recruitment with resistance bands, weights, or manual resistance (Fig 4.13).

There are two ways to perform the shortening strokes:

1. Static compression is applied to an area in the muscle that is hypertonic, contains myofascial trigger points, or appears restricted or tender due to excess tension. Once static compression is applied (only a moderate amount of force is needed), the client is instructed to concentrically contract the affected muscle. Pressure is maintained during the concentric (shortening) phase of the contraction. Pressure can be

maintained or released as the client returns the affected area to the original position. The static compression technique can be applied with a broad base of pressure like the palm or a small area of pressure like a thumb, knuckle, or pressure tool (Fig. 4.14).

2. A more effective method of enhancing the broadening of a muscle during concentric contraction is to use compression broadening strokes during the concentric contraction. The technique begins with the target muscle in a lengthened position. The client is instructed to actively contract (shorten) the affected muscle. During the client's concentric contraction the practitioner performs a compression broadening technique on the muscle (Fig. 4.15). The practitioner releases pressure as the client

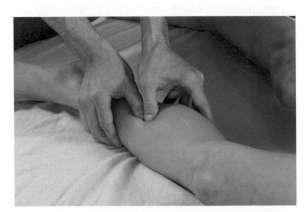

Figure 4.14 Active engagement/shortening with static compression applied to the tibialis posterior (client is actively plantar flexing the foot during compression).

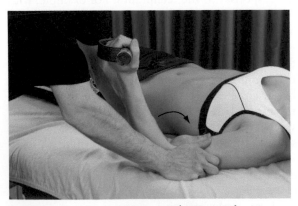

Figure 4.13 Active engagement (shortening) with additional resistance applied to the elbow flexors.

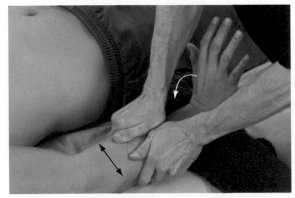

Figure 4.15 Active engagement/shortening with compression broadening applied to the wrist extensors.

returns to the starting position. Then the practitioner again performs a compression broadening technique as the client shortens the affected tissues actively once again. This process is repeated moving along the length of the muscle until the whole muscle has been treated adequately. It is important to make sure the practitioner's movement is coordinated with that of the client's movement so that when the client begins moving, the practitioner begins applying the stroke. When the client reaches the end of the movement, the practitioner should be reaching the end of the stroke.

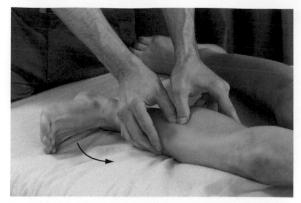

Figure 4.16 Active engagement/lengthening with static compression applied to the tibialis posterior (client is actively dorsiflexing the foot).

Lengthening strokes

Lengthening strokes during active engagement are an effective method of decreasing muscle tightness, reducing irritable myofascial trigger points, and encouraging tissue elongation. Applying simultaneous pressure and stretch to the target tissue helps to lengthen abnormally contracted sarcomeres in the muscle.[29] It is best to perform this technique in the later stages of the rehabilitative process or with individuals whose muscles are in moderately good tone to begin with. The technique is begun with the muscle in its shortest position, in an active muscle contraction. Some muscles, such as the hamstrings, are prone to cramping if contracted in their shortest position. Cramping in a shortened position is most common for multi-articulate muscles (those that cross more than one joint). For these muscles use a more lengthened position to engage the initial contraction. Lengthening strokes are performed in two ways:

1. The technique begins by establishing a moderate level of tension in the muscle with an isometric contraction. This isometric contraction should be engaged close to the shortest position of the muscle as long as that muscle is not prone to cramping in this short position. Static compression is applied to the muscle during the isometric contraction and held throughout the performance of this procedure. A broad contact surface is used initially or for more general applications as it causes less discomfort for the client. For more specific applications of pressure to the target tissue, use a small contact surface.

   The client is then instructed to create an eccentric contraction in the target muscle by slowly releasing, but not letting go of, the contraction. Simultaneously, the practitioner pulls the client's limb in a direction that lengthens the target muscle while applying the static compression (Fig. 4.16). This procedure is similar to the lengthening technique performed with passive movement (pin and stretch) with the only difference being the eccentric contraction in the muscle as opposed to the muscle passively elongating.

2. Reducing muscle tension and enhancing myofascial elongation can be encouraged even more with deep longitudinal stripping performed during the eccentric contraction instead of static compression. The practitioner has the client engage an isometric contraction of the affected muscle from a shortened position as in the procedure above. As with the previous variation, a different initial starting length is used for multi-articulate muscles or any others if muscle cramping is a possibility. The client is then instructed to create an eccentric contraction in the target muscle by slowly releasing, but not letting go of, the contraction. Simultaneously, the practitioner pulls the client's limb in a direction that lengthens the target muscle while applying deep longitudinal stripping on the target muscle (Fig. 4.17). This technique will greatly magnify the effect of deep stripping techniques.

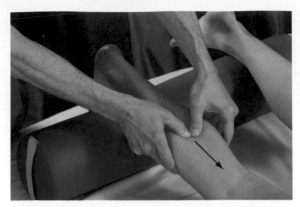

Figure 4.17 Active engagement/lengthening with stripping applied to the gastrocnemius.

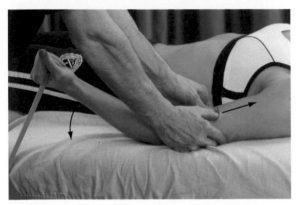

Figure 4.18 Active engagement/lengthening with additional resistance applied to the elbow flexors.

The intensity of muscle contraction can be altered with either of these methods by adding additional resistance. A greater number of muscle fibers are recruited with additional resistance and this makes the pressure level more effective due to increased tissue density. Increase muscular recruitment with resistance bands, weights, or manual resistance. If resistance bands or weights are used for the eccentric contraction, both hands are freed up to perform the longitudinal stripping methods (Fig. 4.18).

MYOFASCIAL APPROACHES

Fascia envelops every soft tissue in the body creating an intricate network of connective tissue that serves important structural and neurological functions. Originally considered by many to be a connective tissue of minor consequence, the importance of fascia in maintaining optimum function in the body has recently gained great interest. As a result, numerous soft-tissue manipulation techniques that focus on fascia have become key tools for soft-tissue clinicians. Much of the credit for the emphasis on therapeutic soft-tissue treatment directed at fascia is due to the pioneering efforts of Ida Rolf.[36] Many of her students have elaborated on her theories to develop new ideas and ways to encourage health in the fascial tissues of the body.[37] Treatment techniques that are specifically aimed at the fascia run from the deep and sometimes painful approaches that were used in the early days of structural integration (Rolfing), to the subtle and often puzzling effects of treatments such as myofascial release.[38]

The key component of all myofascial work is to increase its pliability by applying tensile force to the connective tissue. For many years descriptions of myofascial techniques focused on the mechanical response of the fascia to this pulling force. Proponents of these myofascial techniques emphasized the transformation of fascia from a thicker and gelatinous (gel) state to the more soluble or fluid (sol) state.[36,39] However, many found this explanation challenging because it seemed unlikely that tensile forces applied to fascia during therapeutic treatments could produce this kind of change.

Biomechanical studies have found that the amount of tensile force necessary to produce change in connective tissue would be too great and more likely cause tissue tearing and damage.[40] In addition, tensile force would have to be applied on the fascial tissue for close to 1 hour to make significant changes according to physiological models.[25] Yet numerous clinicians attest to the palpable change in tissue tension felt after only short durations of tensile force on superficial connective tissues. In most of these applications change is felt with tensile force loads much smaller than mechanical models dictate would be necessary for fascial elongation from mechanical stretch alone.[6,38]

New research shows that fascia contains smooth muscle cells and has its own contractile properties and an abundance of specialized sensory receptors.[41,42] These neurological receptors, especially the Ruffini endings, are particularly sensitive to tangential pulling forces applied to the fascia.[25] Tangential forces are those that offer only light pressure loads on the tissue and exert primarily tensile (pulling) force on the fascia. Even when exposed to very light tensile loads, these neural receptors in the fascia modulate activity in the nervous system which then produces a corresponding reduction in muscle tension. The function of fascia is so tightly integrated with muscle tissue that these two are most appropriately considered *myofascial tissues*.[43,44] Therefore when a relaxation is produced in the fascial tissues, there is tension reduction in muscular tissue as well, and thus the palpable change felt by soft-tissue practitioners (Fig. 4.19).

The primary purpose of myofascial techniques is to reduce tension in the fascial and muscular tissues. There are many different myofascial techniques, so this discussion focuses on the elements that are common to most of these methods. Once an area of muscular or fascial restriction is identified, a tangential or pulling force is applied to the connective tissues in the area. This technique is usually performed with minimal or no lubrication so that the practitioner's hands or fingers do not easily glide across the skin but instead pulls across the skin creating greater effect on the fascial layers under the skin.

In some techniques the treating hand glides slowly along the direction of the muscle and fascia being treated (Fig. 4.20). Slow movement is recommended because the lack of lubricant can produce discomfort due to the excess friction. As with the longitudinal stripping methods the practitioner can use a broad contact surface (palm, forearm, knuckles, etc.) for more general applications or a small contact surface (thumbs, fingers, or elbow) for a specific application.

In other myofascial techniques the tangential force applied to the fascia is performed without moving the treatment hand(s). This method is most commonly referred to as myofascial release.[38] To

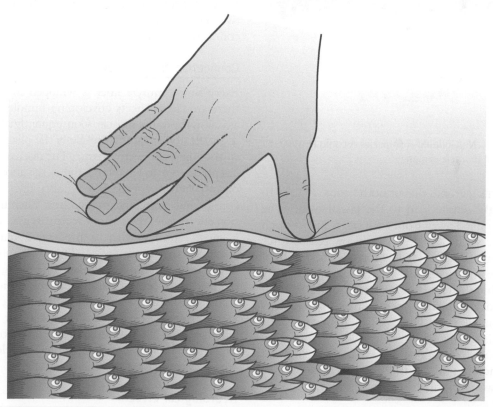

Figure 4.19   Feeling change in myofascial tissues. "Myofascial tissue as a school of fish. A practitioner working with myofascial tissue may feel several of the motor units responding to touch. If the practitioner then responds supportively to their new behavior, the working hand will soon feel other fish joining, and so forth. Figure by Twyla Weixl, Munich, Germany." Reprinted with permission from Schleip R. Fascial plasticity – a new neurobiological explanation. Journal of Bodywork and Movement Therapies. 2003;7(1):11–19.

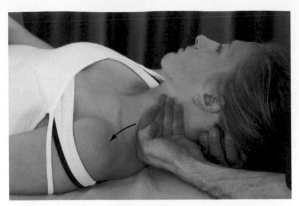

Figure 4.20 Myofascial gliding technique applied with the back of the hand to the lateral neck muscles.

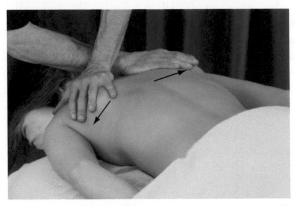

Figure 4.21 Non-gliding myofascial technique applied to the upper thoracic region.

perform this method, one or both hands are used to apply a light tensile load to the fascial tissue. The hands are pulled away from each other just enough to take the slack out and create a low tensile force on the tissue (Fig. 4.21). The force is often so light that it does not seem like anything could possibly be stretching the tissues of the body. Yet fascial elongation and a reduction in muscular hypertonicity result from these methods.[45] The amount of time to hold this tensile force varies, and may range from a few seconds to several minutes. Many practitioners advocate holding the tensile force until a sensation of tissue release is felt by the client or practitioner.[46]

STRETCHING METHODS

Stretching is used extensively as a soft-tissue treatment method. For years clinicians, athletes, and many other rehabilitation specialists have advocated it as a beneficial means for injury prevention and treatment. There seems to be little argument that stretching hypertonic or restricted tissues is a valuable part of injury treatment. However, recent studies into the effects of stretching have been unable to find a correlation between stretching and injury prevention.[47–51] There are likely benefits to stretching as a preventive measure in certain circumstances, but not in all. Stretching is routinely incorporated with massage in the treatment of pain and injury conditions so this discussion of stretching emphasizes its use as a rehabilitative practice more than a preventive one, although the two are closely related.

The primary purpose of any stretching technique is to enhance pliability and flexibility in the soft tissues. Stretching is generally aimed at muscle and fascial tissue, but there is evidence that stretching procedures can enhance elasticity in tendon tissue as well.[52] Stretching procedures can be divided into two separate, but equally important components: connective tissue effects and neurological effects.

Connective tissue effects

Every single muscle fiber is wrapped in fascia and there are fascial sheets enveloping bundles of fibers as well as the entire muscle. Consequently a key factor in the flexibility of any muscle is the pliability of its surrounding connective tissue. The discussion of fascial physiology in Chapter 2 and in the above section on myofascial approaches is also relevant when considering stretching procedures. Eliciting relaxation effects from the sensory receptors in fascial tissue is most effective when a prolonged tensile load is applied to the tissue.[53,54] Stretching produces a tensile load on connective tissues. Holding this tensile load for a certain period reduces tension in the connective tissue and subsequently aids overall myofascial extensibility. There is debate about the ideal length of time to hold a stretch. Several factors related to the ideal time of stretch are discussed below in the section on specific stretching techniques.

Neurological effects

The function of muscle tissue is to generate intramuscular contraction forces in order to create or limit movement in the body. The muscular system is a highly complex feedback system with an extensive array of sensory receptors including the Golgi tendon organs and muscle spindle cells. These two specialized proprioceptors are critically important in understanding various stretching techniques. Both proprioceptors play different roles in helping to manage tension in the muscle and also its ability to elongate during stretching.

The Golgi tendon organ (GTO) is located in the musculotendinous junction (Fig. 4.22). Its primary function is to relay information back to the central nervous system about the amount of contraction force in muscles. When muscle fibers contract, they pull on the tendon, which then transmits the contraction force to the bone. Due to its location in the musculotendinous junction, the GTO is ideally positioned to give the central nervous system information about the level of tension or pulling force that its muscle generates. Its predominant role is to help manage appropriate muscular contraction forces.

Tendons can be pulled either by a muscular contraction or a passive tensile force, such as a stretching procedure. During a strong muscular contraction the muscle pulls on the musculotendinous junction and the GTO is stimulated. It was once thought that the GTO prevented excessive

muscular contraction (and subsequent overcontraction injury) by shutting off a muscle contraction if the contraction stimulus was too strong. However, we have now learned that the GTO does not function in this way and the reflex cessation of overly strong muscular contraction results more from excessive stimulation of free nerve endings (pain receptors).[55]

Another erroneous perception about GTO function that still persists suggests that passive muscle stretching pulls on the musculotendinous junction and stimulates the GTO, thereby causing a corresponding decrease in muscle tension. The GTO is activated by muscle contraction, but in many cases not activated at all by passive stretching.[55] Therefore stimulation of the GTO with passive stretching does not occur and is not a mechanism for increasing stretching effectiveness.

The other muscle proprioceptor that is essential for understanding stretching effectiveness is the muscle spindle cell. Muscle spindle cells are located throughout muscle tissue (Fig. 4.23). Their primary function is to help regulate levels of muscle tension and stretch. While the GTO is receptive to the level of contraction force in a muscle, the spindle cells primarily focus on the degree of muscle stretching. Spindle cell physiology is complex and involves both sensory cells in the spindle as well as motor fibers to the spindle itself that help manage appropriate muscle length. The spindle cell is primarily responsive to the muscle's change in length (how much a muscle lengthens) and the rate of change (how fast it lengthens).

If a muscle elongates either too far or too fast, the muscle spindles report that change to the central nervous system and an automatic reflex muscular contraction ensues to reduce the excess stretch. This reflex is called the myotatic (or stretch) reflex. Its primary function is to prevent muscle tearing that would result from overstretching. Practitioners should be careful with any stretching procedure not to elicit the stretch reflex by stretching the client too far or too fast because the reflex contraction directly reduces the benefit of any stretching procedure.

There is a wide variety of stretching procedures or systems used to increase myofascial flexibility. The most common stretching methods fall under one of three categories: static, ballistic, or active-assisted

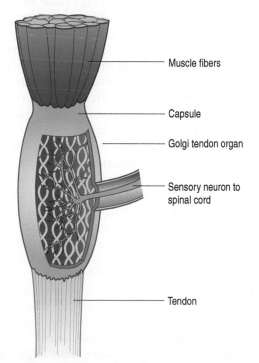

Muscle fibers

Capsule

Golgi tendon organ

Sensory neuron to spinal cord

Tendon

Figure 4.22   Structure of the Golgi tendon organ.

Figure 4.23 Simplified structure of a muscle spindle.

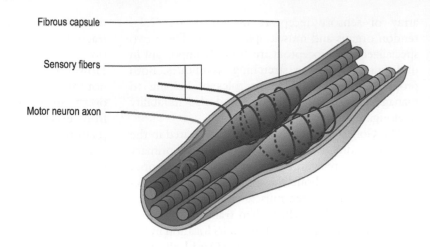

Fibrous capsule

Sensory fibers

Motor neuron axon

stretching. While there are numerous variations of stretching, most techniques are classified as one of these types.[56]

Static stretching

Static stretching is the most common type of stretching procedure. It involves bringing a tissue into a lengthened position and holding it there for some period of time. The ideal length of time to hold a static stretch is debated in the literature and the results still appear inconclusive. Somewhere around 15–20 seconds is a common time frame that achieves good clinical results.[57–60] However, practitioners of hatha yoga are accustomed to holding stretch positions for much longer and there is ample evidence that this centuries-old practice produces enhanced flexibility.

The ideal time frame for a static stretching procedure could be dependent on what muscles are being stretched. Certain muscles are more stretch resistant than others and would therefore benefit from a longer duration of stretch. In his ground-breaking work on muscle function and physiology Vladimir Janda described two categories for many of the major muscles in the body: postural and phasic muscles.[61] Postural muscles are those most associated with maintaining erect posture during locomotion, while phasic muscles have a more important role in large power movements of the body. Postural muscles contain a greater amount of perimysium (fascial connective tissue) and are therefore stiffer than phasic muscles.[54] Consequently, postural muscles could

require a longer duration of static stretch than some phasic muscles to effectively elongate the connective tissue within the muscle.

Ballistic stretching

Ballistic stretching is a practice that has been used to enhance flexibility, especially in the athletic environment. This practice involves bobbing or bouncing into a stretch to encourage tissue elongation in the muscle. Ballistic stretching works by using the momentum of the moving limb to extend past the initial range of motion limitation. There are many who oppose the use of ballistic stretching because the rapid elongation of muscle tissue in the bouncing motion might activate the stretch reflex, which would be counterproductive to the purpose of stretching, potentially causing injury, or reducing the effect.

There are also arguments in favor of ballistic stretching. Many of the movements during athletic activity are sudden muscle lengthening movements and similar to those occurring in ballistic stretching. There is benefit to practicing a form of flexibility enhancement that prepares the body for these movements, especially in athletics. Ballistic stretching has been shown to increase muscle, fascial, and tendon elasticity.[52,62] It is also a very effective stretching method when combined with static stretching. The combination of static and ballistic stretching has been found more effective than either one of them performed alone.[56]

It is argued that ballistic stretching might be effective for people who are less inclined to comply with a stretching routine due to boredom with the activity. Because ballistic stretching involves constant movement, some might find it more interesting to perform and thus use it more often. Consequently, ballistic stretching performed correctly is better than no stretching at all.

Active-assisted methods

In active-assisted stretching the client actively engages specific muscle contractions prior to or during the stretching procedure. There is a variety of active-assisted techniques and they go by different names. There are slight variations in each of these methods, but they are all based on the neurological principles of post isometric relaxation (PIR) and reciprocal inhibition. Experiments that compare active-assisted methods with static or ballistic stretching routinely show the greatest range of motion gains with active-assisted methods.[63,64]

Immediately following an isometric contraction, there is an increased degree of relaxation in that muscle. This immediate reduction in neurological activity is called the PIR.[65] The methods of active-assisted stretching use the window of reduced neurological activity during the PIR to engage a stretch of the target muscle after it has isometrically contracted. Stretching during the PIR is more effective than stretching without the corresponding isometric contraction.[65,66]

The other neurological principle that is of prime importance in active-assisted stretching methods is reciprocal inhibition. When an agonist muscle contracts, there is a neurological inhibition of its antagonist (or opposite) muscle. This reduction in neurological activity in the antagonist muscle is called reciprocal inhibition. Because reciprocal inhibition decreases neurological activity in muscles opposite the ones being contracted, it is helpful to use during stretching procedures. Stretching of the target muscle is enhanced when its opposite muscle is contracted at the same time (Fig. 4.24).

The active-assisted techniques listed below rely on the following two basic stretching methods:

1. Contract–relax (CR): This is a stretching procedure that uses an isometric contraction immediately prior to the stretch. It is also sometimes called contract–relax–stretch or

hold–relax. In a CR procedure the muscle being stretched is the one engaged in the contraction immediately prior to the stretch (Fig. 4.25). There are various lengths of time for holding the isometric contraction. Most recommendations find an isometric contraction between 3 and 7 seconds to be sufficient.[67,68] The length of time to hold the stretch also varies, but a similar amount of time (3 to 7 seconds) is common. Several repetitions of this cycle are more effective than performing the CR stretch just once.[69]

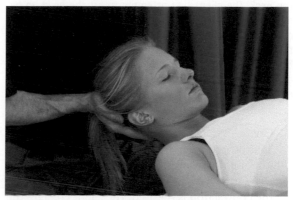

Figure 4.24 Reciprocal inhibition stretching of the anterior neck muscles. The client is using the neck extensors in a contraction first then stretching the neck flexors.

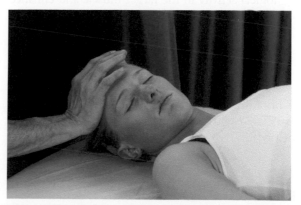

Figure 4.25 Contract–relax (CR) stretch to the right lateral rotator muscles. The client attempts to turn the head to the right while the practitioner resists. When the contraction is released, the practitioner turns the client's head to the left to stretch the right rotator muscles.

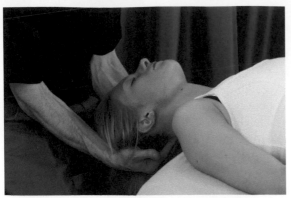

Figure 4.26 Contract–relax–antagonist–contract (CRAC) stretch to the neck flexors on the anterior side of the neck. The client first attempts to lift the head up by contracting the neck flexors. After holding the contraction for several seconds, the client relaxes and then eventually pushes the head into the practitioner's hands by using the neck extensors. The practitioner gradually allows the client to move into full head and neck extension thereby stretching the neck flexors.

2. Contract–relax–antagonist–contract (CRAC): This procedure uses both the PIR and reciprocal inhibition concepts. The target muscle (the one to be stretched) is contracted isometrically. When the contraction is released, the client engages the opposite muscle group to stretch the original target muscle (Fig. 4.26). Using the opposite (antagonist) muscle at the end of the stretch engages reciprocal inhibition to decrease neurological activity in the target muscle and enhance the stretch. CRAC stretching is perhaps the most effective of the various active-assisted methods. Studies that have compared different stretching methods have found the greatest motion gains when using the CRAC variation.[70,71]

A brief description of the various names and terms associated with active-assisted stretching are listed below:

- Proprioceptive neuromuscular facilitation (PNF): This is a system that was originally developed by physical therapists in the 1940s to enhance neurological rehabilitation. It included various movements, especially those involving spiral and diagonal movement patterns, which are more complex than the movement patterns used most often in static stretching.[67] The PNF rehabilitative system is a comprehensive rehabilitative exercise program and the stretching component is only one part of that system. However, the term PNF has become synonymous with just the stretching methods of this system. Some of the early advocates of PNF stretching methods used muscle contractions close to the maximal level. Recent variations have demonstrated stretching results that are just as effective with muscle contractions much lower than the maximum level.[72]

- Muscle energy technique (MET): The osteopathic profession's focus on manual methods of soft-tissue treatment expanded on some of the early concepts used in PNF stretching to promote a similar method, which was called MET. The term muscle energy technique emphasizes the importance of using the client's own muscle contraction energy to enhance the stretching procedure.[68]

- Facilitated stretching: Another name for stretching procedures using the client's energy is facilitated stretching. These methods are very similar to those used in the traditional PNF system with just a few variations.[73]

- Active isolated stretching (AIS): This is an active-assisted stretching procedure that was developed by Aaron Mattes, and is also known as the Mattes method.[74] The cornerstone of this technique is a short duration of stretch (only about 2 seconds). AIS stretching uses reciprocal inhibition, but does not generally use isometric contractions of the target muscle prior to the stretch.

References

1. Fritz S. Mosby's Fundamentals of Therapeutic Massage. 2nd ed. St. Louis: Mosby; 2000.
2. Tappan FM, Benjamin P. Tappan's Handbook of Healing Massage Techniques. 3rd ed. Stamford, CT: Appleton & Lange; 1998.
3. Tiidus PM. Manual Massage and Recovery of Muscle Function Following Exercise – A Literature-Review. J Orthop Sport Phys Therapy. 1997;25(2):107–112.
4. Werner R, Benjamin B. A Massage Therapist's Guide to Pathology. Baltimore: Williams & Wilkins; 1998.

5. McComas A. Skeletal Muscle: Form and Function. Champaign: Human Kinetics; 1996.

6. Cantu R, Grodin A. Myofascial Manipulation: Theory and Clinical Application. Gaithersburg: Aspen; 1992.

7. Guler-Uysal F, Kozanoglu E. Comparison of the early response to two methods of rehabilitation in adhesive capsulitis. Swiss Med Wkly. 2004;134(23–24):353–358.

8. Pettitt R, Dolski A. Corrective neuromuscular approach to the treatment of iliotibial band friction syndrome: a case report. J Athl Train. 2000;35(1):96–99.

9. Pribicevic M, Pollard H. A multi-modal treatment approach for the shoulder: a 4 patient case series. Chiropr Osteopat. 2005;13:20.

10. Stasinopoulos D, Johnson MI. Cyriax physiotherapy for tennis elbow/lateral epicondylitis. Br J Sports Med. 2004;38(6):675–677.

11. Cyriax J. Textbook of Orthopaedic Medicine Volume Two: Treatment by Manipulation, Massage, and Injection. Vol 2. London: Bailliere Tindall; 1984.

12. Cyriax J. Deep massage. Physiotherapy. 1977;63(2):60–61.

13. Chamberlain GL. Cyriax's friction massage: a review. J Orthop Sport Phys Ther. 1982;4(1):16–22.

14. Melham TJ, Sevier TL, Malnofski MJ, Wilson JK, Helfst RH, Jr. Chronic ankle pain and fibrosis successfully treated with a new noninvasive augmented soft tissue mobilization technique (ASTM): a case report. Med Sci Sports Exerc. 1998;30(6):801–804.

15. Lee D. The Pelvic Girdle. 3rd ed. Edinburgh: Churchill Livingstone; 2004.

16. Khan KM, Cook JL, Taunton JE, Bonar F. Overuse tendinosis, not tendinitis – Part 1: A new paradigm for a difficult clinical problem. Physician Sportsmed. 2000;28(5):38+.

17. Nirschl RP. Elbow tendinosis/tennis elbow. Clin Sports Med. 1992;11(4):851–870.

18. Kraushaar BS, Nirschl RP. Tendinosis of the elbow (tennis elbow). Clinical features and findings of histological, immunohistochemical, and electron microscopy studies. J Bone Joint Surg Am. 1999;81(2):259–278.

19. Davidson CJ, Ganion LR, Gehlsen GM, Verhoestra B, Roepke JE, Sevier TL. Rat tendon morphologic and functional-changes resulting from soft-tissue mobilization. Med Sci Sport Exercise. 1997;29(3):313–319.

20. Gehlsen GM, Ganion LR, Helfst R. Fibroblast responses to variation in soft tissue mobilization pressure. Med Sci Sport Exercise. 1999;31(4):531–535.

21. De Bruijin R. Deep transverse friction: its analgesic effect. International Journal of Sports Medicine 1984;5(Suppl): 35–36.

22. Goats GC. Massage – The scientific basis of an ancient art. 2. Physiological and therapeutic effects. Brit J Sport Med. 1994;28(3):153–156.

23. Melzack R, Wall PD. The Challenge of Pain. New York: Basic Books, Inc.; 1983.

24. Cyriax J, Cyriax P. Illustrated Manual of Orthopaedic Medicine. London: Butterworths; 1983.

25. Schleip R. Fascial plasticity – a new neurobiological explanation. Journal of Bodywork and Movement Therapies. 2003;7(1):11–19.

26. Simons D, Travell J, Simons L. Myofascial Pain and Dysfunction: The Trigger Point Manual. Vol 1. 2nd ed. Baltimore: Williams & Wilkins; 1999.

27. Chaitow L. Soft-Tissue Manipulation. Rochester: Healing Arts Press; 1988.

28. Travell JS, D. Myofascial Pain and Dysfunction: The Trigger Point Manual. Vol 1. 1st ed. Baltimore: Williams & Wilkins; 1983.

29. McPartland JM. Travell trigger points – molecular and osteopathic perspectives. J Am Osteopath Assoc. 2004; 104(6):244–249.

30. Simons D. Understanding effective treatments of myofascial trigger points. Journal of Bodywork & Movement Therapies. 2002;6(2):81–88.

31. Al-Shenqiti AM, Oldham JA. Test–retest reliability of myofascial trigger point detection in patients with rotator cuff tendonitis. Clin Rehabil. 2005;19(5):482–487.

32. Gerwin R, Shannon S. Interexaminer reliability and myofascial trigger points. Arch Phys Med Rehabil. 2000; 81(9):1257–1258.

33. McPartland J, Goodridge J. Counterstrain and traditional osteopathic examination of the cervical spine compared. Journal of Bodywork & Movement Therapies. 1997;1(3):173–178.

34. Chaitow L. Positional Release Techniques. 3rd ed. New York: Churchill Livingstone; 2007.

35. D'Ambrogio K, Roth G. Positional Release Therapy. St. Louis: Mosby; 1997.

36. Rolf I. Rolfing. Rochester, VT: Healing Arts Press; 1977.

37. Myers TW. Anatomy Trains. Edinburgh: Churchill Livingstone; 2001.

38. Manheim C. The Myofascial Release Manual. 2nd ed. Thorofare: Slack; 1994.

39. Juhan D. Job's Body. Barrytown, NY: Station Hill Press; 1987.

40. Threlkeld AJ. The effects of manual therapy on connective tissue. Phys Ther. Dec 1992;72(12):893–902.

41. Schleip R. Fascia is able to contract in a smooth muscle-like manner and thereby influence musculoskeletal mechanics. Paper presented at: Fascia Research Congress, 2007; Harvard Medical School, Boston, MA.

42. Spector M. Contractile behavior of musculoskeletal connective tissue cells. Paper presented at: Fascia Research Congress, 2007; Harvard Medical School, Boston, MA.

43. Klingler W, Schlegel C, Schleip R. The role of fascia in resting muscle tone and heat induced relaxation. Paper presented at: Fascia Research Congress 2007; Harvard Medical School, Boston, MA.

44. Huijing PA. Muscle as a collagen fiber reinforced composite: a review of force transmission in muscle and whole limb. J Biomech. 1999;32(4):329–345.

45. Chaitow L, DeLany J. Clinical Application of Neuromuscular Techniques. Vol 1. Edinburgh: Churchill Livingstone; 2000.

46. Barnes J. Myofascial release in treatment of thoracic outlet syndrome. Journal of Bodywork and Movement Therapies. 1996;1(1):53–57.

47. Witvrouw E, Mahieu N, Danneels L, McNair P. Stretching and injury prevention: an obscure relationship. Sports Med. 2004;34(7):443–449.

48. Ingraham SJ. The role of flexibility in injury prevention and athletic performance: have we stretched the truth? Minn Med. 2003;86(5):58–61.

49. Rubini EC, Costa AL, Gomes PS. The effects of stretching on strength performance. Sports Med. 2007;37(3):213–224.

50. Woods K, Bishop P, Jones E. Warm-up and stretching in the prevention of muscular injury. Sports Med. 2007; 37(12):1089–1099.

51. Hart L. Effect of stretching on sport injury risk: a review. Clin J Sport Med. Mar 2005;15(2):113.

52. Witvrouw E, Mahieu N, Roosen P, McNair P. The role of stretching in tendon injuries. Br J Sports Med. 2007; 41(4):224–226.

53. Yahia LH, Pigeon P, DesRosiers EA. Viscoelastic properties of the human lumbodorsal fascia. J Biomed Eng. 1993; 15(5):425–429.

54. Schleip R, Naylor IL, Ursu D, et al. Passive muscle stiffness may be influenced by active contractility of intramuscular connective tissue. Med Hypotheses. 2006;66(1):66–71.

55. Leonard C. Neuroscience of Human Movement. St. Louis: Mosby; 1998.

56. Alter M. Science of Stretching. Champaign, IL: Human Kinetics; 1988.

57. Roberts JM, Wilson K. Effect of stretching duration on active and passive range of motion in the lower extremity. Br J Sports Med. 1999;33(4):259–263.

58. Davis DS, Ashby PE, McCale KL, McQuain JA, Wine JM. The effectiveness of 3 stretching techniques on hamstring flexibility using consistent stretching parameters. J Strength Cond Res. 2005;19(1):27–32.

59. Depino GM, Webright WG, Arnold BL. Duration of maintained hamstring flexibility after cessation of an acute static stretching protocol. J Athl Train. 2000;35(1):56–59.

60. Bandy WD, Irion JM. The effect of time on static stretch on the flexibility of the hamstring muscles. Phys Ther. 1994;74(9):845–850; discussion 850–842.

61. Janda V. Postural and Phasic Muscles in the Pathogenesis of Low Back Pain. Paper presented at: XIth Congress ISRD, 1968; Dublin.

62. LaRoche DP, Connolly DA. Effects of stretching on passive muscle tension and response to eccentric exercise. Am J Sports Med. 2006;34(6):1000–1007.

63. Bonnar BP, Deivert RG, Gould TE. The relationship between isometric contraction durations during hold–relax stretching and improvement of hamstring flexibility. J Sports Med Phys Fitness. 2004;44(3):258–261.

64. Spernoga SG, Uhl TL, Arnold BL, Gansneder BM. Duration of maintained hamstring flexibility after a one-time, modified hold–relax stretching protocol. J Athl Train. 2001;36(1):44–48.

65. Lewit K, Simons DG. Myofascial pain: relief by post–isometric relaxation. Arch Phys Med Rehabil. 1984;65(8): 452–456.

66. Ford P, McChesney J. Duration of maintained hamstring ROM following termination of three stretching protocols. J Sport Rehabil. 2007;16(1):18–27.

67. Sharman MJ, Cresswell AG, Riek S. Proprioceptive neuromuscular facilitation stretching: mechanisms and clinical implications. Sports Med. 2006;36(11):929–939.

68. Chaitow L. Muscle Energy Techniques. 3rd ed. New York: Churchill Livingstone; 2006.

69. Mitchell UH, Myrer JW, Hopkins JT, Hunter I, Feland JB, Hilton SC. Acute stretch perception alteration contributes to the success of the PNF "contract–relax" stretch. J Sport Rehabil. 2007;16(2):85–92.

70. Moore MA, Hutton RS. Electromyographic investigation of muscle stretching techniques. Med Sci Sports Exerc. 1980;12(5):322–329.

71. Etnyre BR, Abraham LD. Gains in range of ankle dorsiflexion using three popular stretching techniques. Am J Phys Med. 1986;65(4):189–196.

72. Feland JB, Marin HN. Effect of submaximal contraction intensity in contract–relax proprioceptive neuromuscular facilitation stretching. Br J Sports Med. 2004;38(4):E18.

73. McAtee R, Charland J. Facilitated Stretching. Champaign, IL: Human Kinetics; 1999.

74. Mattes A. Active Isolated Stretching. Sarasota, FL.: Aaron Mattes; 1995.

Chapter 5

Physiological effects

To achieve successful clinical outcomes in orthopedic massage the practitioner should understand the physiological effects of different treatment methods. There are physiological differences among the various massage techniques, for example the effects of deep transverse friction and effleurage differ in key ways. With such a wide array of techniques, it is impractical to describe the effects of every procedure individually. In fact, despite advances in massage research, the full range of effects for most treatment methods has not been adequately identified. The current understanding is based on clinical experience and established physiological concepts. Consequently, this area is in need of further investigation.

Even with the limited understanding of massage physiology, there must be some awareness of physiological effects for safe and effective massage treatment. This chapter focuses on what is currently known about the physiological effects of massage. As research develops, new techniques and approaches will arise from this improved understanding and established treatment strategies may be revised.

The primary physiological effects of massage can be broken down into several categories. These are classified as fluid mechanics, neuromuscular responses, connective tissue responses, psychological effects, and reflex effects. This chapter looks at each of these categories, and some of the primary treatment techniques used to achieve these effects.

EFFECTS ON FLUID MECHANICS

One of the most commonly described effects of massage is the enhancement of tissue fluid movement. Blood and lymph are the primary tissue fluids affected by massage. These fluids are carried through vessels in the body and their passage is governed by hydraulic movement principles. The application of mechanical pressure on these vessels can either enhance or impede fluid movement. Treatment methods performed in the same direction as the primary flow of fluid enhances fluid movement. Treatments performed in a direction opposing that of fluid movement in the vessels may slow this movement.

There is particular concern about treatments applied to the extremities that move opposite the direction of venous blood return, particularly in the lower extremities. Dangerous levels of fluid pressure can build up in the veins from pushing the blood against the venous valves that keep blood moving proximally. The pressure build-up can dislodge a thrombus and cause serious complications such as an embolism, thereby leading to cardiovascular or cerebral damage.[1]

Tissue fluid movement is primarily encouraged by a pumping action of the vessels, since they have soft and pliable walls. The pumping action results from muscular contraction and movement. The absence of appropriate muscle activity leads to circulatory impairment. The increase of venous pooling and thrombosis from immobilization is an example of circulatory compromise resulting from insufficient movement and fluid pumping.[2–5]

Massage can enhance this process of tissue circulation. The mechanical compression of tissue along with gliding movements encourages the movement of blood and lymph fluid.[6,7] Massage also dilates superficial blood vessels to encourage greater circulation.[8–11] Increased circulation plays an important role in the healing of soft-tissue injury. The body's injury repair processes are reliant on good circulation to remove unwanted tissue debris and replenish nutrient-deprived regions for proper healing.

There is debate in the scientific literature about the role of massage in increasing circulation. Some studies have called into question the idea that massage enhances circulation as much as is frequently reported.[12,13] There is some indication that enhanced circulation may be directly related to the size of the muscle being treated. Yet, in these studies the measurement of blood flow change was by mean blood velocity through large arteries. These studies did not evaluate the contribution of massage to increasing blood flow in small capillaries.

One of the most significant effects of massage is the encouragement of blood flow in smaller capillaries that are restricted due to muscle tightness.[14] This effect is often immediately apparent with the superficial hyperemia and warmth of the skin in the area that has been treated with massage. With this direct indication of an increase in local blood flow, it is difficult to argue that there has not been an increase in local tissue circulation due to the effect of the massage treatment.

Edema can occur in the tissues as a result of an injury such as a sprain or a strain. Excess amounts of fluid can impede the proper healing process, so a reduction in edema is a fundamental goal of most soft-tissue treatments following an injury.[15] Edema can also occur in the tissue because of diseases or pathological processes that impair proper lymphatic drainage.[16] Movement of fluid out of these tissues is enhanced with the application of pressure and gliding movements, and is an essential part of the healing process.[17–20] Massage is an effective treatment for edema reduction. Techniques such as manual lymph drainage have been designed specifically for their effects on

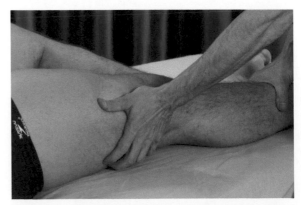

Figure 5.1 Gliding techniques, especially those such as effleurage and sweeping cross fiber, have beneficial effects on enhancing tissue fluid enhancement.

encouraging better flow of lymph fluid and reduction of edema.[16,21,22]

Delayed onset muscle soreness (DOMS) is a common occurrence following bouts of unaccustomed exercise, especially if the exercise involves significant eccentric muscle actions. A primary component of DOMS appears to be an inflammatory reaction in the tissues that results from minor connective tissue tearing.[23,24] The inflammatory reaction creates excess tissue edema. Pressure from edema on local nociceptors is a likely cause of the pain in DOMS. Because of its ability to encourage circulation and remove edema, massage can be helpful in reducing DOMS.[25–27,28–31] However, these findings are still somewhat controversial, as other studies have questioned the role that massage may play in reducing DOMS.[13,32,33]

The most successful means to affect fluid mechanics with massage comes from techniques that involve gliding with pressure. Because of significant circulation effects, most of these gliding techniques are performed in the direction of the heart to prevent backflow pressure against venous valves. Effleurage, which involves long gliding strokes, is the most effective technique for encouraging tissue fluid movement. Sweeping cross fiber techniques that move in a longitudinal/diagonal direction across the muscular fibers also help enhance tissue fluid movement.

Compression broadening techniques, while not moving in a longitudinal direction with most blood and lymph vessels, still enhances tissue fluid movement. The broad pressure application on the tissues during the stroke helps flush the tissues and encourage fluid movement. Deep longitudinal stripping techniques performed with a broad base of pressure, such as the palm, also help improve tissue fluid movement. Because there is a greater degree of pressure with longitudinal stripping, caution is advised if any structures of the circulatory or lymphatic systems appear weakened or compromised. The same will be true of any active engagement methods performed with a broad base of pressure application.

NEUROMUSCULAR EFFECTS

One of the primary reasons for using massage for soft-tissue pain and injury treatment is the reduction of muscle tightness. Muscles become hypertonic because of excess neuromuscular stimulation. Massage reduces this excessive stimulation.[34–37] A variety of conservative treatments are used to address excess muscular tension, and of those procedures massage is one of the most effective.[38]

When muscle tissue is in a heightened state of contraction, the individual muscle fibers are shortened and there is an overlapping of sarcomeres, which makes the muscle feel denser during palpation. The body can maintain this level of contraction in a perpetual state if no other stimulus is introduced. Excess muscle tension produces ischemia, resistance to stretch, and irritation of nociceptors, which bombard the nervous system with sensory information. In turn, this heightened sensory information causes a reactive tightening of muscles and development of the well known pain–spasm–pain cycle.[14,39] Massage breaks the cycle of pain and spasm to reduce the overall neuromuscular tension.

Additional problems with excess neuromuscular activity arise from the muscle spindle cells, one of the primary proprioceptors in the body. The muscle spindle cells are unique among proprioceptors, in that they receive motor signals from the central nervous system through the gamma efferent (motor signal) system. The gamma efferent system is designed to help regulate the proper amount of tension in the muscle tissues.[40] If this system is overactive it causes an increase in muscle tension, as in hypertonic muscles. Excess gamma activity is another aspect of the dysfunctional neuromuscular feedback loop.

Massage can make a beneficial intervention in this dysfunctional process by mechanically stretching the sarcomeres with pressure.[41] When pressure is applied to muscle tissue, the entire fiber is put under a greater tensile load, and this mechanically stretches the muscle tissue. If pressure is held for more than just a few seconds, there is a resetting of the level of resting tension in the muscle by the muscle spindle cells.[42] This change in spindle setting is perceived by both the client and practitioner as a relaxation or softening of the muscle.

Proprioceptors, such as the muscle spindle cells, play another crucial role in the treatment process. The neurological principle of facilitation suggests that when an impulse has traveled along

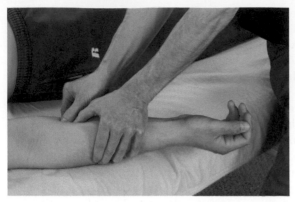

Figure 5.2 Massage techniques, such as deep stripping, greatly enhance elongation of sarcomeres and thereby provide a reduction in neuromuscular tension.

a particular nerve pathway, future impulses are more likely to take that same path.[43] This is the concept behind the learning and improvement of any motor skill. There is a gradual refinement of neuromuscular patterns as the individual practices the complex coordination of motor signals. Likewise, the body may adapt to dysfunctional patterns of motor activity, such as poor posture, simply because it is continually reinforced (facilitated). One of the most powerful effects of soft-tissue manipulation is the ability to re-train the patterns of motor signals in the body, and establish new pathways for facilitation that involve far less chronic tension.[44] Continual reinforcement of reduced muscle tension improves overall muscular patterns, enhances posture and movement, and has beneficial systemic effects as well.[32]

There are many descriptions of the benefits of massage in reducing muscle tension and improving athletic performance. Massage reduces post-activity muscle tension through some of the mechanisms mentioned earlier.[45,46] However, the question of whether or how this tension reduction actually improves sports performance is still controversial. Subjectively, the popularity of massage among athletes suggests that its effects do benefit sports performance.[47,48] More research needs to be performed in this area to understand the complex factors of athletic performance, and how massage may influence those factors.

Massage also produces neuromuscular effects that influence the pain-gate mechanism. Chapter 3 included a discussion of the gate theory of pain, which outlines much of our current understanding of pain sensations in the body.[49] This theory suggests that pain can be reduced or alleviated by pressure or thermal sensations, because the fibers from pressure and thermal receptors transmit signals faster than those from pain receptors. These other sensory signals arrive at the central nervous system before the pain sensations, and in essence 'close the gate' on certain pain signals being reported. Pressure and movement in massage activate proprioceptors in this pain-gate mechanism and reduce painful sensations in the muscle tissue.[50] Massage intervention thereby aids in breaking the pain–spasm–pain cycle.

All of the techniques mentioned in the previous chapter are likely to have a beneficial effect on reducing neuromuscular tension. If the increased neuromuscular tension occurs throughout the muscle, the various gliding techniques, such as effleurage, sweeping cross fiber, and compression broadening, are particularly helpful. Pressure applied to the muscle to reduce tension is magnified with active engagement methods. The increase in pressure level helps stretch a greater number of muscle fibers and their surrounding connective tissue. In many cases, there is greater reduction of neuromuscular tension with active engagement methods than from passive techniques.

If the neuromuscular tension is in a small area, such as a myofascial trigger point, an effective means of addressing that tension is with static compression methods. Broad contact pressure static compression is helpful to reduce overall muscle tension. Following the application of broad contact static compression, more specific compression techniques like those performed with the thumbs, knuckles, elbow, or pressure tools are more appropriate to neutralize the excess neuromuscular activity of myofascial trigger points.[39,51,52]

Because of the active neuromuscular component in various active-engagement stretching methods, these approaches are highly effective in reducing neuromuscular tension. Muscle energy technique (MET), for example, is used frequently for this purpose. MET is highly effective in reducing excess neurological activity because of using the muscle's own neurological energy to aid the relaxation.[53] Neuromuscular tension is also effectively reduced when various methods are combined. An example of combining various approaches to effectively address neuromuscular tension is a combination of static compression, positional release, and muscle energy technique described as integrated neuromuscular inhibition technique, or INIT.[54]

CONNECTIVE TISSUE EFFECTS

Massage affects the connective tissues of the body in numerous ways. Fascia, which is the most prevalent connective tissue in the body, envelops every anatomical structure. This complex fascial network creates a web of connection between every region of the body so that tensile or compressive forces in one area influence those in remote areas.[55] The well-known 'fascial sweater' concept that is described by Ida Rolf illustrates how fascial restriction in one area affects many others.[56] Recent research indicates that tendon is not the only tissue to transmit muscle contraction force. Connective tissue transmits a muscle's contraction force to bones and other adjacent structures.[57,58] Therefore, when massage affects connective tissue tension it also affects tensile loads on muscle and other adjacent structures.

Restriction in free mobility of connective tissues is the origin of many musculoskeletal problems. Tensile loads applied to fascial tissues help elongate and stretch them, and, therefore, reduce the symptoms of many complaints. This is best accomplished

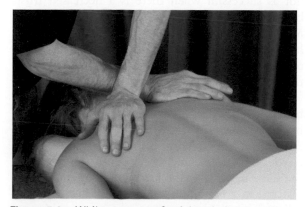

Figure 5.3 While many myofascial techniques apply only superficial pressure, the tensile force applied to the connective tissue can help to release muscle tension even in deeper muscles.

with a low force load that is held for a longer period of time to take advantage of the mechanical property of creep – a slow, gradual tissue elongation when a steady tensile load is applied.[59,60] Connective tissues such as fascia are richly innervated with mechanoreceptors and capable of active contraction.[61,62] Low-level tangential or transverse forces applied to fascia reduce neural excitability and decrease excess muscle tension as well.[41,63]

Connective tissues such as tendons and ligaments also benefit from massage treatments. The most common pathology affecting tendons is tendinosis (commonly called tendinitis). Originally thought to involve an inflammatory reaction in the tendon fibers, research now points to the primary problem as one of collagen degeneration in the tendon tissue.[64–67] Massage is helpful for tendinosis by encouraging fibroblast proliferation, which are essential in the rebuilding of damaged tissue.[68–70] Massage is also beneficial for tendon disorders such as tenosynovitis, which is an inflammation and irritation between the tendon and its surrounding synovial sheath. Adhesions commonly develop between the tendon and its sheath in tenosynovitis. Techniques such as deep transverse friction (DTF) help break dysfunctional adhesions and mobilize the tendon within its sheath, creating less restriction for the tendon.[71]

In some injury conditions, such as muscle strains or ligament sprains, excessive scar tissue impedes the proper healing process when it binds to adjacent fibers during healing. Motion loss in ligament tissue may occur when the ligament is bound to adjacent structures such as bone or joint capsule. Immobilization and lack of movement during the healing process is the usual cause of scar tissue binding in ligament injuries. Massage techniques, especially those such as DTF, can help reduce this scar tissue.[72,73] Scar tissue from soft-tissue injury can also bind nerves and reduce their ability to glide freely beside adjacent tissue.[74,75] When the nerves lose mobility because of soft-tissue binding, neurological symptoms such as pain, paresthesia, numbness, or motor impairment follow. Stretching and massage techniques are valuable in mobilizing the connective tissue that has bound nerves to adjacent structures.[76,77]

Treatment techniques such as the myofascial approaches described in Chapter 4 have the greatest ability to elongate superficial connective tissues throughout the body. However, in many instances the fascial restrictions are in the deeper tissues. The connective tissue surrounding deep muscles may be difficult to access with applications of light pressure used in many myofascial techniques. In those situations, techniques such as the active engagement methods are more effective. The active contraction in the muscle makes the tissue denser, and the pressure is able to penetrate more effectively through the muscle. The result is a greater degree of tensile load applied to the deeper connective tissue layers.

PSYCHOLOGICAL EFFECTS

One of the most commonly reported effects of massage treatment is the overall sense of relaxation felt after the treatment session. The feeling of relaxation is much more than just a reduction in muscle tension. It is a comprehensive psychological response characterized by an overall improved sense of well-being. Numerous factors in massage treatment play a role in enhancing the client's psychological state. However, the effects discussed below are general. There is no established connection between specific massage techniques and their ability to generate or enhance a specific psychological effect.

The massage treatment is a close interaction involving touch between two individuals. The power of touch with therapeutic intent has positive outcomes in a variety of client populations.[78–82] There are other therapeutic interventions that involve touch between a practitioner and the client, but the sense of psychological well-being produced is not as strong. If an individual were receiving an ultrasound treatment, the benefit of the treatment is not likely to be dependent on the person who administers the treatment. This is not true with massage. The interaction between the client and practitioner in the massage environment is of paramount importance and arguably one of the most important therapeutic elements.[83] Unfortunately, this is also one of the most difficult elements to quantify and study through proper research methods.

Our society is currently plagued by stress-induced illnesses. A large majority of the stressors that are manifesting in people's lives have a strong psychological component. Massage is an effective intervention for many stress-induced illnesses such as anxiety or depression.[84–88] One does not need to be experiencing clinically diagnosed anxiety or depression for those beneficial effects to take place. The same mechanisms are at work in each therapeutic session and help enhance various positive psychological states.

While reducing depression and anxiety may not seem to be a primary role of treating orthopedic disorders, attention to the psychological component of soft-tissue disorders is too often an overlooked element in rehabilitation practice. A client is not a machine with a broken part like some current technological health care models espouse. Each individual and their pain complaint exists within a unique psychosocial environment and that environment plays a crucial role in the healing process.[89] Recent developments in psychoneuroimmunology and the study of mind-body medicine emphasize that the psychological and physical components of health cannot be separated when considering optimum health.[90–93] Consequently, anxiety reduction and greater psychological well-being resulting from massage treatment have an important role in the treatment of any orthopedic disorder.

The lack of personalization in the mainstream health care setting can have a detrimental effect on the individual's trust and communication with their health care provider. Health care interventions are not as successful when there is a decreased trust between the client/patient and the practitioner.[94] Massage therapy clients have repeatedly reported high levels of satisfaction in the client/practitioner relationship that contribute significantly to positive therapeutic outcomes.[95,96]

Any soft-tissue manipulation method can have beneficial or detrimental psychological effects based on the way in which it is administered. A roughly administered technique by a disinterested or irritable practitioner does not produce the same benefits as the identical technique administered in a caring and therapeutic manner by a fully engaged and compassionate practitioner. The client must feel trust and safety in the therapeutic environment for beneficial psychological effects to occur. Because the client is usually in some stage of undress during the treatment, there can be increased feelings of vulnerability or power differential between the client and practitioner. The effectiveness of any treatment technique is dependent on the practitioner's ability to gain the client's trust in the treatment process. Massage practitioners tend to spend a greater amount of time with their client's than most other health care providers. Consequently, there is a greater chance of developing a deeper connection and trust between the practitioner and the client. Do not underestimate the power of this relationship as well as the benefits and advantages of this improved trust and connection in a rehabilitative context.

REFLEX EFFECTS

Some of the beneficial effects of massage are not direct physiological responses and are therefore harder to categorize and measure. In a massage treatment sensory signals relating information on touch, pressure, and temperature cause a variety of responses that are regulated by autonomic nervous system (ANS) activity. These ANS mediated responses are called reflex effects.

One of the most powerful reflex effects is massage's influence on the immune system. While more research is clearly needed in this area, numerous studies have demonstrated a positive effect on immune system function.[97–102] Healing from any soft-tissue pain or injury condition is a complex process that requires action from the immune system. With enhanced immune system function there is a greater chance of early and beneficial tissue healing. In addition, massage appears to reduce stress hormone levels, and this effect is connected with the improved immune system function.[43,103] A related reflex effect of massage is its lowering of blood pressure.[32,104] There are both chemical and psychological factors in the massage treatment that appear responsible for decreasing blood pressure. The increase in local tissue circulation discussed earlier may be partially responsible for the blood pressure effects.

A treatment method called connective tissue massage demonstrates one way in which blood pressure changes may occur. Connective tissue massage is a technique that focuses on mobilization of the superficial connective tissue (fascia) throughout the body and is similar to some of the techniques described above in the section on myofascial approaches. Connective tissue treatments increase blood flow to deeply seated organs by triggering cutaneo-visceral reflexes.[105,106] These reflexes cause an increase in blood flow to the affected region, together with suppression of pain sensations.[107] There is also a beta-endorphin release that is linked with the sensation of pain relief.[108] While many of these effects have been studied specifically with the techniques of connective tissue massage, they are likely with many other massage techniques as well. In addition, the practitioner should bear in mind that it is difficult to predict exactly how massage may produce some of these reflex effects.

Any discussion of reflex effects of massage treatment would not be complete without mention of the many different treatment systems that use specific reflex points in precise locations on the body. The Asian bodywork systems such as acupressure, shiatsu, and tui-na are examples of these systems that use specific reflex points. The physiological models these systems use are entirely different from Western anatomy and physiology. The considerable differences in theoretical models pose difficulty for many Western-trained clinicians in understanding the reflex processes in how these systems work.[109] According to these systems, a number of maladies that are remote from the site of treatment can be affected by compression on these points.[110–112] Most of the treatment procedures in these systems use static compression techniques on precise locations (usually corresponding to acupuncture points) to achieve a therapeutic response.

Several other treatment systems are based on reflex points. These include Chapman's neurolymphatic reflex points, Bennett's neurovascular reflex points, and the various autonomic nervous system effects from myofascial trigger points.[113] There is some common ground in the physiological effects that these different systems produce. For example, there appears to be a relationship between acupuncture points and myofascial trigger points.[114] When many of these systems of 'points' are mapped onto the body, a considerable overlap is evident.

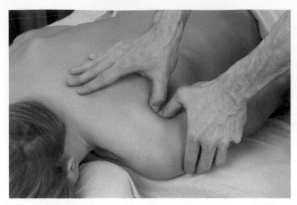

Figure 5.4 Static compression techniques are used in many reflex systems such as acupressure, tui-na or shiatsu.

Another reflex effect from soft-tissue manipulation is the viscerosomatic reflex. A viscerosomatic reflex is one that involves reflex actions through the central nervous system between visceral (organ) and somatic (usually muscular) tissues. These reflexes occur because nerve fibers to and from abdominal viscera come off the spinal cord at the same level as sensory or motor fibers for back and abdominal muscles. Because of their close proximity, reflex arcs develop between visceral and somatic fibers so there can be interactions between the two. In a viscerosomatic reflex, excessive sensory stimuli from a dysfunctional abdominal organ may travel to the spinal cord and spill over in a reflex arc to muscular tissues whose motor fibers originate at the same level. The excessive sensory stimuli from the dysfunctional organ create increased motor signals and subsequent increases in muscle tension.

The reverse process is also a viscerosomatic reflex (although some call this a somatic-visceral reflex). Sensory signals from exceedingly tight muscles may spill over in the spinal cord to afferents associated with organ function. The spillover creates a dysfunctional level of neural stimulation to the organ resulting in an eventual organ disorder. Massage can have a positive outcome in reducing viscerosomatic reflex activity. A reduction in sensory stimulation can occur in this area if the muscles are treated and their overall neuromuscular activity is reduced. Massage can interrupt viscerosomatic reflexes and reduce excessive input to the central nervous system.[115]

Choosing specific treatment techniques to maximize reflex effects can be challenging because these effects are difficult to predict. It is more valuable for the clinician to bear in mind that all of the above effects are possible results from therapeutic procedures (the exception is if the individual is using a system that is specific for particular reflex effects, such as shiatsu). In this way, the practitioner should have a better understanding of what reflex processes might occur as a result of treatment.

References

1. Werner R, Benjamin B. A Massage Therapist's Guide to Pathology. Baltimore: Williams & Wilkins; 1998.
2. Partsch H, Blattler W. Compression and walking versus bed rest in the treatment of proximal deep venous thrombosis with low molecular weight heparin. J Vasc Surg. 2000;32(5):861–869.
3. Junger M, Diehm C, Storiko H, et al. Mobilization versus immobilization in the treatment of acute proximal deep venous thrombosis: a prospective, randomized, open, multicentre trial. Curr Med Res Opin. 2006;22(3): 593–602.
4. Slipman CW, Lipetz JS, Jackson HB, Vresilovic EJ. Deep venous thrombosis and pulmonary embolism as a complication of bed rest for low back pain. Arch Phys Med Rehabil. 2000;81(1):127–129.
5. Kuipers S, Schreijer AJ, Cannegieter SC, Buller HR, Rosendaal FR, Middeldorp S. Travel and venous thrombosis: a systematic review. J Intern Med. 2007; 262(6):615–634.
6. Callaghan MJ. The role of massage in the management of the athlete: a review. Br J Sports Med. 1993;27(1):28–33.
7. Cafarelli E, Flint F. The Role of Massage in Preparation For and Recovery From Exercise: An Overview. Sport Med. 1992;14(1):1.
8. Goats GC. Massage – The Scientific Basis of an Ancient–Art. 2. Physiological and Therapeutic Effects. Brit J Sport Med. 1994;28(3):153–156.
9. Hansen TI, Kristensen JH. Effect of massage, shortwave diathermy and ultrasound upon 133Xe disappearance rate from muscle and subcutaneous tissue in the human calf. Scand J Rehabil Med. 1973;5(4):179–182.
10. Hovind H, Nielsen SL. Effect of massage on blood flow in skeletal muscle. Scand J Rehabil Med. 1974;6(2): 74–77.

11. Wakim KG. Physiologic effects of massage. In: Licht S, ed. Massage, Manipulation, and Traction. Huntington, NY: R.E. Krieger; 1976.

12. Shoemaker JK, Tiidus PM, Mader R. Failure of manual massage to alter limb blood-flow – measures by Doppler ultrasound. Med Sci Sport Exercise. 1997;29(5):610–614.

13. Tiidus PM, Shoemaker JK. Effleurage massage, muscle blood-flow and long-term postexercise strength recovery. Int J Sport Med. 1995;16(7):478–483.

14. Travell JS, D. Myofascial Pain and Dysfunction: The Trigger Point Manual. Vol 1. 1st ed. Baltimore: Williams & Wilkins; 1983.

15. AAOS. Athletic Training and Sports Medicine. 2nd ed. Park Ridge: American Academy of Orthopaedic Surgeons; 1991.

16. Chikly B. Silent Waves: Theory and Practice of Lymph Drainage Therapy. Scottsdale, AZ: I.H.H. Publishing; 2002.

17. Kriederman B, Myloyde T, Bernas M, et al. Limb volume reduction after physical treatment by compression and/or massage in a rodent model of peripheral lymphedema. Lymphology. 2002;35(1):23–27.

18. Ladd MP, Kottke FJ, Blanchard RS. Studies of the effect of massage on the flow of lymph from the foreleg of the dog. Arch Phys Med. 1952;33:604–612.

19. Leduc O, Leduc A, Bourgeois P, Belgrado JP. The physical treatment of upper limb edema. Cancer. 1998; 83(12 Suppl American):2835–2839.

20. Wakim KG, Tin GM, Krusen FH. Influence of centripetal rhythmic compression on localized edema of an extremity. Arch Phys Med. 1955;36:98–103.

21. Haren K, Backman C, Wiberg M. Effect of manual lymph drainage as described by Vodder on oedema of the hand after fracture of the distal radius: a prospective clinical study. Scand J Plast Reconstr Surg Hand Surg. 2000; 34(4):367–372.

22. Johansson K, Albertsson M, Ingvar C, Ekdahl C. Effects of compression bandaging with or without manual lymph drainage treatment in patients with postoperative arm lymphedema. Lymphology. 1999;32(3):103–110.

23. Lieber RL, Friden J. Mechanisms of muscle injury after eccentric contraction. J Sci Med Sport. 1999;2(3):253–265.

24. Vickers AJ. Time course of muscle soreness following different types of exercise. BMC Musculoskelet Disord. 2001;2(1):5.

25. Ernst E. Does postexercise massage treatment reduce delayed-onset muscle soreness – a systematic review. Brit J Sport Med. 1998;32(3):212–214.

26. Rodenburg JB, Steenbeek D, Schiereck P, Bar PR. Warm-up, stretching and massage diminish harmful effects of eccentric exercise. Int J Sport Med. 1994;15(7):414–419.

27. Smith LL, Keating MN, Holbert D, et al. The effects of athletic massage on delayed-onset muscle soreness, creatine-kinase, and neutrophil count – a preliminary-report. J Orthop Sport Phys Therapy. 1994;19(2):93–99.

28. Zainuddin Z, Newton M, Sacco P, Nosaka K. Effects of massage on delayed-onset muscle soreness, swelling, and recovery of muscle function. J Athl Train. 2005; 40(3):174–180.

29. Cheung K, Hume P, Maxwell L. Delayed onset muscle soreness: treatment strategies and performance factors. Sports Med. 2003;33(2):145–164.

30. Farr T, Nottle C, Nosaka K, Sacco P. The effects of therapeutic massage on delayed onset muscle soreness and muscle function following downhill walking. J Sci Med Sport. 2002;5(4):297–306.

31. Hilbert JE, Sforzo GA, Swensen T. The effects of massage on delayed onset muscle soreness. Br J Sports Med. 2003;37:72–75.

32. Field TM. Massage therapy effects. Amer Psychol. 1998;53(12):1270–1281.

33. Weber MD, Servedio FJ, Woodall WR. The effects of 3 modalities on delayed-onset muscle soreness. J Orthop Sport Phys Therapy. 1994;20(5):236–242.

34. Braverman DL, Schulman RA. Massage techniques in rehabilitation medicine. Phys Med Rehabil Clin N Am. 1999;10(3):631–649, ix.

35. Morelli M, Seaborne DE, Sullivan SJ. H-reflex modulation during manual muscle massage of human triceps surae. Arch Phys Med Rehabil. 1991;72(11):915–919.

36. Nordschow W, Bierman W. Influence of manual massage on muscle relaxation: effect on trunk flexion. Phys Ther. 1962;42:653.

37. Sullivan SJ, Williams LR, Seaborne DE, Morelli M. Effects of massage on alpha motoneuron excitability. Phys Ther. 1991;71(8):555–560.

38. Liebenson C. Active muscular relaxation techniques. Part I. Basic principles and methods. J Manipulative Physiol Ther. 1989;12(6):446–454.

39. Mense S, Simons DG. Muscle Pain: Understanding Its Nature, Diagnosis, & Treatment. Baltimore: Lippincott Williams & Wilkins; 2001.

40. Leonard C. Neuroscience of Human Movement. St. Louis: Mosby; 1998.

41. Schleip R. Fascial plasticity – a new neurobiological explanation. Part 2. Journal of Bodywork and Movement Therapies. 2003;7(2):104–116.

42. Korr IM. Proprioceptors and somatic dysfunction. J Am Osteopath Assoc. 1975;74(7):638–650.

43. Fritz S. Mosby's Fundamentals of Therapeutic Massage. 2nd ed. St. Louis: Mosby; 2000.

44. Juhan D. Job's Body. Barrytown, NY: Station Hill Press; 1987.

45. Rinder AN, Sutherland CJ. An investigation of the effects of massage on quadriceps performance after exercise fatigue. Complement Ther Nurs Midwifery. 1995; 1(4):99–102.

46. Viitasalo JT, Niemela K, Kaappola R, et al. Warm underwater water-jet massage improves recovery from intense physical exercise. Eur J Appl Physiol Occup Physiol. 1995;71(5):431–438.

47. Hemmings B, Smith M, Graydon J, Dyson R. Effects of massage on physiological restoration, perceived recovery, and repeated sports performance. Brit J Sport Med. 2000;34(2):109–114.

48. Nannini L, Myers D, Glotzbach B, Poland P. The Centennial Olympic Games and massage therapy: the first official team.

Journal of Bodywork and Movement Therapies. 1997; 1(3):130–133.

49. Melzack R, Wall PD. The Challenge of Pain. New York: Basic Books, Inc.; 1983.

50. Bowsher D. Modulation of nociceptive input. In: Wells PE, Frampton V, Bowsher D, eds. Pain Management and Control in Physiotherapy. London: Heinemann Medical; 1988.

51. Simons D. Understanding effective treatments of myofascial trigger points. Journal of Bodywork & Movement Therapies. 2002;6(2):81–88.

52. Huguenin L. Myofascial trigger points: the current evidence. Physical Therapy in Sport. 2004;5:2–12.

53. Mitchell F. Elements of Muscle Energy Technique. In: Basmajian J, Nyberg R, eds. Rational Manual Therapies. Baltimore: Williams & Wilkins; 1993.

54. Chaitow L. Muscle Energy Techniques. New York: Churchill Livingstone; 1996.

55. Myers TW. Anatomy Trains. Edinburgh: Churchill Livingstone; 2001.

56. Rolf I. Rolfing. Rochester, VT: Healing Arts Press; 1977.

57. Monti RJ, Roy RR, Hodgson JA, Edgerton VR. Transmission of forces within mammalian skeletal muscles. J Biomech. 1999;32(4):371–380.

58. Huijing P. Muscular force transmission: a unified, dual or multiple system? A review and some explorative experimental results. Arch Physiol Biochem. 1999; 107(4):292–311.

59. Cantu R, Grodin A. Myofascial Manipulation: Theory and Clinical Application. Gaithersburg: Aspen; 1992.

60. Chaitow L, DeLany J. Clinical Application of Neuromuscular Techniques. Vol 1. Edinburgh: Churchill Livingstone; 2000.

61. Schleip R. Fascial plasticity – a new neurobiological explanation. Journal of Bodywork and Movement Therapies. 2003;7(1):11–19.

62. Schleip R. Fascia is able to contract in a smooth muscle-like manner and thereby influence musculoskeletal mechanics. Paper presented at: Fascia Research Congress, 2007; Harvard Medical School, Boston, MA.

63. LeMoon K. Connective tissue contractility is the central mediating factor in myofascial pain syndrome: a fasciagenic pain model. Paper presented at: Fascia Research Congress, 2007; Harvard Medical School, Boston, MA.

64. Almekinders LC, Temple JD. Etiology, diagnosis, and treatment of tendinitis – an analysis of the literature. Med Sci Sport Exercise. 1998;30(8):1183–1190.

65. Gibbon WW, Cooper JR, Radcliffe GS. Distribution of sonographically detected tendon abnormalities in patients with a clinical diagnosis of chronic achilles tendinosis. J Clin Ultrasound. 2000;28(2):61–66.

66. Kraushaar BS, Nirschl RP. Tendinosis of the elbow (tennis elbow). Clinical features and findings of histological, immunohistochemical, and electron microscopy studies. J Bone Joint Surg Am. 1999;81(2):259–278.

67. Nirschl RP. Elbow tendinosis/tennis elbow. Clin Sports Med. 1992;11(4):851–870.

68. Brosseau L, Casimiro L, Milne S, et al. Deep transverse friction massage for treating tendinitis (Cochrane Review). Cochrane Database Syst Rev. 2002(1): CD003528.

69. Cook JL, Khan KM, Maffulli N, Purdam C. Overuse tendinosis, not tendinitis part 2. Applying the new approach to patellar tendinopathy. Physician Sports Med. 2000;28(6):31+.

70. Davidson CJ, Ganion LR, Gehlsen GM, Verhoestra B, Roepke JE, Sevier TL. Rat tendon morphologic and functional changes resulting from soft-tissue mobilization. Med Sci Sport Exercise.1997;29(3): 313–319.

71. Cyriax J. Textbook of Orthopaedic Medicine Volume Two: Treatment by Manipulation, Massage, and Injection. Vol 2. London: Baillière Tindall; 1984.

72. Chamberlain GL. Cyriax's friction massage: a review. J Orthop Sport Phys Therapy. 1982;4(1):16–22.

73. Cyriax J. Deep massage. Physiotherapy. 1977;63(2):60–61.

74. Gallant S. Assessing adverse neural tension in athletes. J Sport Rehabil. 1998;7(2):128–139.

75. Turl SE, and George KP. Adverse neural tension – a factor in repetitive hamstring strain. J Orthop Sport Phys Therapy. 1998;27(1):16–21.

76. Butler D. Mobilisation of the Nervous System. London: Churchill Livingstone; 1991.

77. Shacklock M. Clinical Neurodynamics. Edinburgh: Elsevier; 2005.

78. Weze C, Leathard HL, Grange J, Tiplady P, Stevens G. Evaluation of healing by gentle touch. Public Health. 2005;119(1):3–10.

79. Wilkinson DS, Knox PL, Chatman JE, et al. The clinical effectiveness of healing touch. J Altern Complement Med. 2002;8(1):33–47.

80. Collinge W, Wentworth R, Sabo S. Integrating complementary therapies into community mental health practice: an exploration. J Altern Complement Med. 2005;11(3):569–574.

81. Smith MC, Stallings MA, Iner S, Burrall M. Benefits of massage therapy for hospitalized patients: a descriptive and qualitative evaluation. Altern Ther Health Med. 1999;5(4):64–71.

82. Sharpe PA, Williams HG, Granner ML, Hussey JR. A randomised study of the effects of massage therapy compared to guided relaxation on well-being and stress perception among older adults. Complement Ther Med. 2007;15(3):157–163.

83. Hyland ME. Reports by some massage therapists of a sense of 'special connection' that is sometimes experienced with clients/patients. Forsch Komplement Med (2006). 2006;13(6):335–341.

84. Ferrell–Torry AT, Glick OJ. The use of therapeutic massage as a nursing intervention to modify anxiety and the perception of cancer pain. Cancer Nurs. 1993; 16(2):93–101.

85. Field T, Grizzle N, Scafidi F, Schanberg S. Massage and relaxation therapies' effects on depressed adolescent mothers. Adolescence. 1996;31(124):903–911.

86. Kim MS, Cho KS, Woo H, Kim JH. Effects of hand massage on anxiety in cataract surgery using local anesthesia. J Cataract Refract Surg. 2001;27(6):884–890.

87. Richards KC, Gibson R, Overton-McCoy AL. Effects of massage in acute and critical care. AACN Clin Issues. 2000;11(1):77–96.

88. Zeitlin D, Keller SE, Shiflett SC, Schleifer SJ, Bartlett JA. Immunological effects of massage therapy during academic stress. Psychosom Med. 2000;62(1):83–84.

89. Waddell G. The Back Pain Revolution. Edinburgh: Churchill Livingstone; 1998.

90. Jacobs GD. The physiology of mind–body interactions: the stress response and the relaxation response. J Altern Complement Med. 2001;7(Suppl 1):S83–92.

91. Ray O. How the mind hurts and heals the body. Am Psychol. 2004;59(1):29–40.

92. Ray O. The revolutionary health science of psychoendoneuroimmunology: a new paradigm for understanding health and treating illness. Ann N Y Acad Sci. 2004;1032:35–51.

93. Gilbert MD. Weaving medicine back together: mind–body medicine in the twenty-first century. J Altern Complement Med. 2003;9(4):563–570.

94. Illingworth P. Trust: the scarcest of medical resources. J Med Philos. 2002;27(1):31–46.

95. Stewart D, Weeks J, Bent S. Utilization, patient satisfaction, and cost implications of acupuncture, massage, and naturopathic medicine offered as covered health benefits: a comparison of two delivery models. Altern Ther Health Med. 2001;7(4):66–70.

96. Cherkin DC, Deyo RA, Sherman KJ, et al. Characteristics of licensed acupuncturists, chiropractors, massage therapists, and naturopathic physicians. J Am Board Fam Pract. 2002;15(5):378–390.

97. Hernandez-Reif M, Field T, Ironson G, et al. Natural killer cells and lymphocytes increase in women with breast cancer following massage therapy. Int J Neurosci. 2005;115(4):495–510.

98. Hernandez-Reif M, Ironson G, Field T, et al. Breast cancer patients have improved immune and neuroendocrine functions following massage therapy. J Psychosom Res. 2004;57(1):45–52.

99. Diego MA, Field T, Hernandez-Reif M, Shaw K, Friedman L, Ironson G. HIV adolescents show improved immune function following massage therapy. Int J Neurosci. 2001;106(1–2):35–45.

100. Ironson G, Field T, Scafidi F, et al. Massage therapy is associated with enhancement of the immune system's cytotoxic capacity. Int J Neurosci. 1996;84(1–4): 205–217.

101. Field T, Diego MA, Hernandez–Reif M, Deeds O, Figuereido B. Moderate versus light pressure massage therapy leads to greater weight gain in preterm infants. Infant Behav Dev. 2006;29(4):574–578.

102. Birk TJ, McGrady A, MacArthur RD, Khuder S. The effects of massage therapy alone and in combination with other complementary therapies on immune system measures and quality of life in human immunodeficiency virus. J Altern Complement Med. 2000;6(5):405–414.

103. Field T. Touch Therapy. Edinburgh: Churchill Livingstone; 2000.

104. Cady SH, Jones GE. Massage therapy as a workplace intervention for reduction of stress. Percept Mot Skills. 1997;84(1):157–158.

105. Ebner M. Connective Tissue Manipulation: Theory and Therapeutic Application. 3rd ed. Malabar, FL: R.E. Krieger; 1975.

106. Gifford J, Gifford L. Connective tissue massage. In: Wells PE, Frampton V, Bowsher D, eds. Pain: Management and Control in Physiotherapy. London: Heinemann Medical; 1988.

107. Goats GC, Keir KA. Connective tissue massage. Br J Sports Med. 1991;25(3):131–133.

108. Kaada B, Torsteinbo O. Increase of plasma beta-endorphins in connective tissue massage. Gen Pharmacol. 1989;20(4):487–489.

109. Oschman J. Energy Medicine: The Scientific Basis. Edinburgh: Churchill Livingstone; 2000.

110. Yeh ML, Chen CH, Chen HH, Lin KC. An intervention of acupressure and interactive multimedia to improve visual health among Taiwanese schoolchildren. Public Health Nurs. 2008;25(1):10–17.

111. Somma C, Luchetti M. Shiatsu. J Altern Complement Med. 2007;13(6):679–680.

112. Wu HS, Lin LC, Wu SC, Lin JG. The psychologic consequences of chronic dyspnea in chronic pulmonary obstruction disease: the effects of acupressure on depression. J Altern Complement Med. 2007;13(2): 253–261.

113. Chaitow L. Soft-Tissue Manipulation. Rochester: Healing Arts Press; 1988.

114. Melzack R. Myofascial trigger points: relation to acupuncture and mechanisms of pain. Arch Phys Med Rehabil. 1981;62(3):114–117.

115. Beal MC. Viscerosomatic reflexes: a review. J Am Osteopath Assoc. 1985;85(12):786–801.

SECTION **2**

A regional approach to pathology and treatment

SECTION CONTENTS

The next section examines the most commonly occurring soft-tissue pathologies the orthopedic massage practitioner is likely to see. Each of these disorders is presented as a separate condition that has unique clinical signs and symptoms. However, in many cases the client's condition is not limited to a single discrete pathology. Several problems can co-exist and they may involve a complex interaction of clinical factors. Biomechanics, nutrition, chemical exposure, and psychosocial stress are just a few of the additional factors that should be considered when evaluating and treating any orthopedic disorder. For that reason, the client must be viewed in a multi-dimensional manner, and not simply as a body with a condition.

The soft-tissue massage treatment methods described in the following chapters have been developed through years of research and clinical practice. Numerous practitioners were consulted in developing these treatment guidelines. Methods are suggested that have demonstrated positive results and are based on sound physiological principles. At the present time the field of orthopedic massage is limited on research literature that has evaluated these therapeutic procedures. Hopefully in years to come, research scientists and funding sources will be attracted to this therapeutic approach and can help validate the clinical efficacy of these methods.

It is difficult to teach a complex psychomotor skill such as massage through a book. Quality massage treatment requires a wide variety of skills. Proper training in basic and advanced skills of soft-tissue manipulation is essential to be a safe and effective orthopedic massage practitioner. There are numerous ways to learn and develop these skills including traditional schooling, continuing education courses, and multimedia options such as DVDs. However, a word of caution is necessary for those unfamiliar with massage training. Do not dismiss these skills as easy or too simple to warrant the time devoted to practice and mastery. High-quality massage treatment is a lot harder to perform than it looks.

Under each of the conditions described in the following chapters, a variety of treatment methods are presented. There are important considerations regarding when to use the techniques most effectively and when they should be modified. These concepts are discussed in the treatment subsections *Rehabilitation protocol considerations*. As you consider different treatment options keep in mind the legal scope of practice in your jurisdiction. Depending on your professional training and licensure status, some of the treatments recommended in this section may fall outside your legal scope of practice. You should not attempt to perform any technique or method that is out of your scope of practice, simply because it is included in the suggestion of treatments.

In presenting treatment suggestions a deliberate attempt is made to provide effective guidelines, but steer clear of giving a rigid treatment routine for these conditions. Massage techniques are frequently taught in a routine because it is an easy way to convey a set of movement skills. Yet, overemphasis on a specific treatment routine can cause the practitioner to look for overly simplistic solutions at the expense of greater clinical versatility.

Chapter **6**

Foot, ankle, and lower leg

The foot and ankle provide the fundamental base of support for bipedal locomotion. As a result this region is built for the challenges of movement, stability, and transmission of high force loads from body weight. The skeletal structure of the foot, ankle, and leg handle the majority of compressive loads during locomotion, which can amount to several times the body weight.[1] Soft tissues of the foot also handle considerable force loads. Consider the role of the lateral ankle ligaments in maintaining ankle stability or the plantar fascia in upholding the longitudinal arch. Other tissues, such as the tibialis posterior have a primary role in preventing overpronation of the foot. All these tissues are subjected to chronic overuse in our daily activities and numerous soft-tissue pathologies can result.

There are particularly high demands placed on this region of the body during athletics or other activities that require high force loads or long periods of locomotion, which can lead to numerous overuse soft-tissue disorders. However, it does not take excessive overuse or athletic activity to develop significant problems in this region. Something as simple as improper shoes can play a role in many lower extremity soft-tissue pathologies.[2–4] For many of these conditions, massage is one of the very best interventions to restore normal and healthy tissue function.

INJURY CONDITIONS

ANKLE SPRAINS

Description

There are three separate joints to consider when looking at ankle sprains. Technically, the ankle is the joint between the talus and the distal articulation of the tibia and fibula. This articulation is also called the talocrural joint (Fig. 6.1). The distal articulation between the tibia and fibula is also part of the ankle and can be involved in ankle sprains. The joint below the talocrural joint where the talus articulates with the calcaneus is the sub-talar joint. Sprains may occur to the ligaments that span any of these joints.

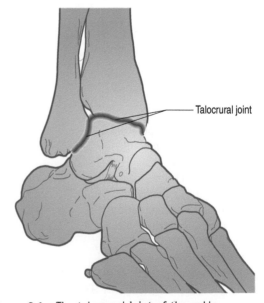

Figure 6.1   The talocrural joint of the ankle.

The ankle (talocrural) joint is a simple hinge joint. It relies strongly on the congruence of bones for its stability. However, there is a complex webbing of ligamentous structures that aids in stability of the ankle. There are three primary ligaments on the lateral side of the ankle that aid stability and prevent excessive inversion and rotational stresses at the ankle. They are the anterior talofibular, calcaneofibular, and posterior talofibular (Fig. 6.2).

On the medial side of the ankle the ligaments are designed to prevent excessive eversion as well as rotational stresses. There are four ligaments that aid in stability on the medial side of the ankle. They are the posterior tibiotalar, tibiocalcaneal, tibionavicular, and the anterior tibiotalar. These four ligaments create a strong triangular-shaped ligamentous restraint. Their fibers are blended together, and therefore they are often referred to simply as the deltoid ligament – referring to the Greek letter Delta that is shaped like a triangle.

The distal tibiofibular joint is called a syndesmosis. A syndesmosis joint is one that is tightly bound by ligaments and permits very little movement. It is crucial that the tibia and fibula stay tightly bound together at this joint to create the proper articular surface for the talus. The ligaments of this syndesmosis joint are not often sprained, but they should be considered as a possible source of injury with ankle sprains.

The ankle has different degrees of stability on each side. This stability is determined by the structural integrity of the ligaments that span the joint. The weaker the ligaments are, the more likely they are to be injured from an ankle sprain. Ligaments are weaker on the lateral side of the ankle than on the medial side.[5] The deltoid ligament group is particularly strong and this is one reason why medial ankle sprains are so much less common than lateral ankle sprains.

Lateral ankle sprains

Sprains to the lateral ligaments of the ankle are the most common lower-extremity injury seen by health care providers.[6] It is estimated that 85% of all ankle injuries involve ligament sprains.[7] The anterior talofibular ligament is the most frequently injured, and the calcaneofibular is the second. The posterior talofibular ligament is rarely injured.[6,7]

A typical cause for this injury involves a twisting motion of the foot where the foot is excessively inverted. Inversion occurs at the sub-talar joint, and the lateral ankle ligaments are quite vulnerable as they cross that joint. Injuries are likely to be worse if the foot is both inverted and plantar flexed simultaneously. The severity of this condition is graded at three levels: grade one sprain is mild, grade two is moderate, and grade three is severe.

Swelling and pain usually accompany the onset of a lateral ankle sprain. Ecchymosis (bruising) is common after the initial injury as well. The bruising may settle into the lateral or medial aspect of the heel. Depending upon the severity of the injury, the client may have a difficult time bearing weight on the affected side. Swelling routinely stays in the region for long periods (sometimes weeks) after the initial injury.

Medial ankle sprains

Medial ankle sprains are far less common than lateral ankle sprains. The strength of the deltoid ligament group is one of the primary reasons for fewer sprains to the medial side of the ankle. The deltoid ligament complex is designed to prevent excessive eversion. However, this ligament group is assisted by the fibula.

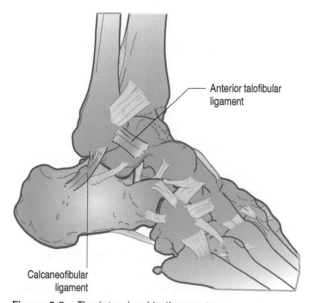

Anterior talofibular ligament

Calcaneofibular ligament

Figure 6.2 The lateral ankle ligaments.

The fibula extends farther distally than the tibia and, as a result, prevents excessive eversion of the foot. When a sprain does occur to the deltoid ligament group, it is usually a severe injury, and could involve fractures or ligament avulsions as well. An avulsion is an injury in which the ligament tears away from its attachment site. It can also take a small chunk of bone with it and if so this is called an avulsion fracture.

Syndesmosis sprains

Sprains to the distal tibiofibular syndesmosis are not very common. However, when they do occur they are generally slower to heal than sprains to the ligaments on either side of the ankle.[8] As the syndesmosis is superior to the other ligaments of the ankle, a sprain to the ligaments at this joint may be referred to as a high ankle sprain. These injuries ordinarily occur when the foot is exposed to a rotational stress or extremes of dorsiflexion.[9,10] During rotational stress or extreme dorsiflexion, the distal tibia and fibula are forced apart, causing a sprain to the ligaments.

Treatment

Traditional approaches

Ankle sprains are generally treated conservatively. A frequent guideline applied to acute injuries such as an ankle sprain is the acronym PRICE (Protection, Rest, Ice, Compression and Elevation).[11] In this instance, protection should mean preventing excessive movements in the direction of ligamentous weakness and instability. Ankle sprains used to be treated with immobilization, such as casting. However, recent studies supported by clinical experience conclude that early mobilization is more effective for helping ligament injuries heal because it stimulates collagen production.[12–14]

In the beginning of rehabilitation, the primary goals are to decrease pain, increase pain-free active range of motion, and protect the injured site from further damage. As the condition improves, greater effort is made to increase range of motion, improve flexibility, and enhance proprioceptive awareness in the area. Once the injured ligament has significantly improved, rehabilitative exercises are begun that strengthen the area to prevent injury recurrence.[14] These procedures should follow the rehabilitation protocol described in Chapter 1.

While some advocate that it is best not to perform significant exercise with the ligament until it has fully healed, lack of exercise can decrease the client's ability to achieve the best functional recovery. Experts argue that waiting until a ligament is fully healed would require waiting months for an athlete to return to their sport.[15] The majority of people are back to activity long before complete healing of the ligament. Active movement exercises, such as attempting to draw the letters of the alphabet in the air with the foot, are commonly used. Because this movement activity is performed in a non-weight-bearing position, it can be used without much pain for many ankle sprains relatively soon.[16]

Sprains usually heal within several weeks, depending upon their severity. The more severe the sprain, the longer is the period of recovery. However, if pain from an ankle sprain appears to linger long after the sprain should have healed, there is cause for concern, and the practitioner should consider the possibility of other complications. Persistent pain after injury can be the result of tissue impingement, insufficient rehabilitation, osteochondral injury, peroneal tendon damage, or chronic instability.[17]

Soft-tissue manipulation

General guidelines   Massage can be a valuable part of the treatment approach for ankle sprains. The practitioner should thoroughly assess the problem and first determine no other serious pathology that may need medical attention. In the early stages of injury, the primary interventions focus on relieving pain and restoring pain-free range of motion. Often this involves active movements performed within the client's pain tolerance. With regard to massage treatment of a ligament sprain, the appropriate time period after which treatment can commence has yet to be determined. Physical-assessment procedures help establish the severity of the injury. Practitioners should avoid treating the region if it is still in an acute inflammatory stage.

The acute injury stage covers the first 48–72 hours after injury. As the swelling begins to subside (and this may be helped with ice or other anti-inflammatory methods), light stroking in a proximal direction aids the lymphatic drainage in the area. Lymphatic drainage reduces excess tissue fluid, and contributes to a decrease in pain. Discomfort following a sprain is often a result of excess fluid in the area that presses on nerve endings and fills the interstitial spaces.

It is common for swelling to stay in the region of an ankle sprain for several weeks post injury. Waiting until all the visible swelling is gone misses the ideal window of opportunity for the best contribution to injury rehabilitation. The techniques described below can be delivered in moderation even if some chronic swelling persists.

Once the initial swelling has subsided, more vigorous treatments may be incorporated. Deep friction massage specifically to the site of the injury is beneficial for repairing the ligament tissue damage. Deep transverse friction (DTF) massage is used to realign scar tissue in the damaged ligament (or tendon). In addition, DTF plays a role in mobilizing the ligament and preventing it from adhering to adjacent tissues. Deep friction also has a fundamental role in collagen synthesis in repairing the damaged tissue.[18] DTF is normally performed in a direction that is perpendicular to the direction of the ligament's fibers.

In addition to the foot, the lower leg muscles are treated, especially if they are in some degree of protective spasm following the injury. For example, after an inversion sprain there is usually tightness in the peroneal muscles, as they are likely to become hypertonic. Not everyone experiences the same rate of injury healing. A severe injury that is several years old can be bound down with a great amount of scar tissue. It could take this individual a longer time to regain proper functional movement than someone who has a very recent sprain.

Stretching is incorporated along with soft-tissue manipulation. After an inversion ankle sprain, it is helpful to stretch the peroneal muscles (moving the foot into inversion). Too much passive stretching, especially at the early stages of the injury, can over-stretch the ligaments. Stretching in the later stages is an important part of developing a healthy and functional repair of the injury site.

Following a ligament injury, it is important to achieve early mobilization of the area for the most beneficial healing to occur. Because passive movement runs the risk of overstretching the damaged tissue, active movement is preferable, especially in the early stages. The client is unlikely to perform any movement that hurts too much, so active movement is self-limiting and not likely to cause further damage.

Suggested techniques and methods

A. Deep friction Collagen synthesis and ligament repair is enhanced with deep friction. Apply friction directly to affected ankle ligaments if it is a medial or lateral ankle sprain (Fig. 6.3). A cycle of friction along with other techniques is used. Apply friction for several minutes and then use joint range-of-motion movements along with treatment of nearby and associated tendons and muscles. Repeat this sequence 3 or 4 times. The location of syndesmosis sprains are difficult to reach with DTF, but the technique can be applied to the anterior ankle region because pressure on structures in this area can also press on the affected syndesmosis tissues.

B. Deep longitudinal stripping Muscles often become hypertonic in reaction to the injury. This technique helps reduce overall muscle tension in the region. Apply deep longitudinal stripping to muscles in the region. For lateral ligament injuries, treat the peroneal muscles (Fig. 6.4). For medial sprains the muscles of the deep posterior compartment, tibialis posterior, flexor hallucis longus and flexor digitorum longus are addressed.

C. Superficial myofascial and lymphatic drainage techniques Reducing local edema is helpful,

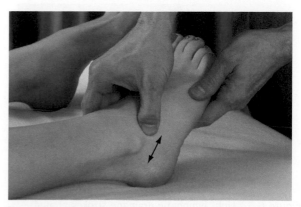

Figure 6.3 Deep transverse friction to medial and lateral ankle ligaments.

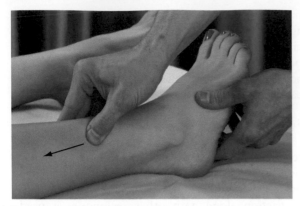

Figure 6.4 Deep stripping to the peroneal muscles.

especially prior to some of the other treatments. Use the back side of the fingers to apply very light pressure with strokes moving in a proximal direction (Fig. 6.5). This technique is effective both before and after some of the other applications such as DTF.

D. Stretching and mobilization Enhancing joint mobility as the ligaments heal is a primary goal of treatment. Only gentle stretches or joint movements should be applied so no further tissue damage is caused. Gently stretching the damaged ligament in the direction of its primary tensile loads will help the ligament remodel; for lateral ankle sprains, the direction of stretch is inversion, for medial sprains it is eversion, and dorsiflexion is best for syndesmosis sprains. Because ligaments are the primary tissues being stretched, long (at least 20 seconds) static stretches are more effective than short duration stretches.

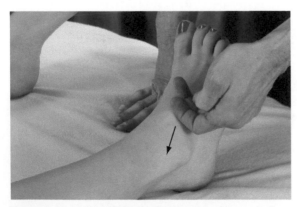

Figure 6.5 Light lymphatic drainage strokes around the ankle for ankle sprain.

Rehabilitation protocol considerations

- The primary focus in treating sprains is to assist in modeling an effective tissue repair.

- Another important goal is to decrease the onset of dysfunctional biomechanical muscular patterns.

- The more severe the ankle injury, the less intense the DTF applications should be. The severity of the sprain is determined with physical assessment.

- If the sprain is old (more than 6 months), excessive scar tissue may have accumulated in the area causing a thick degree of fibrosis. In this situation DTF applications can last considerably longer and be more aggressive. Instability should not be an issue in the joint because the ligament injury has healed. However, excessive scar tissue will need to be mobilized. The longer excessive scar tissue and adhesion build-up has been present in the tissues, the longer its resolution is going to take.

- As the injury progresses, greater degrees of movement and weight-bearing are incorporated with the soft-tissue treatment. It is also valuable to work on all the other lower extremity tissues (especially the lower leg) as they may have developed altered biomechanics as compensation for the injured joint.

- Proper movement and proprioception are important factors for preventing re-injury.

Cautions and contraindications Before treating an ankle sprain, identify the severity of the injury and make sure a more serious complication is not present. If the sprain is severe, a fracture or ligament avulsion can exist. These conditions should be ruled out before beginning massage treatment; referring the client may be necessary. If there is tenderness over the posterior distal portion of the medial or lateral malleolus, and the client is unable to bear weight, they should be referred for evaluation for a fracture or avulsion injury.[15] Swelling can exist with an ankle sprain for a long period, but if there is excessive swelling in the region, deep or vigorous treatments should not be attempted.

Pain reported by the client is a good guide for intensity of the treatment. Treatment approaches, whether they are specific massage applications or movement of the injured area, should be performed within the client's pain tolerance. As the condition improves, friction massage can become more vigorous and greater range of motion can be attempted.

MORTON'S NEUROMA

Description

Morton's neuroma, also called an interdigital neuroma or Morton's metatarsalgia, is a nerve injury in the distal region of the foot. A neuroma is an enlarged and irritated section of nerve tissue.[19] Morton's neuroma affects the medial and lateral plantar nerves or their terminal branches, the plantar digital nerves. This neuroma is most likely to develop between the heads of the third and fourth metatarsals, although it can occur between other metatarsals. Neuromas result from pressure on the nerve. In Morton's neuroma the nerve pressure can come from several different factors.

The medial and lateral plantar nerves are branches of the tibial nerve. They divide from the tibial nerve as they are exiting the tarsal tunnel on the medial side of the ankle. However, there is a communicating branch that converges between the medial and lateral plantar nerves near the heads of the third and fourth metatarsals (Fig. 6.6). This connecting branch is not present in everyone.[20] Lack of this connecting branch reduces the risk of developing Morton's neuroma.

Because the nerves converge between the metatarsal heads, the nerve diameter is greater here.[21] With a greater nerve diameter, there is an increased chance of pressure on the nerve by other structures, such as the metatarsal heads. There is less space between the third and fourth metatarsal heads than between the others, and the smaller space plays a role in the onset of Morton's neuroma as well.[20]

Another factor leading to neuroma development is the lack of mobility of the nerves in this region. The affected nerves are on the underside of the foot and they pass underneath (on the plantar side of) the transverse metatarsal ligaments that span between heads of the metatarsals.[22] The nerves can be irritated by tension against the transverse metatarsal ligaments. This would happen in a situation where the distal end of the nerve was being stretched. The distal region of the medial and lateral plantar nerves is stretched most during dorsiflexion with toe extension. Examples of this

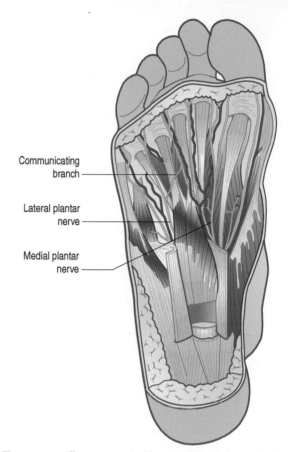

Communicating branch

Lateral plantar nerve

Medial plantar nerve

Figure 6.6 The communicating branch of the medial and lateral plantar nerves.

movement are the end of the push-off phase during normal gait, or squatting down while keeping the heels lifted off the ground and the weight on the forefoot (Fig. 6.7).[23]

Nerve injuries commonly occur as a result of excess neural tension (exaggerated pulling forces on the nerve in various positions).[24–27] Irritation of nerve tissues is exaggerated in areas where the nerves either branch or converge because there is less mobility at that location.[25,28] That is the case with Morton's neuroma, and it can play a role in the onset of the problem.

A person with Morton's neuroma usually feels sharp, shooting pain sensations in the forefoot or into the toes. The pain is likely to be aggravated by wearing narrow toe box shoes that force the metatarsal heads together. This condition is more common in women than in men.[21] A primary reason may be the wearing of high heel shoes. Not only do these shoes have a

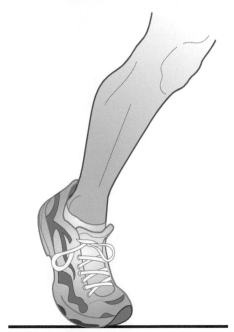

Figure 6.7   Bowstringing of the plantar nerves during push-off.

narrow toe box, but the elevation of the heel shoves the foot into the front of the shoe increasing compression of the metatarsal heads even further.[3]

Treatment

Traditional approaches

Morton's neuroma is usually treated with conservative methods. A primary aspect of treatment is to reduce nerve compression by the metatarsal heads. Changing to a shoe with a wider toe box may be the simplest means of treating this problem, and often all that is needed.

In addition to changing shoes, orthotics are sometimes advocated for Morton's neuroma. Rigid orthotics that limit dorsiflexion may be helpful if the primary problem is aggravated by positions of toe hyperextension with dorsiflexion. A typical orthotic device is a domed pad that sits under the heads of the metatarsals. This pad spreads the metatarsal heads apart inside the shoe and relieves pressure on the irritated nerve.

Anesthetic or corticosteroid injections may be used in the area to reduce pain or inflammation of the nerve. However, repeated corticosteroid injections can cause additional problems such as fat pad atrophy.[23,29] As a result these approaches are being used less. Surgical removal of the neuroma (neurectomy) is an option if conservative measures fail.

Soft-tissue manipulation

General guidelines   Morton's neuroma will sometimes develop as a result of previous injury that has left scar tissue in the area. If this is the case, massage may be beneficial in breaking up fibrous scar tissue that is binding the nerve.[23] Other forms of massage are useful for treating Morton's neuroma, but techniques that put direct pressure on the region near the metatarsal heads should be avoided.

The neuroma is aggravated from pressure by the metatarsal heads, so it is best to use approaches that separate the metatarsal heads. These massage techniques are most effective when they are performed in conjunction with the other therapies, such as changing footwear.

It is important to address neural tension as excess tension in the nervous system can contribute to this problem. The practitioner should treat the tissues adjacent to sciatic nerve, along its length and branches in the lower extremity where additional restrictions might occur. Areas of potential nerve binding or restriction include the ankle, calf, hamstring, and gluteal regions. Valuable mobilization techniques are those that encourage flexibility and pliability as they enhance neural mobility. Metatarsal spreading and mobilization is relatively simple, and is something the client can do at home.

Suggested techniques and methods

A. Metatarsal spreading techniques Tightness in the intrinsic muscles in the foot can further aggravate the nerve compression. Metatarsal spreading techniques reduce soft-tissue binding and stretch the intrinsic foot muscles. Use the thumbs on the plantar surface of the foot in sweeping arcs across the metatarsal heads to encourage separation (Fig. 6.8).

B. Metatarsal mobilization Individual metatarsal mobilization techniques help flexibility and movement between metatarsals so they are less likely to squeeze nerve tissue. Grasp the forefoot with both hands. Begin with four metatarsals in one hand and one in the other. Pull and stretch the metatarsals in each hand away from each other in multiple directions. Then perform the same movements on the gap between the next two metatarsals so that

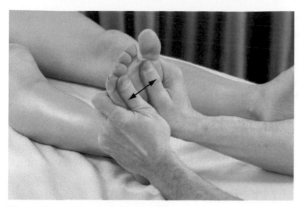

Figure 6.8   Metatarsal spreading.

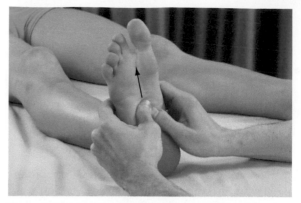

Figure 6.10   Deep stripping to plantar surface of the foot.

two are in one hand and three in the other (Fig. 6.9). Continue the process of stretching the tissues between metatarsals until spaces between all of them have been treated.

C. Deep stripping techniques Mobility of the medial and lateral plantar nerve branches are enhanced with stripping techniques performed to the plantar surface of the foot. These stripping techniques can be performed from the toes toward the heel or vice versa (Fig. 6.10).

D. Neural stretching Neural movement that focuses on dorsiflexion and toe extension helps encourage full nerve mobility of the sciatic nerve and its distal branches. After performing some of the other mobilization techniques described above, pull the foot into simultaneous dorsiflexion with toe extension. This movement is performed at a moderate pace without stopping to hold the stretch at the end of the movement. The neural stretching movement can be repeated 5–10 times

in one set and then repeated for several sets with a short period of rest between sets (Fig. 6.11). Knee extension and hip flexion can be added into each stretch to enhance sciatic nerve mobilization.

Rehabilitation protocol considerations

- If the Morton's neuroma is severe, use caution because the neural tissue may be sensitive to tension or compression.

- As the condition improves, more vigorous stretching or mobilization can be applied.

- These techniques are most effective when combined with changes in footwear that alleviate nerve compression by the metatarsal heads.

- In the early stages the client may be encouraged to avoid movements of dorsiflexion with toe extension (as in the push-off stage of gait), especially if it aggravates symptoms. In the later

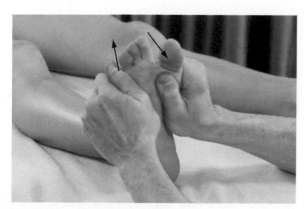

Figure 6.9   Metatarsal mobilization.

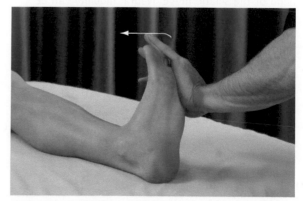

Figure 6.11   Neural stretching of the plantar nerves for Morton's neuroma.

stages of the condition as it improves, these movements and positions are encouraged to further help with nerve mobilization.

- Nerves are notoriously slow in healing so the client may be improving, although the symptoms are still prevalent. Encourage the client to pay close attention to the levels of irritability of neural structures. A visual analog scale or some other measure for pain sensation may be valuable.

Cautions and contraindications A neuroma is an enlarged and irritated section of nerve. Avoid treatments that aggravate the client's symptoms as this could put unnecessary force on the irritated nerve. There can be a palpable mass of the nerve tissue just adjacent to the metatarsal heads so palpate this region carefully. Exercise caution with techniques that increase pressure on the metatarsal heads from the side of the foot. These methods can also aggravate the neuroma and increase the client's symptomatic complaints.

Box 6.1 Clinical Tip

Assessment techniques for peripheral nerve disorders use a number of neurodynamic tests to evaluate mobility in the nervous system. The same techniques that are used for the evaluation of neural tension can be used in treatment as neural mobilization (stretching) techniques. For example, the neural stretching technique mentioned in D under Morton's neuroma describes a position of dorsiflexion and toe extension to stretch the distal end of the sciatic nerve. Neural mobility can be enhanced even farther by using additional components of the neurodynamic evaluation procedure called the straight-leg raise test.
In this procedure the hip is flexed with the knee in extension to give the greatest amount of tensile stretch to the sciatic nerve.

PLANTAR FASCIITIS

Description

Plantar fasciitis is the most common cause of painful feet encountered in clinical practice and occurs more in women than in men.[30] The primary cause of this condition is excessive tension on the attachment of the plantar fascia into the anterior calcaneus. The plantar fascia plays a crucial role in maintaining stability and contributing to shock absorption in the foot. As a result, high tensile forces on the tissue can cause an irritation at its attachment sites.

The foot is composed of many joints, but becomes a stiff spring when the muscles acting on it become taut. The plantar fascia is an important part of this spring mechanism, because it is essentially a tension cable between the heel and toes. It acts like a mechanical pulley device called a Spanish windlass (Fig. 6.12).[31]

In the windlass mechanism tension on the 'cable', which in this case is the plantar fascia, is increased as the second segment (the phalanges) are extended. At the end of the push-off phase of gait there is increased tension generated in the foot to propel the body forward.[32] Because of the windlass design in the foot, the tension is greatest when the toes are in hyperextension. There is also increased tension on the plantar fascia from normal weight bearing. Downward-directed pressure on the longitudinal arch from weight bearing increases tension along the plantar fascia.[33] The increased tension pulls on each end of the plantar fascia.

The plantar fascia attaches distally into the fascia that crosses the metatarsal heads and extends

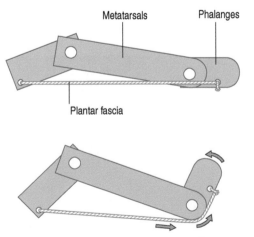

Figure 6.12 The plantar fascia seen as a Spanish windlass.

into the toes. Proximally its attachment is on the anterior calcaneus. Because the attachment site on the anterior calcaneus is so much smaller than the attachment region across the metatarsal heads, there is more force per square millimeter applied to the attachment site at the calcaneus. This concentrated force leads to the development of plantar fasciitis.

When a tendon or connective tissue such as the plantar fascia inserts into a bone it does not stop right at the bone. It has fibrous continuity with the bony matrix.[34] Therefore, excessive tensile stress on that site also affects the bone. As a result of the tensile stress placed on the bony attachment site, an exostosis (bone spur) can develop.[35] Therefore, plantar fasciitis is usually painful at the calcaneal attachment site. The planta fascia pulls on the periosteum, which is one of the most pain sensitive tissues in the body.

A frequent cause of plantar fasciitis is biomechanical dysfunction in the foot. While improper footwear can contribute, overpronation appears to be a major cause.[36,37] When the individual overpronates, the plantar fascia must take on greater shock absorption in the lower extremity. The increased tensile stress on the plantar fascia leads to fiber breakdown with resultant stress on the calcaneal attachment site. Overpronation often accompanies a flat foot (pes planus), so the presence of pes planus in the client is a good indicator that plantar fasciitis could occur. A pes cavus (high arch) foot is also a common factor in plantar fasciitis.[38] In pes cavus there is increased tension in the toe flexor muscles, and the higher arch may generate greater tensile stresses on the plantar fascia.

The plantar fascia has fascial connections with the gastrocnemius and soleus muscles. Keeping these muscles, the plantar fascia, and the corresponding connective tissues in a shortened position for long periods commonly aggravates the symptoms. Tissue shortening is most evident when the client first gets up in the morning and walks across the floor. The pain sensations are intense at that time. At night the client sleeps with their feet in a plantar flexed position. The soft tissues adapt to this shortened position, and then vertical weight bearing puts a strong tensile load on them when first standing and exaggerates the pain.

Treatment

Traditional approaches

The primary goal of plantar fasciitis treatment is to reduce tensile stress at the calcaneal attachment site of the plantar fascia. Reducing tensile stress gives the irritation site a chance to heal. Rest from further offending activities is also a crucial part of the rehabilitation strategy. Orthotics are used to change faulty biomechanical patterns in the foot, and take pressure off the plantar fascia. Orthotics are also useful if the client has either pes cavus or pes planus that is contributing to the plantar fascia overload.

Corticosteroid injections into the plantar fascia have been used to address inflammatory effects. However, these injections can have detrimental effects. Injections can leak into the fat pad causing fat pad degeneration and rupture of the plantar fascia.[39-41]

The tension night splint is used to treat plantar fasciitis with very good results.[42-44] This is a brace worn on the foot to maintain the foot in a position of dorsiflexion during the night (Fig. 6.13). The long period of dorsiflexion stretches the gastrocnemius and soleus muscles as well as some of the flexor muscles on the bottom surface of the foot. Prolonged dorsiflexion also conditions the plantar fascia to tensile stress and prevents the aggravation of tensile forces on the attachment site at the calcaneus.

Ice applications are routinely used to treat plantar fasciitis. Ice is used to reduce inflammatory activity associated with the chronic irritation of the fascia's attachment site. However, there is some question as to how much inflammation is actually occurring in this condition. Plantar fasciitis may result more from collagen degeneration (as in tendinosis) as opposed to inflammatory activity.[45]

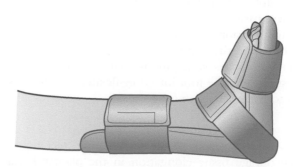

Figure 6.13   The tension night splint.

Extracorporeal shock wave therapy is a new treatment that is being used to treat plantar fasciitis. The focus of shock wave therapy is on bone spurs that develop at the fascial attachment site. However, several reviews of shock wave therapy indicate that this treatment does not have consistent effectiveness.[46,47]

Soft-tissue manipulation

General guidelines   Massage techniques are valuable in treatment of plantar fasciitis as long as they are performed within proper rehabilitation protocol guidelines. Treatment focuses on the dysfunctional plantar fascia as well as other supporting soft tissues that biomechanically support it. The primary treatment goal is to reduce the chronic tensile load on the attachment site. Reducing the tensile load at the attachment site reduces stress on both the soft tissues and the bones to which they attach.

Muscles such as the tibialis posterior, which play a prominent role in dynamic foot stability, should be treated to reduce hypertonicity. Fatigue from eccentric overload of the tibialis posterior can cause overpronation and subsequent plantar fasciitis overload.[31] Massage assists the effectiveness of a tension night splint by reducing tightness in the connective tissues and muscles of the plantar surface of the foot and posterior calf.

Practitioners should also treat the muscles of the entire lower extremity when addressing plantar fasciitis. Biomechanical compensations as a result of the foot pain have effects on other areas as well. The effects of these compensations may not be limited to the lower extremity, so watch for bony or soft-tissue changes throughout the body.

Stretching the gastrocnemius and soleus muscles is very important in plantar fasciitis treatment. Stretching several times during the day is best if possible. Wearing a tension night splint will stretch these tissues during the night, and reduce accumulated tension on the plantar fascia attachment. Stretching that emphasizes elongating the plantar surface tissues is helpful as well. To stretch these tissues, pull the foot into dorsiflexion and the toes into hyperextension.

Suggested techniques and methods

A. Longitudinal stripping   Stripping techniques encourage tissue elongation in the plantar fascia and the flexor muscles on the bottom surface of

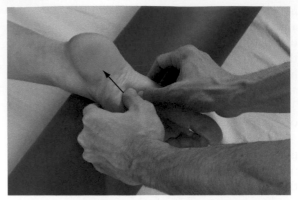

Figure 6.14   Deep stripping on plantar surface of the foot (toward the calcaneus).

the foot. Perform a stripping technique with the thumbs, fingers, or other smaller contact surface from one end of the plantar fascia to the other (Fig. 6.14). Performing longitudinal stripping methods toward the calcaneus reduces additional tensile stress on the plantar fascia and is less painful for the client.

B. Deep transverse friction   Fibroblast activity can be increased in the plantar fascia with friction techniques. Apply friction with the thumb or fingers near the calcaneal attachment of the plantar fascia, but not right on the insertion (Fig. 6.15). Do not press directly on the anterior calcaneus when performing the deep-friction treatments because there is potential for a bone spur. Because it is not known whether a bone spur is present or not without an X-ray, assume that one is present and avoid treatments that would aggravate the tissues there.

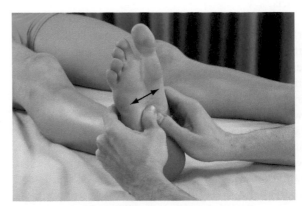

Figure 6.15   Friction treatment to plantar fascia (away from calcaneus).

C. Compression broadening and deep longitudinal stripping The triceps surae are an integral part of the kinetic chain of tightness in plantar fasciitis, and reducing tightness in them is an important part of treatment. Apply compression broadening and deep stripping methods to the triceps surae group (gastrocnemius and soleus) to reduce tightness (Figs 6.16 & 6.17). Perform deep stripping techniques with a broad contact surface first for more general applications and then follow up with a small contact surface for more specific applications. Stretching can follow these techniques.

D. Deep stripping techniques Attention should also focus on the deep posterior compartment muscles. These muscles help the mechanical function of the plantar fascia. With the client in a side-lying position, use the thumb or fingertips to strip in a proximal direction along the medial border of the tibia to reduce tightness in the

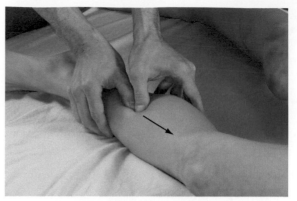

Figure 6.18 Deep stripping to deep posterior compartment muscles along tibial border.

tibialis posterior and other deep posterior compartment muscles (Fig. 6.18).

E. Active engagement lengthening techniques A greater penetrating effect of pressure is achieved with active engagement techniques. Use the same initial position for the client as in (D). Have the client move their foot in full dorsiflexion and plantar flexion in a slow repeated motion. During the dorsiflexion, perform a short specific stripping technique to the deep posterior compartment muscles (Fig. 6.19). Only move a few inches proximally with each stroke during the dorsiflexion. Repeat this process until the entire length of the tibia has been treated. Moving proximally, this treatment also addresses the soleus attachments along the proximal tibia.

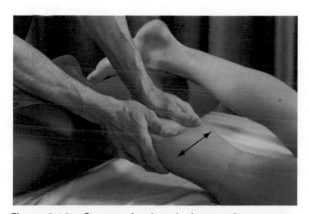

Figure 6.16 Compression broadening to triceps surae.

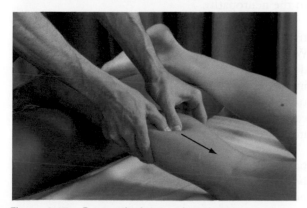

Figure 6.17 Deep stripping to triceps surae.

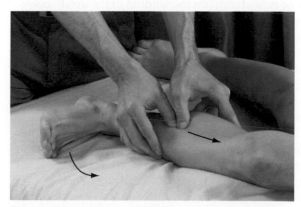

Figure 6.19 Active engagement lengthening to deep posterior compartment muscles.

Rehabilitation protocol considerations

● Be careful with the level of pressure applied with any of the techniques on the bottom surface of the foot. The client's pain is a good guide. If the treatment is too painful, reduce pressure.

● In early stages of the treatment when the plantar surface of the foot is very painful, focus treatment on the supportive structures of the plantar fascia (techniques C, D, & E).

● Ice applications are helpful after treatment to reduce post-treatment soreness.

● Stretching affected tissues is a crucial aspect of plantar fasciitis treatment and should be incorporated throughout the treatment process as tolerated by the client.

Cautions and contraindications Pressure that is too painful for the client should not be used. Be careful about applying pressure near the attachment site of the plantar fascia on the anterior calcaneus. If a bone spur is present in this area, additional pressure over the spur is painful and could cause further tissue damage as well.

TARSAL TUNNEL SYNDROME

Description

There is a soft-tissue tunnel on the medial side of the ankle called the tarsal tunnel. It is similar in structure to the carpal tunnel in the wrist. The flexor retinaculum creates the roof of the tunnel and the calcaneus and medial malleolus create the floor (Fig. 6.20). The tunnel contains the tendons of the tibialis posterior, flexor digitorum longus, and flexor hallucis longus muscles. There are tendon sheaths surrounding these tendons as they course through the tunnel to reduce their friction in the area.[23] Also within the tunnel are the posterior tibial nerve, artery, and vein. Tarsal tunnel syndrome is a compression or tension neuropathy of the tibial nerve in the tunnel.

The tibial nerve enters the tarsal tunnel after leaving the calf in the deep posterior compartment of the leg. Shortly after the nerve leaves the tarsal tunnel it divides into the medial and lateral plantar nerves. Sometimes this division occurs within the tarsal tunnel, making the nerve more susceptible to compression and tension neuropathies.[25]

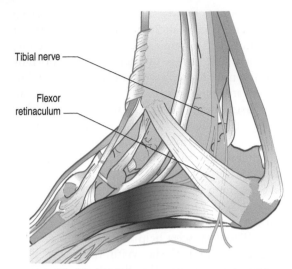

Figure 6.20 Medial view of the ankle showing the tarsal tunnel.

Tibial nerve

Flexor retinaculum

Tarsal tunnel syndrome usually develops as a compression neuropathy of the tibial nerve under the flexor retinaculum. Overuse of the tibialis posterior and flexor tendons cause swelling in the tendon sheaths (tenosynovitis) that in turn compress the tibial nerve. Space-occupying lesions such as small tumors or excess fluid that gathers in the tarsal tunnel can also press on the nerve in this region.[23,35]

Certain biomechanical factors increase the incidence of tarsal tunnel syndrome. Overpronation of the foot can cause tarsal tunnel syndrome due to excessive eversion of the foot. As the foot turns into greater eversion during overpronation, there is increased tension on the posterior tibial nerve. The increased tension injures the nerve and leads to the neuropathy.

Excess supination can also play a part in tarsal tunnel syndrome by compressing the tibial nerve. When the foot is over supinating there is a greater degree of inversion at the sub-talar joint. Increased inversion compresses the contents of the tarsal tunnel. Even a minor degree of nerve compression can become symptomatic as pressure in the area is increased from the foot inversion.

The symptoms of tarsal tunnel syndrome include pain near the medial side of the ankle or along the bottom surface of the foot. The pain is usually sharp or shooting in nature, and can extend all the way into the toes.[48] Pain may be felt proximal to the tarsal tunnel, but is much less common than distal projecting pain. Paresthesia is felt in the foot and in some cases motor function and weakness in the foot muscles supplied by the nerve may be evident.

Treatment

Traditional approaches

One of the primary aims of treatment for tarsal tunnel syndrome is biomechanical correction of the foot mechanics that have led to the problem. Tarsal tunnel syndrome occurs as an overuse activity, so treatment begins with an effort to reduce or eliminate offending activities that are contributing to the problem.

Orthotics are used for this purpose. For example, if the primary problem involves overpronation, an orthotic that is built up on the medial side can prevent the foot rolling into excessive eversion. If the individual is over supinating and has a calcaneal varus angulation, a lateral heel wedge is used to correct the foot mechanics.[48]

Anti-inflammatory medications such as non-steroidal anti-inflammatory drugs (NSAIDs) are used to reduce swelling of the synovial sheaths of the flexor tendons in the tarsal tunnel.[35] Corticosteroid injections into the region of the tarsal tunnel are also used to address inflammation in the area, although there is some controversy about the safety and effectiveness of this procedure.[49]

If conservative treatment is unsuccessful, surgery is an option. The surgical approach divides the flexor retinaculum to allow greater space for the structures underneath in the tunnel. There are detrimental biomechanical effects to cutting the flexor retinaculum, so conservative approaches are preferred.

Soft-tissue manipulation

General guidelines Massage can be beneficial for nerve pathologies such as tarsal tunnel syndrome. Yet, improperly applied massage techniques can cause further damage in the region. Because this condition involves a nerve compression pathology, avoid putting additional compression directly over the tarsal tunnel, except under certain circumstances described below. Massage approaches typically used for this problem are indirect, meaning they are aimed at reducing the factors that lead to tarsal tunnel syndrome, but do not specifically address the damaged

nerve. For example, tenosynovitis in the deep flexor muscles of the foot and toes may be compressing the nerve. Massage treatment aims to reduce the tenosynovitis and thereby decrease nerve compression by the irritated tendons.

Adverse tension throughout the sciatic nerve can contribute to irritation of the tibial nerve in the tarsal tunnel. Therefore, it is helpful to encourage full mobility of the entire sciatic nerve. Stretching and neural mobilization procedures that are directed at the entire length of the sciatic nerve from the lumbar region to the toes is beneficial in tarsal tunnel syndrome.[50]

Tension in the tendons traveling through the tunnel can contribute to nerve compression, so these tendons should be stretched. One of the particular challenges to stretching the tibialis posterior is that the foot is limited in how much it can evert because the fibula stops eversion prior to a complete stretch of the tibialis posterior. Therefore, this muscle is susceptible to accumulated tension, because it can never fully lengthen. The tendons that course through the tarsal tunnel are stretched in dorsiflexion and some degree of eversion. However, if eversion or dorsiflexion increase the pain or paresthesia sensations, do not continue stretching as the nerve is most likely being overstretched.

Suggested techniques and methods

A. Deep longitudinal stripping Deep posterior compartment muscles are treated with longitudinal stripping techniques. Reducing tension in these muscles decreases stress on the tendons and lessens the chance that they will irritate the tibial nerve. (See Fig. 6.18 and Treatment D under Plantar fasciitis.)

B. Active engagement lengthening Greater effectiveness of pressure on the deep posterior compartment muscles is achieved with active engagement techniques. (See Fig. 6.19 and Treatment E under Plantar fasciitis.)

C. Gentle deep friction or thumb stroking Direct pressure on a nerve compression is usually contraindicated, but is beneficial in some cases. While massaging a dysfunctional nerve may seem counterintuitive there are some potential physiological benefits. The theory is that direct massage of the impaired nerve region moves fluid away from the tunnel, improves intraneural fluid pressures, and blood flow.[26] This technique may also reduce

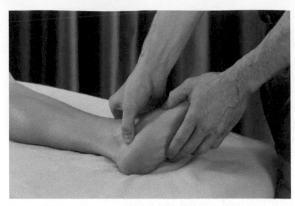

Figure 6.21 Direct massage of the tarsal tunnel region (circular friction or thumb gliding).

sensitivity of the nerve as well. Apply gentle pressure and friction to the tarsal tunnel region (Fig. 6.21). Stretching and neural mobility should be encouraged immediately after these friction techniques.

D. Neural stretching Enhancing neural mobility is a crucial aspect of treating any nerve compression syndrome. Use the same neural stretching technique that is described for Morton's neuroma. (See Fig. 6.11 and Treatment C under Morton's neuroma.)

E. Deep stripping Neural mobility is further enhanced with deep stripping to the plantar surface of the foot. (See Fig. 6.14 and Treatment A under Plantar fasciitis.)

Rehabilitation protocol considerations
- The greater the level of nerve damage, the more sensitive the region to treatment and the greater the symptoms that the client reports. Gauge treatment pressure and intensity with the client's symptoms so that the region is not stressed.

- In nerve compression pathologies, aggravating the client's neurological sensations is not advised. If symptoms increase, it means the nerve is being aggravated and that is not conducive to nerve healing.

- Nerve tissue is considerably slower than other tissues in healing time, so allow ample time for symptoms to abate. Encourage the client to closely monitor symptoms to watch for even small signs of improvement.

- Because neural mobility is an important aspect of rehabilitation for this condition, stretching

should be an integral part of the treatment from the start.

- In order for treatments to have the ideal opportunity for success correction of dysfunctional biomechanics or other offending activities must be encouraged throughout treatment.

Cautions and contraindications   Use caution with massage applications performed directly over the tarsal tunnel (see C above), as they can aggravate the compression. Avoid techniques that significantly elevate symptoms. Likewise, avoid movement activities of the foot that either compress or stretch the aggravated structures, to the point of causing an increase in pain. Tibial nerve irritation can result from a space-occupying mass or lesion in the tarsal tunnel. If palpation of the region reveals a mass or cyst-like tissue in the tunnel, the client should be referred to a physician for a more comprehensive evaluation.

RETROCALCANEAL BURSITIS

Description

Retrocalcaneal bursitis produces pain on the posterior side of the heel. The retrocalcaneal bursa, as its name implies, is located directly behind the calcaneus. There are actually two bursae posterior to the calcaneus, and either one can be implicated (Fig. 6.22). The subcutaneous bursa, which sits just under the skin and superficial to the Achilles tendon, is generally the bursa irritated in this condition. It is usually the one referred to as the retrocalcaneal bursa. However, the subtendinous bursa that sits between the Achilles tendon and the calcaneus is also called the retrocalcaneal bursa.

Retrocalcaneal bursitis results from repeated compression of the bursa by footwear. The heel counter is the portion of the shoe that wraps around the posterior side of the heel and causes bursitis. This condition is a component of Haglund's syndrome. Haglund's syndrome is a swelling in the posterior heel region that can include: retrocalcaneal bursitis, thickening of the Achilles tendon, a convexity of the soft tissues at the Achilles tendon insertion, and a prominent calcaneal projection. The prominent calcaneal projection is an exostosis (bone spur), caused by constant tensile stress from the Achilles tendon insertion or pressure from the shoe's heel counter.

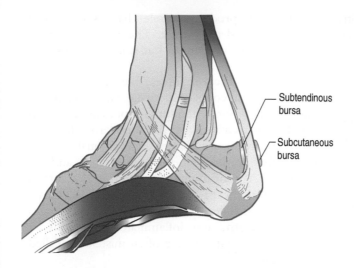

Subtendinous
bursa

Subcutaneous
bursa

Figure 6.22   Medial view of the ankle showing retrocalcaneal bursae.

The spur is also called Haglund's deformity or a *pump bump*.[51,52] While direct pressure on the bursa is the most common cause of retrocalcaneal bursitis, there can be several other causes. Repeated tensile stress at the insertion site of the Achilles tendon can also cause bursitis.[53]

Treatment

Traditional approaches

As with any bursitis condition, an important aspect of treatment is to remove compression and friction on the bursa. Changing footwear and reducing or eliminating offending activities is the best strategy. Heel lifts that reduce tension on the Achilles tendon have also been suggested.[35]

Because bursitis is an inflammatory condition, various anti-inflammatory medications are frequently used. Corticosteroid injections may be used for the inflamed bursa, but caution is warranted because of potential damage to surrounding structures, especially the Achilles tendon[54,55] If conservative measures are not successful in treating bursitis, surgery can be used. However, it is not common.[52]

Soft-tissue manipulation

General guidelines   If retrocalcaneal bursitis is present, avoid direct massage of the area. The additional compressive force of massage aggravates the inflamed bursa. However, reducing tension on the gastrocnemius and soleus muscles through

massage and stretching helps, because tensile stress at the Achilles tendon insertion is a primary component of this problem. The most important part of treatment is relieving compression on the affected bursa. Change of footwear is an important means of reducing posterior heel compression.

Suggested techniques and methods

A. Compression broadening and longitudinal stripping techniques   Reducing tension on the Achilles tendon can lessen irritation of the insertion site and decrease a Haglund's deformity. Reducing the Haglund's deformity decreases compressive forces on the posterior heel by the shoe. Muscle tension is decreased using compression broadening and stripping techniques for the triceps surae group. (See Figs 6.16 & 6.17 and Treatment C under Plantar fasciitis.)

B. Stretching   Muscle tightness is also reduced in this area through proper and frequent stretching for the gastrocnemius and soleus muscles.

Rehabilitation protocol considerations

- Reducing compressive forces on the bursa is important. The treatment strategies described provide indirect benefits by decreasing irritation at the insertion site.

- In rare cases retrocalcaneal bursitis can result from a systemic infection and not from mechanical compression. In those cases soft-tissue interventions and relief of compression on the bursa may not be enough to address the condition. If the inflamed bursa is resistant to treatment or the bursitis appears for no apparent reason, consider a systemic disorder and refer to a physician for evaluation.

Cautions and contraindications   Do not pressure directly on the bursa with massage or soft-tissue manipulation as it may aggravate the inflammatory condition. Some thickening of the Achilles tendon can occur from chronic overuse, but is not necessarily evidence of an inflammatory disorder (see the discussion of Achilles tendon disorder below). In those cases it is still appropriate to treat the Achilles tendon and triceps surae muscles to reduce tension, which could aid the bursitis treatment.

ACHILLES TENDINOSIS

Description

The Achilles tendon is the strongest tendon in the body. It has to be strong because of the extreme tensile forces from the gastrocnemius and soleus muscles during locomotion. With each plantar flexion of the foot, these muscles have to propel the weight of the body forward, so very strong contraction forces are required. They also produce very high loads during eccentric muscle activity such as stepping down or landing from a jump.

Tendons exposed to high tensile loads are continually repairing themselves to maintain optimal strength. Achilles tendinosis develops as the tendon is unable to repair the tendon and keep up with the demands placed on it. Adequate blood supply is needed in tendons to enhance tissue repair and bring proper nutritional supply to the tendon fibers. The blood supply to the tendon is poor throughout, but appears worst in the distal portion of the Achilles tendon. As a result, this is the region of the tendon that is most susceptible to overuse injury.[56-58]

Several factors in the client's history may indicate the presence of Achilles tendinosis. Sudden changes in activity level, inadequate stretching, training errors, rigid training surfaces, mechanical alignment problems, or certain systemic diseases play a role in its onset.[59] It was mentioned in Chapter 2 that often tendon overuse problems are not inflammatory in nature (tendinitis), but involve collagen degeneration (tendinosis) as the primary pathology. The Achilles tendon is one of the few that produces visible changes in its size when subjected to overuse. There can be fibrous thickening in the tendon, but it is not necessarily inflamed.

To reduce friction forces, the tendon is surrounded by a connective tissue layer called the paratenon.[31] Some tendons, especially those in the distal extremities that travel underneath a retinaculum, are surrounded by an additional synovial sheath that lies between the tendon fibers and the paratenon. An inflammatory condition that affects the synovial sheath is called tenosynovitis. However, the Achilles tendon does not have this synovial sheath, and inflammatory reactions in the Achilles paratenon are often mistakenly called tenosynovitis.[60]

Dysfunctional biomechanical patterns often play a role in the development of Achilles tendinosis. During normal foot pronation there is a whip-like force on the tendon from the point of foot contact through the push-off phase. If an individual overpronates, this whipping action is much more pronounced, and can lead to collagen degeneration in the tendon.[35,61]

Certain medications play a role in the onset of Achilles tendinosis. A group of antibiotics called fluoroquinolones can lead to tendon disorders. The fluoroquinolones appear to cause the greatest damage to tendons under high tensile load, such as the Achilles tendon. Use of these antibiotics can predispose an individual to either tendinosis or complete tendon ruptures.[62-64] Previous corticosteroid injections in the Achilles tendon are also related to tendon weakening and should be investigated in the client history.[65,66]

Treatment

Traditional approaches

A key factor in Achilles tendinosis treatment is to reduce the load on the tendon. A heel lift placed in the shoe is an effective means of reducing tendon load. Orthotics are used to correct biomechanical dysfunction, such as the whipping action of the tendon. Activity modifications that reduce tendon load are also important to include in treatment.

Anti-inflammatory medication is often used to treat Achilles tendinosis. However, there can be limits to the effectiveness of this approach, because the condition does not appear to be an inflammatory problem in most cases.[67] Despite their widespread use, anti-inflammatory medications do not appear very effective in addressing the primary problems in tendinosis conditions.[68]

Non-steroidal anti-inflammatory drugs (NSAIDS) are the most common type of anti-inflammatory treatment for tendinosis. Corticosteroid injections were formerly a common treatment for tendinosis with the idea that it was an inflammatory problem. This treatment is now strongly discouraged, due to evidence that steroid injections can cause tendon ruptures.

Soft-tissue manipulation

General guidelines A critical factor in treating Achilles tendinosis is to reduce tension on the tendon fibers. A variety of massage techniques applied to the triceps surae assist in this process. Deep transverse friction (DTF) is applied to the Achilles tendon to enhance fibroblast proliferation and promote faster healing of the tendon tissue.[69,70]

Short periods of friction massage application are followed with passive and active movement and other circulatory enhancing massage techniques. Refer to the discussion of deep friction massage in Chapter 4 for standard guidelines regarding friction massage applications and combining this approach with other techniques.

The process of collagen reformation in a damaged tendon is not fast. This is especially true in a tendon like the Achilles that is continually exposed to tensile forces while it is in the healing process. A recovery period of several months is not unreasonable to get a full return to function.[71]

Suggested techniques and methods

A. Sweeping cross fiber This technique reduces overall tension in the triceps surae group which lessens the pulling force on the Achilles tendon. It can be performed in conjunction with effleurage when first beginning treatment of this region. Use a broad sweeping motion with the thumb and hand that moves diagonally across the fibers of the triceps surae group (Fig. 6.23). This is a moderately superficial technique so it is best to perform it at the outset of the treatment to encourage tissue warming and begin enhancing pliability.

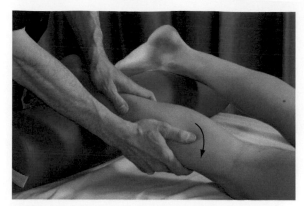

Figure 6.23 Sweeping cross fiber to triceps surae.

B. Compression broadening Additional muscle mobilization and relaxation of the triceps surae is achieved with compression broadening techniques (see Fig. 6.16). This technique uses more pressure than the sweeping cross fiber technique so it begins to address some of the deeper fibers of the muscle group.

C. Deep stripping Muscle relaxation and tissue pliability are enhanced with the deep stripping technique. Perform deep stripping techniques with a broad contact surface first for more general applications and then follow that up with a small contact surface for more specific applications (see Fig. 6.17).

D. Active engagement (shortening movements) After superficial applications, tension in deeper muscle fibers is addressed with active engagement methods. The client is in a prone position. Instruct the client to begin a slow but steady movement of the foot in full dorsiflexion and plantar flexion. During the plantar flexion (the concentric or shortening phase for the triceps surae muscles), perform a compression broadening technique to the triceps surae muscles. Remove pressure as the client lengthens the muscle during dorsiflexion and repeat the compression broadening technique on each plantar flexion until the entire muscle group is treated (Fig. 6.24).

E. Active engagement (lengthening movements) Deep fibers of the triceps surae are most effectively addressed for elongation and enhanced pliability with active engagement lengthening movements. The client is in the same position as in D (see above) and the technique begins with

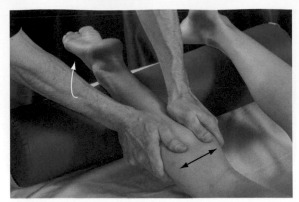

Figure 6.24 Active engagement shortening to triceps surae.

the same repetitive slow flexion and extension movement. Perform a deep stripping technique as the triceps surae is lengthening during dorsiflexion (Fig. 6.25). This technique can be somewhat painful or intense for the client so pressure level should be gentle until the client's pressure tolerance has been determined.

F. Deep friction Friction techniques encourage fibroblast proliferation and tendon healing. Apply friction techniques longitudinally or in a transverse direction with the thumb or fingers (Fig. 6.26). Friction techniques are best performed while the tendon is on stretch.

G. Stretching Tissue elongation is an essential aspect of effective treatment. Stretch the gastrocnemius by moving the foot in dorsiflexion while the knee is extended. To stretch the soleus, simply dorsiflex the foot. The soleus does not cross the

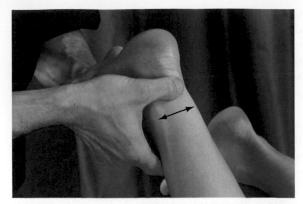

Figure 6.26 Deep transverse friction to Achilles tendon.

knee joint so the position of the knee is not as important for soleus stretching.

Rehabilitation protocol considerations

- Collagen degeneration that causes tendinosis can develop over a long period and takes a long time to heal. Do not expect rapid treatment results (although that can occur in some cases).

- Orthotics or shoe inserts that decrease tension on the Achilles tendon are likely to speed the soft-tissue healing process.

- Fibrous thickening of the tendon can linger long after the primary symptoms of pain have abated.

Box 6.2 Clinical Tip

Due to the shape and location of the Achilles tendon, performing deep transverse friction on this tendon can be awkward sometimes. There are a few ways to address this positional challenge. Instead of trying to apply friction with the tip of the finger or thumb as is often done, use the interphalangeal joint of the thumb as the contact point and perform the transverse friction with the thumb's joint. This prevents rapidly flicking on and off the tendon as the transverse friction is applied. Research has indicated that tendinosis is effectively treated with longitudinal friction. Applying longitudinal friction to the Achilles tendon is much easier and prevents rapidly slipping off the edge of it during transverse movements.

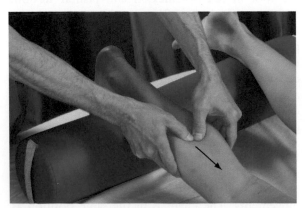

Figure 6.25 Active engagement lengthening to triceps surae.

Cautions and contraindications   Achilles tendinosis can sometimes be a symptom of other systemic disorders such as Reiter's syndrome. Perform a comprehensive assessment to investigate if the client's symptoms are predominantly mechanical or if there are symptoms that indicate some type of systemic disorder. Use caution in applying friction to the site of primary discomfort. This is likely to be the site of greatest collagen breakdown in the tissue. Excessive pressure and friction in the area can cause the client pain during treatment. There can be a fine line in determining how much discomfort is an acceptable amount. It is often a matter of trial and error and will vary from individual to individual.

ANTERIOR COMPARTMENT SYNDROME

Description

The lower leg is composed of four separate compartments: the anterior, lateral, superficial posterior and deep posterior. Each compartment is separated from the others by strong fascial walls. The tibia and fibula also contribute part of the unyielding borders for these fascial compartments (Fig. 6.27). A compartment syndrome can occur in any of the limbs, but usually it develops in the lower leg, and especially in the anterior compartment.

Anterior compartment syndrome results from swelling of the muscles within the compartment.

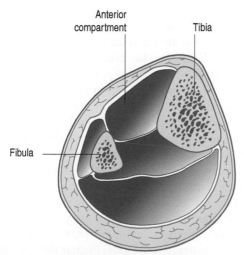

Figure 6.27   Cross section of the leg showing the fascial compartments.

Because the compartment walls are strong and unyielding, there is no extra room for the expanding muscles. As a result there is a pressure increase inside the compartment and the muscles press on other structures inside the compartment. During anterior compartment syndrome, there may be as much as a 20% increase in muscle mass.[72]

The anterior compartment of the lower leg contains three muscles: tibialis anterior, extensor digitorum longus, and extensor hallucis longus. It also contains the tibial artery and vein, as well as the deep peroneal nerve. Increased pressure inside the compartment can impair these structures. Pressure on the vascular structures can cause ischemia, possible color changes in the limb, and sensations of coldness in the extremity or the feet. Lack of circulation is a serious concern in compartment syndromes. Prolonged ischemia from compression of the vascular structures can lead to tissue necrosis. In severe cases, the necrosis can be damaging enough to warrant amputation of the limb.

Compression injury to the nerves that run through the compartment is also a primary concern. Symptoms of numbness, tingling, or loss of dorsiflexor function result from nerve compression. Sharp or shooting pain sensations on the dorsal surface of the foot may also be reported. Compression of the deep peroneal nerve in the anterior compartment can also occur from pressure on the nerve against the head of the fibula.[73]

The pain sensations of anterior compartment syndrome are often mistaken for shin splints. However, there are some distinct differences between the conditions. For example, shin splints rarely cause neurological sensations, as the deep peroneal nerve is not affected in shin splints. Treatment for these two problems is quite different, and an untreated compartment syndrome can be a serious condition. The primary indicator of a compartment syndrome is pain that is out of proportion to what is likely for shin splints.[74]

Anterior compartment syndrome occurs as either an acute or chronic condition. If it is an acute condition, it usually results from a direct blow to the anterior shin. However, it can occur along with a fracture or other acute trauma, such as a muscle strain. Several authors have reported acute compartment syndromes occurring directly after severe muscle strains to the muscles in the lower leg.[75,76]

As a result of the acute trauma, the muscles swell, become ischemic, and increase pressure levels within the compartment. It is not mandatory that an individual have a direct blow to cause the acute compartment syndrome. An excessive bout of activity can also cause the acute compartment syndrome.[77]

The chronic compartment syndrome is much more common. This condition is also called exertional compartment syndrome (ECS), because the primary cause is repetitive exertion and overuse of the lower leg muscles. It results from exercise on an unyielding surface, improper footwear, or activity that is out of proportion to what the individual has conditioned for.

A chronic compartment syndrome can develop into an acute compartment syndrome if the individual engages in a greater than normal level of activity or sustains a direct blow to the muscles in the compartment. A chronic compartment syndrome can also develop from an acute injury. One author reported a case of chronic compartment syndrome developing after an individual had sustained a direct blow to the lower leg.[78] The direct blow did not initiate an acute compartment syndrome, but some time later the individual developed symptoms of chronic ECS that had never been felt before.

The pain from a compartment syndrome increases as activity progresses. Because the compartmental pressure is increasing during activity, the pain continues to get worse. Even after stopping the activity, pain from an ECS can continue to increase for a short time.

Treatment

Traditional approaches

In a chronic ECS it is important to reduce the factors that lead to overuse injury. This may include the use of orthotics, changes in footwear, and modifying activity levels. Usually when activity is halted, the chronic ECS will subside. However, individuals often cannot cease their activity altogether. If this is the case, these other biomechanical modifications are increasingly important. NSAIDS are also sometimes used, but their effectiveness in dealing with this problem is minimal.[79]

The principle of RICE (Rest, Ice, Compression, and Elevation) is used as a standard approach for the treatment of acute injuries. However, compartment syndrome is one of those that are exceptions to the rule. Ice and elevation will both have a detrimental effect on the reduced circulation that is already present in the compartment. Compression is certainly contraindicated, as the pressure levels in this area are already too high.

Surgical treatment of anterior compartment syndrome may be necessary, especially for acute cases. If there is an acute compartment swelling and it is not treated soon enough, tissue necrosis can occur. If left unchecked, this can eventually lead to limb amputation. Surgical treatment may also be used for chronic compartment syndromes that do not respond to conservative treatment. The surgical procedure for treating a compartment syndrome will attempt to reduce compression in the compartment by cutting a longitudinal incision along the fascial wall and allowing the muscles to bulge and protrude out of the compartment.[80,81] This procedure is called a fasciotomy. Once the incision is made it is not immediately closed. It can be left open for about 48–72 hours to let the swollen tissues subside.[75]

Soft-tissue manipulation

General guidelines Massage treatment is not a good option for an acute compartment syndrome. This injury causes an immediate increase in compartmental pressure, and waiting any length of time to reduce that pressure can be dangerous. An individual with symptoms of an acute compartment syndrome should be immediately referred to a physician for appropriate evaluation and the possibility of surgery.

Chronic ECS can be effectively treated with massage. However, do not perform treatment at the time symptoms are aggravated. The practitioner should wait until symptoms have subsided before beginning soft-tissue manipulation. Because various biomechanical factors including muscle hypertonicity can contribute to a chronic compartment syndrome, reduction of excess muscle tension is a primary goal of massage treatment. Various forms of massage have a positive effect on chronic anterior compartment syndrome.[82]

Stretching methods reduce hypertonicity in the anterior compartment muscles. Plantar flexion stretches that elongate the dorsiflexors are the most helpful. Use the client's comfort level as a guide because stretching of the anterior compartment muscles is often painful when the condition is aggravated.

Lower extremity biomechanical dysfunctions can contribute to overuse of the muscles in the anterior compartment. Stretching and massage treatment for these other muscles is highly advised. Stretches should address all the muscles of the lower leg that act on the foot, as well as other lower extremity muscles such as the hamstrings and quadriceps.

Suggested techniques and methods These treatment techniques assume a chronic and not acute compartment syndrome.

A. Sweeping cross fiber Superficial muscle relaxation and tissue pliability is enhanced with this technique. The thumb applies a sweeping stroke to the anterior compartment muscles that travels diagonally across the fiber direction of the anterior compartment muscles (Fig. 6.28). Longitudinal gliding (effleurage) and broad sweeping cross fiber strokes reduce muscular tension and encourage tissue fluid movement, reducing compartmental pressure.

B. Deep longitudinal stripping Tension reduction in the anterior compartment muscles is further enhanced with deep stripping techniques. Stripping can begin with a broad contact surface, such as the heel of the hand or back side of the fist. Following broad contact surface applications, more specific stripping is performed with the finger tips or thumb (Fig. 6.29). Stripping techniques are performed from distal to proximal to follow the direction of venous return.

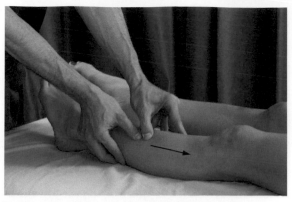

Figure 6.29 Deep stripping to the anterior compartment muscles.

C. Deep broadening Spreading fibers of the anterior compartment muscles helps decrease tension and can reduce overuse that leads to an increase in compartmental pressure. Begin with the thumbs against the lateral tibial border. Apply a moderate amount of pressure through the thumbs and then slowly move laterally until the anterior and lateral leg region has been covered (Fig. 6.30). Start in one location and then gradually treat the entire length of the lower leg with successive strokes.

D. Active engagement shortening movements Deeper tissues can be reached for tension reduction with active engagement techniques after the deep broadening methods. Instruct the client to repeatedly dorsiflex and plantar flex the foot and a slow, steady pace. Use the same deep broadening stroke with the thumbs as in C during the dorsiflexion (Fig. 6.31). Pressure is removed as the client plantar

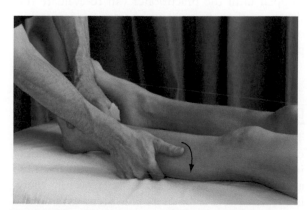

Figure 6.28 Sweeping cross fiber to anterior compartment muscles.

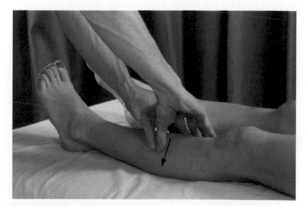

Figure 6.30 Deep broadening to anterior/lateral compartment muscles.

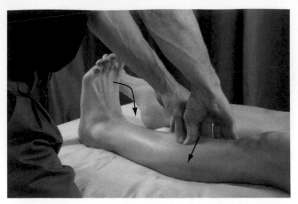

Figure 6.31 Active engagement shortening to anterior compartment muscles.

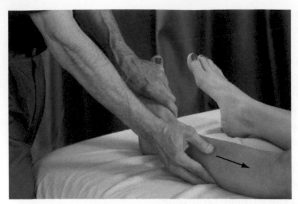

Figure 6.32 Active engagement lengthening to anterior compartment with additional resistance. Practitioner is gradually moving client's foot into plantar flexion as client pulls foot against practitioner's hand.

flexes the foot and resumes with the next dorsiflexion. Continue this process until the entire anterior compartment region has been treated.

E. Active engagement lengthening movements This technique can follow the shortening movements and is effective for enhancing flexibility and tension reduction in the anterior leg muscles. The same position is used as in D (see above). The client begins the repetitive slow dorsiflexion and plantar flexion movement. Perform a deep stripping technique on the anterior leg muscles as the client is plantar flexing the foot. Pressure is relieved as the foot is dorsiflexed and resumes again on the next plantar flexion. Due to the foot's position in relation to gravity there are relatively few anterior, leg-muscle fibers recruited to plantar flex the foot during the stripping technique. This technique is more effective if additional resistance is added during the plantar flexion to recruit more fibers (Fig. 6.32).

Rehabilitation protocol considerations

- Appropriate pressure level and choice of technique are dependent on the severity of the condition.

- Perform a comprehensive assessment to determine the severity of the compartment syndrome symptoms.

- Active engagement methods are best performed if the condition is not severe to begin with or in the later stages of the rehabilitation process when the client has improved significantly.

- Use caution when performing the active engagement methods. Active dorsiflexion can increase pressure levels in the anterior compartment and this can provoke greater discomfort.[83] If there is too much discomfort to perform the active engagement strokes, passive engagement methods can be used or simply stick with techniques A, B, and C.

Cautions and contraindications Recognition of the compartment syndrome's severity is very important in its treatment. If this condition is acute, massage should not be performed and the individual should be immediately referred to a physician for possible surgical intervention. If at any time during the treatment symptoms are increased, there is cause for concern that the treatment may be aggravating the problem. If this occurs, the current course of treatment should be stopped until the practitioner can re-evaluate the situation. If an acute compartment syndrome has occurred, the generally accepted rehabilitation principle of RICE does not apply to this condition.

SHIN SPLINTS

Description

The term shin splints is not clinically specific as it can encompass a number of different pathologies, including periostitis, muscle strain, stress fracture, and compartment syndromes.[84] However, there is a recent effort to be more consistent with terminology for these overuse leg conditions. In most cases the term applies to periostitis and muscle irritation resulting from overuse. Shin splints occur in two different regions. Both result from repetitive overuse of the lower extremity, making them common injuries in activities such as running or dancing.

The first type of shin splint is called anterior or lateral shin splints. Pain from this type of shin splints is felt in the anterior region of the lower leg, generally at the proximal one-third of the anterolateral region of the tibia. These shin splints are associated with overuse of the tibialis anterior and other anterior compartment muscles. The client feels pain throughout the anterior shin muscles and there is usually a history of lower extremity overuse affecting the dorsiflexor muscles. Eccentric overload is usually responsible for the onset of symptoms. Walking or running down a steep hill is a good example of eccentric overload of the dorsiflexors.

Anterior shin splints result from excessive tensile stress on the tibialis anterior attachment site along the tibial border. Constant tensile stress at the attachment of the tendon into the periosteum of the bone causes periosteal irritation, and therefore this problem is called periostitis. Although there are descriptions of shin splints as the muscle pulling away from the bone, they are erroneous. There is no evidence of tendon avulsion being a component of this condition.

The second type of shin splint produces pain in the medial and distal tibial region. Due to its location it is called posterior or medial shin splints. This condition is also called medial tibial stress syndrome (MTSS). As with the anterior shin splints, this problem also involves periostitis, although in this case it is from the tibialis posterior and soleus attachments.

The tibialis posterior is the primary muscle involved in MTSS. It works eccentrically during normal gait mechanics to prevent overpronation. Foot overpronation places excessive loads on the tibialis posterior, and tensile stress is concentrated at its origin site on the tibia. One study found the emphasis on a forefoot running stride to be the primary factor in a case of MTSS.[85] Landing on the forefoot puts excessive tensile stress on the tibialis posterior muscle. When the running stride was corrected the shin splint pain was relieved.

The soleus muscle is also a causative factor in MTSS.[86] The majority of symptoms in MTSS are felt in the distal one-third of the tibia, and a number of anatomy references suggest that the tibialis posterior does not attach that low on the tibia.[87] However, another study found that ten different specimens all had a portion of the tibialis posterior in the lower third of the tibia.[88] Based on these conflicting reports, both muscles can be involved in this condition.

Medial tibial stress syndrome can be a precursor to stress fractures in the tibia. Excessive use of the tibialis posterior or soleus muscles can cause a bowing of the tibia that leads to uneven stresses on the bone.[10] Therefore, stress fractures should always be considered as a possible cause of pain for individuals suspected of having shin splints.

Treatment

Traditional approaches

Treatment for both types of shin splints is similar. Rest from offending activities is paramount to reducing tensile stress on the attachment sites. If the offending activities can be reduced or avoided, this is often enough to alleviate the problem. Orthotics are sometimes used to correct biomechanical distortions in the client's gait pattern. Ice applications are recommended to reduce pain and resulting inflammation after activity. Anti-inflammatory medications are also recommended in some cases to reduce the inflammatory reaction of the periostitis.

Soft-tissue manipulation

General guidelines Both types of shin splints involve muscular overuse so massage is highly effective in this condition's management. For anterior shin splints, attention should focus on reducing chronic tightness in the muscles of the anterior compartment of the lower leg. The treatment techniques used to address anterior shin splints are the same as those described in the section above on anterior compartment syndrome. Pressure applied during these treatments should be within the client's tolerance levels. Treatment approaches for MTSS are slightly different and described below.

Stretching is an important component of treatment for either type of shin splints. For anterior shin splints, stretching emphasizes pulling the foot into plantar flexion as far as possible. Adding flexion of the toes also stretches the extensor digitorum and extensor hallucis longus muscles.

Stretching for MTSS is a challenge because the tibialis posterior is unable to fully stretch. It is primarily an inverter of the foot, so moving the foot into eversion is an effective stretching position. However, eversion is limited by the lateral malleolus of the fibula, and the strong deltoid ligament on the medial side of the foot. The stripping techniques and active engagement methods described below will encourage greater elongation in the tibialis posterior. Pulling the foot as far as possible into dorsiflexion stretches the soleus. If the knee is flexed, there is a greater emphasis on stretching the soleus than the gastrocnemius, with which it shares a common tendon.

Suggested techniques and methods   Treatment techniques for anterior/lateral shin splints are the same as those described for anterior compartment syndrome in the previous section. All of these treatment techniques pertain to MTSS.

A. Deep stripping Tension is reduced in deep posterior compartment muscles with specific stripping techniques. With the client in a side-lying position, use the thumb or fingertips to strip in a proximal direction along the medial border of the tibia (Fig. 6.18 under the description for Plantar fasciitis treatment).

B. Active engagement lengthening movements More effective access to these deep posterior compartment muscles is possible with active engagement techniques. Use the same initial position for the client as in A. Have the client move their foot in full dorsiflexion and plantar flexion in a slow repeated motion. During the dorsiflexion, perform a short specific stripping technique to the deep posterior compartment muscles (Fig. 6.19 under the description for Plantar fasciitis treatment). Only move a few inches proximally with each stroke during the dorsiflexion. Repeat this process until the entire length of the tibia has been treated. Moving proximally, this treatment also addresses the soleus attachments along the proximal tibia.

C. Active engagement with resistance Deep muscles in the posterior compartment are addressed more effectively when engaged with additional

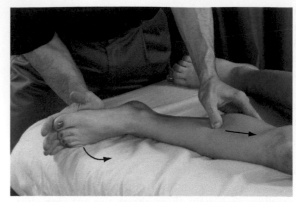

Figure 6.33   Active engagement lengthening to deep posterior compartment with additional resistance. Practitioner is gradually moving client's foot into dorsiflexion as client pushes against practitioner's hand.

resistance. This technique is effective for treating the deep posterior compartment muscles in the later stages of rehabilitation. The client is in a side-lying position just as in A and B (see above). Instruct the client to hold the foot in a plantar flexed position while resistance is offered (creating an initial isometric contraction). Instruct the client to slowly let go of the contraction as the client's foot is slowly pushed into dorsiflexion. While pushing the client's foot into dorsiflexion, perform a deep longitudinal stripping technique along the tibial border just as in B (see above) (Fig. 6.33). This technique can be painful for the client so the stripping techniques should be applied gently.

Rehabilitation protocol considerations   For both anterior and posterior shin splints:

- Shin splint pain is most pronounced around 12–36 hours after activity that initiated the problem. Massage can increase soreness if performed during the peak period so alter treatment intensity based on the severity of symptoms.

- Strengthening and conditioning of the region greatly reduces the likelihood of developing shin splints. Once the condition has developed, leave strengthening or conditioning activities until after the condition's symptoms have substantially reduced.

- Active engagement techniques and engagement with resistance can feel painful, especially for

MTSS. Use these techniques in the later stages of rehabilitation when the condition has already made considerable improvement.

Cautions and contraindications Both types of shin splints described here are effectively treated with massage. Yet there are situations where a more serious underlying condition, such as a stress fracture, can be present. Massage could decrease some of the symptoms, but offers little benefit for healing the stress fracture itself. Always consider the possibility of a more serious condition, such as a compartment syndrome or stress fracture, causing the symptoms attributed to shin splints. Proper assessment of the client's initial condition and ongoing status helps manage the condition appropriately.

Box 6.3   Clinical Tip

There are a variety of different positions that can be use to treat the deep posterior compartment muscles, such as the tibialis posterior. The side lying position described with the active engagement techniques is effective because it allows for easy access to the muscle as well as easy movement of the foot. Another very effective position to treat the tibialis posterior is with the client supine, hip flexed, and knee flexed with the foot flat on the treatment table (this is sometimes called the hook-lying position). In this position, gravity assists the technique by pulling the superficial posterior calf muscles, gastrocnemius and soleus, away from the tibial border. With the muscles being pulled away from the tibia by gravity, there is easier access for the treatment hand to get to the deep posterior compartment muscles.

POSTURAL DISORDERS

The next section includes a number of structural and postural disorders of the foot and ankle. These disorders are not considered injury conditions, as are the prior conditions in this chapter. However, they can produce considerable stress on other tissues or structures and contribute to their dysfunction. For some of these conditions there are massage treatment approaches that are helpful. In other cases massage is beneficial in addressing some of the symptoms resulting from the condition, but may not change the condition much itself.

HALLUX VALGUS

Description

A valgus angulation is one in which the distal end of a bony segment deviates in a lateral direction. In this condition the distal end of the hallux is forced in a lateral direction (Fig. 6.34). There are several factors that can cause a hallux valgus deformity including biomechanical, structural, or genetic disorders, lax ligaments, weak muscles, improper footwear, or abnormal bone structure.[89] Wearing shoes with a narrow toe region is considered the primary cause of this disorder.[90]

When the foot is in a shoe with a narrow toe region, the distal end of the hallux is forced toward the midline of the foot (a lateral direction in relation to the midline of the body). As the distal end of the hallux is pushed laterally (toward the foot's midline), the proximal end pushes the first metatarsal head medially against the edge of the shoe, resulting in callus formation and subcutaneous inflammation.[91] This callus formation is also called a bunion. Some sources call the hallux valgus deviation a bunion, so terminology is not always consistent in this condition.[92]

A hallux valgus deformity can contribute to numerous lower extremity biomechanical problems. The hallux has a primary role in maintaining foot

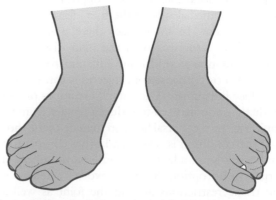

Figure 6.34 The hallux valgus deformity.

stability and absorbing forces during normal gait. When the distal hallux deviates laterally it is no longer able to carry out that crucial mechanical function. The loss of optimum foot mechanics from the hallux valgus deviation can lead to shin splints, myofascial trigger points, stress fractures, or over-pronation. Some of these disorders can also create or increase a valgus deviation in the hallux. Over-pronation, for example, puts a heavy biomechanical load on the distal hallux and metatarsophalangeal joint. If pronation is excessive it can gradually force the distal hallux into its deviated position.

There is a noticeable gender difference in hallux valgus occurrence. It is far more common in women than in men. However, it is unclear if this difference is caused by structural or physiological differences or if it is caused by the different type of shoes worn by men and women.[90]

There is a strong genetic pattern of hallux valgus occurrence. What is not clear is if the condition is more common within a family because of structural factors, sociological and cultural norms of particular shoes, or if there is just a genetic propensity for the condition that is exacerbated by outside factors. The condition does occur more commonly within families in the absence of particular shoes, indicating more important structural genetic factors.

Treatment

Traditional approaches

It is difficult to reverse a hallux valgus disorder because gradual pressure on the forefoot over time is responsible for the change in hallux angulation. In order to reverse the process it would be necessary to pull the distal hallux in the opposite direction (toward the medial side of the foot) for prolonged periods all day. In some cases there is inflammatory activity associated with the joint disorder. In those cases non-steroidal anti-inflammatory drugs (NSAIDS) or corticosteroid injections can be used to reduce inflammatory activity.[93] Orthotics or pads inside the shoe are used to reduce pressure from the bunion at the metatarsal head on the side of the shoe.

If the condition is severe and other conservative methods are not adequate to address the disorder, surgery is an option. Surgery involves a release of soft-tissue restrictions around the joint as well as a procedure called an osteotomy, which involves cutting a portion of the bone to aid in realignment.[94] Changing footwear is also an important part of treatment. It is not going to reverse the valgus drift of the hallux, but can sometimes prevent the condition from becoming worse.

Soft-tissue manipulation

General guidelines Massage can sometimes reduce foot pain and the discomfort that results from a hallux valgus deformity. The disorder cannot be reversed without more intensive interventions. Massage applications to the metatarsophalangeal joint can reduce fibrosity in that joint and make the joint more pliable. The hallux can then be stretched back toward its normal direction more easily. These techniques are helpful for encouraging motion in the intended direction of correction. However, lasting change is unlikely unless there is a constant force that pulls the hallux back into its normal alignment position for long periods every day.

Suggested techniques and methods

A. Deep friction Mobility of joint tissue is enhanced with friction techniques to the metatarsophalangeal joint. Apply the deep friction treatments in multiple directions to the joint tissue to enhance mobility (Fig. 6.35). Friction treatments can have longer duration than those that are used to treat scar tissue from torn muscles or tendons. Fibrous adhesion around the joint develops over time so longer and more aggressive bouts of friction are beneficial for joint mobilization.

B. Stretching of the hallux The position of the hallux can be altered somewhat by stretching the

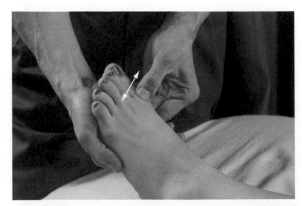

Figure 6.35   Deep friction to metatarsophalangeal (MTP) joint to address hallux valgus.

tissues that span the joint. After soft-tissue mobilization techniques such as the deep friction techniques mentioned in A (see above), pull the hallux back toward a position of proper alignment. Fibrous scar tissue is likely contributing to holding the hallux in the deviated position. Long-duration stretches (at least 20 seconds) are most effective in flexibility enhancement for this fibrous tissue.[95,96] This stretching method can enhance flexibility, but correction of this postural disorder is unlikely without something pulling the hallux back in a neutral position for long periods.

Rehabilitation protocol considerations

- Hallux valgus deformities occur over a long period. Therapeutic interventions of short duration (such as a massage treatment) can reduce pain symptoms and encourage greater mobility, but are limited in their effectiveness in reversing the postural disorder.

- A hallux valgus condition that is of recent onset is more likely to benefit from soft-tissue treatment than one developed over a long time.

Cautions and contraindications Depending on the severity of the condition, callus formation (bunion) around the metatarsal head can be painful. Use caution with friction techniques in this area. The client's pain tolerance is an appropriate guide. Massage can be used to improve mobility after surgical procedures, such as the metatarsal osteotomy. Wait an appropriate period after the surgery before attempting massage and consult with the surgeon about any necessary precautions for that client's surgical procedure.

MORTON'S FOOT

Description

The hallux is usually longer than all the other toes. Morton's foot, also called Morton's toe or Grecian foot is a postural condition in which the second toe appears longer than the hallux. It is a common anatomical variation and appears in about 40% of the population.[97] It results from either a short first metatarsal or a long second metatarsal. This postural condition does not necessarily produce problematic symptoms. A large number of people have a Morton's foot and never have symptoms.

The condition becomes an issue for some people when it adversely affects gait and contributes to other lower-extremity conditions. If the second metatarsal is longer than the first, there is a change in weight distribution throughout the forefoot. The second metatarsal head takes a greater percentage of weight bearing due to its increased length. Calluses can then form underneath the second metatarsal head. If the individual is not doing an excessive amount of activity, the result of Morton's foot is usually not a problem. However, for the individual that is performing multiple foot strikes in occupational or recreational activities, the accumulated stress on the metatarsal head can lead to other disorders.

Another problem results if, in addition to a long second metatarsal, there is a short first metatarsal and shortened hallux. A primary biomechanical function of the hallux is to help resist overpronation during normal foot mechanics. If the hallux is shorter due to metatarsal or phalangeal length, it may not be able to adequately resist foot pronation. Other lower-extremity disorders such as shin splints, stress fractures, or plantar fasciitis could result.

Treatment

Traditional approaches

Morton's foot is a congenital bone structure of the foot and typically does not cause a problem. If a problem does result from altered foot mechanics, orthotics are common treatments.

Soft-tissue manipulation

General guidelines Morton's foot is a congenital bone structure so massage treatment will not change this condition. However, massage can be effective in addressing some of the detrimental ramifications resulting from the condition. Myofascial trigger points resulting from biomechanical compensation can occur in the peroneal muscles, knee extensors, as well as gluteus medius and minimus.[97] Static compression techniques, deep longitudinal stripping, and stretching techniques should be applied to trigger points identified in lower extremity muscles. Any of the techniques for muscular tension reduction described earlier in this chapter are helpful for addressing biomechanical strain from the Morton's foot.

Cautions and contraindications Other than general precautions there are no major contraindications for working on a client with Morton's foot.

PES PLANUS

Description

Pes planus is a postural disorder of the foot more commonly known as *flat foot*. It results from a dropped or fallen longitudinal arch (Fig. 6.36). The primary function of the longitudinal arch is to aid in propulsion of the foot and shock absorption during foot strike. A detrimental effect of pes planus is that it decreases the shock-absorbing capability of the longitudinal arch. Pes planus results from weakness or laxity in those soft tissues that support the longitudinal arch including the tibialis posterior and intrinsic foot muscles, plantar fascia, tarsal, deltoid, and calcaneonavicular ligaments.[98]

Of these, the tibialis posterior is considered the primary dynamic structural support for the arch. When other support tissues are weakened, even greater load is placed on the tibialis posterior to maintain the arch. Fatigue and dysfunction of the muscle is a common cause of pes planus and can lead to other problems such as shin splints, stress fractures, and plantar fasciitis.[91]

The condition can appear earlier in life as a congenital deformity, but is often the result of age, increasing weight, and gradual loss of residual strength in the soft tissues that support the arch. Pes planus does not always lead to other disorders of the lower extremity. Many people have pes planus and experience no symptoms.

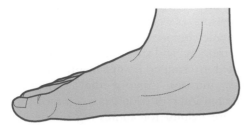

Figure 6.36 Pes planus (flat foot).

Treatment

Traditional approaches

Pes planus is most commonly treated with orthotics. The orthotic is designed to support the longitudinal arch and take stress off the soft tissues, such as the tibialis posterior. If the pes planus involves a severe case of bone deformity, surgery is sometimes used to correct the disorder.

Soft-tissue manipulation

General guidelines Pes planus results from weakening of structures that support the longitudinal arch. Massage reduces symptoms from the soft-tissue stress. However, massage treatment will not restore the arch to its proper form on its own. Some form of postural re-education is necessary; biomechanical interventions such as orthotics and strengthening and conditioning exercises in the foot are beneficial.

Suggested techniques and methods The techniques listed in the descriptions under plantar fasciitis or medial tibial stress syndrome are helpful for reducing symptoms resulting from pes planus.

Rehabilitation protocol considerations

- Massage treatment for pes planus is primarily for symptom management and not for corrective measures and can be performed at any time throughout the rehabilitation process.

- The primary protocol consideration is for the practitioner to remember that soft-tissue therapy can change biomechanical relationships that are being addressed with other procedures, such as orthotics.

Cautions and contraindications As long as working on the foot and leg region is appropriate there are no major cautions or contraindications for working on a client with pes planus

PES CAVUS

Description

Pes cavus is a postural disorder characterized by a high longitudinal arch in the foot that does not flatten with weight bearing (Fig. 6.37). In pes cavus there is a shortening of soft tissues that support the longitudinal arch, such as the plantar

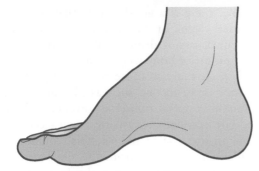

Figure 6.37   Pes cavus (high arch).

fascia and tibialis posterior muscles. Bone deformities can also cause or result from this foot disorder.[99] Intrinsic foot muscles, as well as the tibialis anterior and posterior, can be hypertonic and maintain the distorted position of the arch. The plantar fascia is in a shortened position causing increased tensile loads at its attachment points, especially at the anterior calcaneus.[91] Due to the altered pull of muscular imbalance lateral foot pain is frequently reported in clients with pes cavus.[100]

There are numerous causes of pes cavus. This postural disorder is often caused by neuromuscular disorders such as muscular dystrophy or Charcot–Marie–Tooth disease.[101,102] The condition can also be congenital. It is normal to see an increased incidence of other foot, ankle, or leg disorders that the pes cavus has contributed to, such as metatarsal stress fractures, plantar fasciitis, or Morton's neuroma. In some cases the condition results from traumatic injury that causes alterations in tarsal bone position.

Numerous biomechanical problems result from the high longitudinal arch. With increased arch height, there is greater weight-bearing pressure on the metatarsal heads. Increased pressure in this region can lead to Morton's neuroma, metatarsal stress fractures, or other biomechanical distortions such as claw-toe deformity.[103]

Treatment

Traditional approaches

If there is a progressive underlying disease or disorder that has produced the pes cavus, treatment options may be limited. In less severe cases orthotics can be helpful in correcting improperly distributed pressure levels on the foot. Physical therapy is used to stretch tight muscles and strengthen weak ones with the overall goal of addressing muscle imbalance to restore a proper arch. If the condition is severe, surgery may be necessary to correct the dysfunctional alignment. Surgical procedures may involve efforts to re-position bones or surgically release the plantar fascia, which has become shortened and fibrous.[103]

Soft-tissue manipulation

General guidelines   Pes cavus usually involves a combination of some leg and foot muscles that are tight, and others that have become weakened. Various conditioning activities will be necessary to strengthen the weakened muscles, but massage is a valuable treatment approach for addressing the hypertonic muscles. The exact pattern of muscle tightness and weakness can differ among clients, but these general guidelines can help in a majority of cases.

There is usually greater weakness in the tibialis anterior and peroneus brevis muscles. These are the muscles that benefit from strengthening procedures. Tibialis posterior and peroneus longus tend more towards hypertonicity, so these muscles benefit from massage treatment.

Suggested techniques and methods

A. Longitudinal stripping to plantar surface of the foot   Tension in soft tissues that shorten the arch is addressed with deep stripping techniques to the plantar surface of the foot. This technique is described in A under Plantar fasciitis and pictured in Figure 6.14.

B. Deep stripping and active engagement techniques   Reduction of muscle tension that leads to pes cavus is also achieved with active engagement techniques that focus on the tibialis posterior. These techniques are described in D and E under Plantar fasciitis and illustrated in Figures 6.18 and 6.19.

C. Deep stripping to peroneal muscles   Peroneal muscles can aid in pulling the arch in a higher position. Stripping techniques that emphasize the peroneal muscles reduce tension on the arch. This technique is virtually the same as that described in B under Anterior compartment syndrome and pictured in Figure 6.29. The only difference is emphasis of the stripping technique on the lateral region of the lower leg to address the peroneus longus and not as much on the anterior compartment.

Rehabilitation protocol considerations

- If another health professional is treating the client for biomechanical distortions associated with the pes cavus condition, consider the impact of massage treatment on those other procedures and adjust treatment accordingly.

Cautions and contraindications   It is generally safe to use soft-tissue therapy on a pes cavus condition as long as there are no other major contraindications that would be cause for concern. If the client's pes cavus condition is the result of some neuromuscular disorder or systemic disease, consult with the client's health care provider. It is unlikely that massage would have adverse effects on other treatments, but it is better to first clarify that before treatment.

CALCANEAL VALGUS

Description

A valgus angulation is one in which the distal end of a bony segment deviates in a lateral direction. In this condition the distal calcaneus deviates laterally (Fig. 6.38). Excessive eversion of the sub-talar joint produces the valgus angulation. Calcaneal valgus is a contributing factor to overpronation (discussed later in this chapter). However, it is only one component of the dynamic postural distortion of overpronation.

The best position to view calcaneal valgus is looking at the client's foot from behind. The wear pattern on the underside of the shoe can also provide evidence of calcaneal valgus. If there is a more concentrated wear pattern on the medial side of the

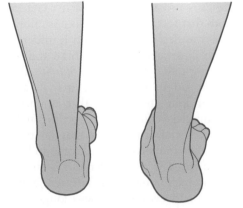

Figure 6.38   Calcaneal valgus.

shoe's sole, there is a good chance that the client has calcaneal valgus, or they may be overpronating.

A calcaneal valgus disorder places a disproportionate amount of body weight on the medial side of the foot. It can also cause additional problems in the foot or lower leg such as plantar fasciitis, stress fractures, tarsal tunnel syndrome, and shin splints. The compensatory pattern with calcaneal valgus is an increase in medial tibial rotation.[104] Knee disorders resulting from the tibial rotation can also be traced to the calcaneal valgus.

Treatment

Traditional approaches

The most common method of addressing calcaneal valgus is with orthotics. These inserts attempt to correct the biomechanical deviation, and are valuable in addressing the other disorders resulting from the valgus angulation. Orthotics are available from a variety of sources. Orthotics bought off the shelf in a pharmacy or medical supply store may be all that is needed to correct the client's postural challenge. In other cases over-the-counter products may not be as effective because they are not designed for that client's unique foot structure. In some cases, an improper orthotic can make the condition worse, so it is advisable to refer the client to a specialist in foot care and orthotics.

Soft-tissue manipulation

General guidelines   The calcaneal valgus angulation is usually a complex biomechanical dysfunction with multiple factors. The primary muscular components involve weakness and overstretching in the foot inverters, such as tibialis anterior and posterior. There is also a corresponding shortness in the foot everters, such as the peroneal group, which is not necessarily due to tightness of the peroneal muscles. Calcaneal valgus is due more to alignment issues in the calcaneus that are exacerbated by weight bearing, rather than muscle tightness.

Although calcaneal valgus generally does not develop due to muscle tightness, soft-tissue treatment is still beneficial for hypertonicity that develops in other muscles due to the condition. If orthotics are used, massage can reduce overload on foot and ankle muscles that start to adjust to the new position.

Suggested techniques and methods

A. Deep stripping Stripping is applied to the peroneal muscles to reduce tension and aid muscular balance around the ankle joint. This technique is virtually the same as that described in B under anterior compartment syndrome and pictured in Figure 6.29. The only difference is emphasis of the stripping techniques on the lateral compartment of the leg to address the peroneal muscles.

B. Active engagement techniques After initial treatment to reduce tension in lateral compartment muscles, active engagement can further reduce tightness in the affected tissues. The tibialis anterior and posterior are usually somewhat overstretched in this postural disorder. However, being under high mechanical demand and held at longer than their normal resting length can cause them to develop myofascial trigger points. Techniques for addressing the tibialis posterior are described in D and E under Plantar fasciitis and demonstrated in Figures 6.18 and 6.19. Effective techniques for the tibialis anterior are listed in B and E under Anterior compartment syndrome and illustrated in Figures 6.29 and 6.32 respectively.

C. Stretching techniques After soft-tissue manipulation, stretching of the peroneal muscles is suggested.

Rehabilitation protocol considerations
- Massage treatment can alter biomechanical function in the foot and ankle region. In some cases orthotics have been prescribed and/or specifically designed for that client's foot condition. Massage is not likely to alter the biomechanical changes with the orthotics significantly, but consider it as a possibility if symptoms change significantly after the massage treatment.

Cautions and contraindications Other than general precautions there are no major contraindications for working on a calcaneal valgus foot posture.

CALCANEAL VARUS

Description

Calcaneal varus is a postural disorder in which the distal portion of the calcaneus deviates in a medial direction (Fig. 6.39). It is best viewed from

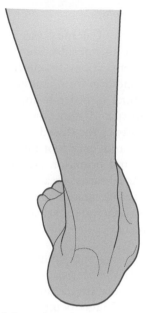

Figure 6.39 Calcaneal varus

the posterior side of the heel. The wear pattern on the bottom of the shoe often gives clues to calcaneal varus. Calcaneal varus produces excessive wear on the lateral aspect of the sole. Calcaneal varus is also a component of excessive supination and that may be the cause for the wear pattern as well.

Calcaneal varus can produce a number of soft-tissue problems throughout the foot and lower leg because of the altered shock absorbency and force loading on the foot. As with calcaneal valgus, varus angulations in the calcaneus can cause plantar fasciitis, shin splints, stress fractures, tarsal tunnel syndrome, or other lower extremity disorders. The varus angulation of the calcaneus and increased supination of the foot during gait also makes the individual more susceptible to lateral ankle sprains.

Treatment

Traditional approaches

Calcaneal varus is commonly treated with orthotics, just like calcaneal valgus. The same principles and concepts related to orthotic use and selection as described in that section apply for calcaneal varus as well. It is best to refer the client to a specialist in foot care and orthotics.

Soft-tissue manipulation

General guidelines Calcaneal varus is a chronic postural disorder that results from a number of factors. Treatment is most effective when it addresses the condition from multiple approaches. While this postural disorder is not created solely through soft-tissue dysfunction, treating soft-tissue components of the disorder is helpful.

The muscles producing foot inversion, such as tibialis anterior and posterior, are in a shortened position in calcaneal varus. Treatment should focus on encouraging elongation in these muscles. Stretching approaches are a valuable adjunct after massage treatment.

Suggested techniques and methods

A. Deep stripping to peroneal muscles These muscles are under greater stretch and increased length in calcaneal varus. Trigger points and muscular dysfunction can develop in the muscles as a result of being held in chronic stretch. Deep stripping technique is virtually the same as that described in B under Anterior compartment syndrome and pictured in Figure 6.29. The only difference is emphasis of the stripping techniques on the lateral compartment of the leg to address the peroneal muscles.

B. Active engagement techniques Treatment of tibialis anterior and posterior is emphasized for this condition. These muscles are in a shortened position in calcaneal varus, so the aim of treatment is to encourage elongation. Techniques for addressing the tibialis posterior are described in D and E under Plantar fasciitis and demonstrated in Figures 6.18 and 6.19. Effective techniques for the tibialis anterior are listed in B and E under Anterior compartment syndrome and illustrated in Figures 6.29 and 6.32 respectively.

C. Stretching techniques Following massage treatment with stretching of the tibialis anterior and posterior is encouraged.

Rehabilitation protocol considerations

- Soft-tissue work is valuable, but will have limited effectiveness without more forceful postural change, such as orthotics or changes in footwear. Massage treatment can be performed simultaneously with orthotic usage, but note that changes in muscle balance around the foot may require alteration of the orthotic.

Cautions and contraindications Other than general precautions there are no major contraindications for massage treatment on a calcaneal valgus foot posture.

EXCESSIVE SUPINATION

Description

The postural disorders presented so far in this section have all been evaluated primarily in static positions. The next two disorders, excessive supination and overpronation, are distinctly different in that they are dynamic postural disorders. That means they are more accurately evaluated in active movement as opposed to a static position. The concept of *acture* (active posture) presented by Chaitow and Delany is appropriate for these conditions.[105]

Supination is motion around an oblique or diagonal axis and is a combination of inversion, adduction and plantar flexion. When the foot is in a position that includes all three of these combined movements it is fully supinated. A foot with excessive supination bears more weight on the lateral edge (Fig. 6.40). A primary component of

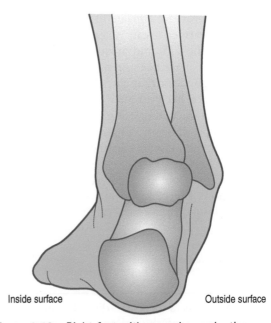

Inside surface   Outside surface

Figure 6.40 Right foot with excessive supination viewed from behind.

excessive supination is subtalar inversion. Therefore, an individual with calcaneal varus is likely to have excessive supination during the weight-bearing phase of gait. Indication of excessive supination is evident with a wear pattern on the outside lateral edge of the shoe.

The ability of the foot to supinate and pronate is particularly important for adapting to variations in ground surface. In the dynamic movement of gait the foot is in a slight degree of supination during the swing-through phase of the normal gait and begins to pronate immediately after contacting the ground.[91] If, however, the foot stays more supinated during the weight-bearing phase of gait, this is considered excessive supination.

Treatment

Traditional approaches

Traditional treatment approaches for excessive supination focus on biomechanical corrections through the use orthotics. Because of the biomechanical similarity between the conditions, the treatment strategies are virtually the same as those described in the section under calcaneal varus.

Soft-tissue manipulation

As with the traditional approaches to treatment, soft-tissue manipulation and rehabilitation protocol considerations are virtually the same as those described under the section on calcaneal varus.

Cautions and contraindications Other than general precautions there are no major contraindications for working on a calcaneal valgus foot posture.

OVERPRONATION

Description

Pronation is a dynamic movement of the foot that includes dorsiflexion, eversion, and abduction. A foot with overpronation bears more weight on the medial edge (Fig. 6.41). There is a natural degree of pronation as the foot moves through the different phases of weight-bearing during normal gait. The term pronation is sometimes inappropriately used to signify dysfunctional foot mechanics.

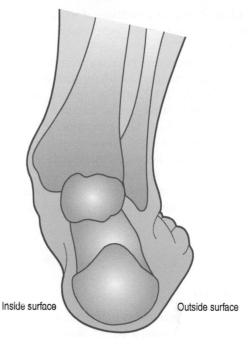

Inside surface　　　Outside surface

Figure 6.41 Right foot with overpronation viewed from behind.

Pronation is a normal part of movement, but excessive pronation is called *overpronation* or *hyperpronation*. Overpronation occurs when an individual moves either too far or too fast through the phases of pronation, placing more weight on the medial side of the foot during gait.

Unless there is a severe, acute injury, overpronation develops as a gradual biomechanical distortion. Several factors contribute to developing overpronation, including tibialis posterior weakness, ligament weakness, excess weight, pes planus, genu valgum, subtalar eversion, or other biomechanical distortions in the foot or ankle. Overpronation often includes a combination of factors.[91]

Tibialis posterior weakness is one of the primary factors leading to overpronation. Pronation is primarily controlled by the architecture of the foot and eccentric activation of the tibialis posterior.[106] If the tibialis posterior is weak, the muscle cannot adequately slow the natural pronation cycle.

Obesity is another cause of overpronation. The architecture of the foot is not designed to carry disproportionate weight. As a result, the excessive weight causes subtalar eversion and forces the longitudinal arch to collapse. A static calcaneal valgus is evident during examination of the foot, and this valgus angulation causes overpronation during the gait cycle.

Overpronation can be a contributing factor in other lower extremity disorders, such as foot pain, plantar fasciitis, ankle injuries, medial tibial stress syndrome, periostitis, stress fractures, and myofascial trigger points. Overpronation increases the degree of internal tibial rotation, thereby contributing to various knee disorders such as meniscal injury or ligament sprains.

The effects of the postural deviation are exaggerated in athletes due to the increase in foot strikes while running and the greater impact load experienced. When running, three to four times the body weight is experienced with each foot strike.[31] If overpronation exists, the shock force is not adequately absorbed by the foot and is transmitted further up the kinetic chain.

Treatment

Traditional approaches

The primary focus for overpronation treatments is correcting the dynamic position of the foot during the weight-bearing phase of gait. This is usually

---

Box 6.4 Case Study

Background

Nina is a 33-year-old entrepreneur who owns a baking shop. Owning a baking business means she spends a great deal of time on her feet. Her bakery has a concrete floor which seems to really make her feet hurt after long days. She has been complaining recently of increasing pain in her lower leg and foot, especially after long days at work. Her feet also feel stiff and somewhat painful upon first waking up and walking on them in the morning. She has recently started wearing running shoes at work and mentioned that the change in footwear has helped some, but the problem is still bothering her.

Observation of Nina's posture shows a slight degree of genu valgum and calcaneal valgus bilaterally. Physical examination reveals tenderness to palpation along the distal medial border of the tibia and the plantar surface of the foot. When these regions are palpated, it reproduces the primary pain and discomfort Nina has been experiencing. There are no signs of neurological disorder present. Stretching of the posterior calf muscles and plantar foot muscles by moving the foot in dorsiflexion creates a mild sensation of discomfort. This motion is one of the things she does during work that seems to help a little.

Questions to consider

- Nina's leg and foot discomfort appears to be related to her long hours of work while standing on a concrete floor. Because she is not able to change that significantly right now, what suggestions outside of soft-tissue manipulation might be helpful to reduce some of her symptoms?
- What do you think is the primary cause of her pain and discomfort? Name specific tissues or structures that you think are involved.
- If massage treatment is directed at muscles of the lower leg and foot to reduce overuse stress, how often do you think she should come for this treatment?
- If you think massage treatment is appropriate for her, what techniques do you suggest for her at this stage of her injury condition?
- What role should stretching play in the management of her condition? Consider stretching that you might perform in the treatment room as well as stretching that she could perform on her own.
- If this condition appeared to be primarily an overuse disorder and she did not choose to have any treatment for the problem, what are some of the possible detrimental outcomes?
- Do you think thermal modalities will be of use to her? If so, which ones and when should she use them.

accomplished with orthotics. The treatment strategies for overpronation are virtually the same as those described in the section under calcaneal valgus.

Soft-tissue manipulation

Soft-tissue treatment for overpronation emphasizes numerous muscles and soft tissues of the lower extremity. Massage treatment alone is not sufficient to create the needed biomechanical corrections of overpronation. The primary focus of massage treatment is to support and enhance other approaches such as orthotics and footwear changes. To address this condition follow the treatment suggestions and rehabilitation protocol considerations that are described in the section under calcaneal valgus.

Cautions and contraindications Other than general precautions there are no major contraindications for working on a client with overpronation.

References

1. Clarke TE, Frederick EC, Cooper LB. Effects of shoe cushioning upon ground reaction forces in running. Int J Sports Med. 1983;4(4):247–251.
2. Dixon SJ, Collop AC, Batt ME. Surface effects on ground reaction forces and lower extremity kinematics in running. Med Sci Sports Exerc. 2000;32(11):1919–1926.
3. Snow RE, Williams KR. High heeled shoes: their effect on center of mass position, posture, three-dimensional kinematics, rearfoot motion, and ground reaction forces. Arch Phys Med Rehabil. 1994;75(5):568–576.
4. Robbins S, Waked E. Hazard of deceptive advertising of athletic footwear. Br J Sports Med. 1997;31(4): 299–303.
5. Attarian DE, McCrackin HJ, DeVito DP, McElhaney JH, Garrett WE, Jr. Biomechanical characteristics of human ankle ligaments. Foot Ankle. 1985;6(2):54–58.
6. Garrick JG. The frequency of injury, mechanism of injury, and epidemiology of ankle sprains. Am J Sports Med. 1977;5(6):241–242.
7. Liu SH, Jason WJ. Lateral ankle sprains and instability problems. Clin Sports Med. 1994;13(4):793–809.
8. Wuest TK. Injuries to the distal lower extremity syndesmosis. J Am Acad Orthop Surg. 1997;5(3): 172–181.
9. Smith AH, Bach BR. High ankle sprains. Physician Sportsmed. 2004;32(12).
10. Panjabi M, White A. Biomechanics in the Musculoskeletal System. New York: Churchill Livingstone; 2001.
11. Bleakley CM, O'Connor S, Tully MA, Rocke LG, Macauley DC, McDonough SM. The PRICE study (Protection Rest Ice Compression Elevation): design of a randomised controlled trial comparing standard versus cryokinetic ice applications in the management of acute ankle sprain [ISRCTN13903946]. BMC Musculoskelet Disord. 2007;8(1):125.
12. Eiff MP, Smith AT, Smith GE. Early mobilization versus immobilization in the treatment of lateral ankle sprains. Am J Sports Med. 1994;22(1):83–88.
13. Kannus P. Long-term results of conservatively treated medial collateral ligament injuries of the knee joint. Clin Orthop. 1988(226):103–112.
14. Safran MR, Zachazewski JE, Benedetti RS, Bartolozzi AR, 3rd, Mandelbaum R. Lateral ankle sprains: a comprehensive review part 2: treatment and rehabilitation with an emphasis on the athlete. Med Sci Sports Exerc. 1999; 31(7 Suppl):S438–447.
15. Garrick JG, Schelkun P. Managing ankle sprains. Physician Sportsmed. 1997;25(3).
16. Prentice W. Rehabilitation Techniques in Sports Medicine. St. Louis: Mosby; 1990.
17. Bassewitz H, Shapiro M. Persistent pain after ankle sprain. Physician Sportsmed. 1997;25(12).
18. Hammer WI. Functional Soft-Tissue Examination and Treatment by Manual Methods. 3rd ed. Boston: Jones and Bartlett; 2007.
19. Blauvelt C, Nelson, F. A Manual of Orthopaedic Terminology. 3rd ed. St. Louis: C.V. Mosby Company; 1985.
20. Levitsky KA, Alman BA, Jevsevar DS, Morehead J. Digital nerves of the foot: anatomic variations and implications regarding the pathogenesis of interdigital neuroma. Foot Ankle. 1993;14(4):208–214.
21. Mollica MB. Mortons neuroma – getting patients back on track. Physician Sportsmed. 1997;25(5):76.
22. Moore K, Dalley A. Clinically Oriented Anatomy. 4th ed. Philadelphia: Lippincott Williams & Wilkins; 1999.
23. Dawson D, Hallett M, Wilbourn A. Entrapment Neuropathies. 3rd ed. Philadelphia: Lippincott–Raven; 1999.
24. Breig A. Adverse Mechanical Tension in the Central Nervous System. Stockholm: Almqvist & Wiksell; 1978.
25. Butler D. Mobilisation of the Nervous System. London: Churchill Livingstone; 1991.
26. Shacklock M. Clinical Neurodynamics. Edinburgh: Elsevier; 2005.
27. Petty N, Moore A. Neuromusculoskeletal Examination and Assessment. Edinburgh: Churchill Livingstone; 1998.
28. Wu KK. Morton's interdigital neuroma: a clinical review of its etiology, treatment, and results. J Foot Ankle Surg. 1996;35(2):112–119; discussion 187–188.
29. Basadonna PT, Rucco V, Gasparini D, Onorato A. Plantar fat pad atrophy after corticosteroid injection for an interdigital neuroma – A case report. Amer J Phys Med Rehabil. 1999;78(3):283–285.
30. Pyasta RT, Panush RS. Common painful foot syndromes. Bull Rheum Dis. 1999;48(10):1–4.
31. Nordin M, Frankel V. Basic Biomechanics of the Musculoskeletal System. 2nd ed. Malvern: Lea & Febiger; 1989.

32. Fuller EA. The windlass mechanism of the foot. A mechanical model to explain pathology. J Am Podiatr Med Assoc. 2000;90(1):35–46.

33. Huang CK, Kitaoka HB, An KN, Chao EY. Biomechanical evaluation of longitudinal arch stability. Foot Ankle. 1993;14(6):353–357.

34. Juhan D. Job's Body. Barrytown, NY: Station Hill Press; 1987.

35. Torg J, Shephard R. Current Therapy in Sports Medicine. 3rd ed. St. Louis: Mosby; 1995.

36. Fu F, Stone D. Sports Injuries: Mechanisms, Prevention, Treatment. Baltimore: Williams & Wilkins; 1994.

37. Kwong PK, Kay D, Voner RT, White MW. Plantar fasciitis. Mechanics and pathomechanics of treatment. Clin Sports Med. 1988;7(1):119–126.

38. Gill LH. Plantar Fasciitis: Diagnosis and Conservative Management. J Am Acad Orthop Surg. 1997;5(2): 109–117.

39. Acevedo JI, Beskin JL. Complications of plantar fascia rupture associated with corticosteroid injection. Foot Ankle Int. 1998;19(2):91–97.

40. Sellman JR. Plantar fascia rupture associated with corticosteroid injection. Foot Ankle Int. 1994;15(7): 376–381.

41. Roberts WO. Plantar fascia injection. Physician Sportsmed. 1999;27(9):101–102.

42. Wapner KL, Sharkey PF. The use of night splints for treatment of recalcitrant plantar fasciitis. Foot Ankle. 1991;12(3):135–137.

43. Mizel MS, Marymont JV, Trepman E. Treatment of plantar fasciitis with a night splint and shoe modification consisting of a steel shank and anterior rocker bottom. Foot Ankle Int. 1996;17(12): 732–735.

44. Batt ME, Tanji JL, Skattum N. Plantar fasciitis: a prospective randomized clinical trial of the tension night splint. Clin J Sport Med. 1996;6(3):158–162.

45. Lemont H, Ammirati KM, Usen N. Plantar fasciitis: a degenerative process (fasciosis) without inflammation. J Am Podiatr Med Assoc. 2003;93(3):234–237.

46. Ho C. Extracorporeal shock wave treatment for chronic plantar fasciitis (heel pain). Issues Emerg Health Technol. Jan 2007(96(part 1)):1–4.

47. Rompe JD, Furia J, Weil L, Maffulli N. Shock wave therapy for chronic plantar fasciopathy. Br Med Bull. 2007;81–82:183–208.

48. Radin EL. Tarsal tunnel syndrome. Clin Orthop. 1983(181):167–170.

49. Jackson DL, Haglund BL. Tarsal tunnel syndrome in runners. Sports Med. 1992;13(2):146–149.

50. Turl SE, and George KP. Adverse neural tension – a factor in repetitive hamstring strain. J Orthop Sport Phys Therapy. 1998;27(1):16–21.

51. Pavlov H, Heneghan MA, Hersh A, Goldman AB, Vigorita V. The Haglund syndrome: initial and differential diagnosis. Radiology. 1982;144(1):83–88.

52. Stephens MM. Haglund's deformity and retrocalcaneal bursitis. Orthop Clin North Am. 1994;25(1):41–46.

53. Rufai A, Ralphs JR, Benjamin M. Structure and histopathology of the insertional region of the human Achilles tendon. J Orthop Res. 1995;13(4):585–593.

54. Fredberg U. Local corticosteroid injection in sport – review of literature and guidelines for treatment. Scand J Med Sci Sports. 1997;7(3):131–139.

55. Shrier I, Matheson GO, Kohl HW, 3rd. Achilles tendonitis: are corticosteroid injections useful or harmful? Clin J Sport Med. 1996;6(4):245–250.

56. Carr AJ, Norris SH. The blood supply of the calcaneal tendon. J Bone Joint Surg Br. 1989;71(1):100–101.

57. Kraushaar BS, Nirschl RP. Tendinosis of the elbow (tennis elbow). Clinical features and findings of histological, immunohistochemical, and electron microscopy studies. J Bone Joint Surg Am. 1999;81(2):259–278.

58. Ahmed IM, Lagopoulos M, McConnell P, Soames RW, Sefton GK. Blood supply of the Achilles tendon. J Orthop Res. Sep 1998;16(5):591–596.

59. Malone T, McPoil T, Nitz A. Orthopedic and Sports Physical Therapy. 3rd ed. St. Louis: Mosby; 1997.

60. Cailliet R. Foot and Ankle Pain. 2nd ed. Philadelphia: F.A. Davis Company; 1983.

61. Clement DB, Taunton JE, Smart GW. Achilles tendinitis and peritendinitis: etiology and treatment. Am J Sports Med. 1984;12(3):179–184.

62. Harrell RM. Fluoroquinolone-induced tendinopathy: what do we know? South Med J. 1999;92(6):622–625.

63. Huston KA. Achilles tendinitis and tendon rupture due to fluoroquinolone antibiotics. N Engl J Med. 1994;331(11):748.

64. McGarvey WC, Singh D, Trevino SG. Partial Achilles tendon ruptures associated with fluoroquinolone antibiotics: a case report and literature review. Foot Ankle Int. 1996;17(8):496–498.

65. Fadale PD, Wiggins ME. Corticosteroid injections: their use and abuse. J Am Acad Orthop Surg. 1994;2(3): 133–140.

66. Halpern AA, Horowitz BG, Nagel DA. Tendon ruptures associated with corticosteroid therapy. West J Med. 1977;127(5):378–382.

67. Maffulli N, Khan KM, Puddu G. Overuse tendon conditions: time to change a confusing terminology. Arthroscopy. 1998;14(8):840–843.

68. Almekinders LC, Temple JD. Etiology, diagnosis, and treatment of tendinitis – an analysis of the literature. Med Sci Sport Exercise. 1998;30(8):1183–1190.

69. Davidson CJ, Ganion LR, Gehlsen GM, Verhoestra B, Roepke JE, Sevier TL. Rat tendon morphologic and functional changes resulting from soft-tissue mobilization. Med Sci Sport Exercise. 1997;29(3):313–319.

70. Gehlsen GM, Ganion LR, Helfst R. Fibroblast responses to variation in soft tissue mobilization pressure. Med Sci Sport Exercise. 1999;31(4):531–535.

71. Khan KM, Cook JL, Taunton JE, Bonar F. Overuse tendinosis, not tendinitis – Part 1: A new paradigm for a

difficult clinical problem. Physician Sportsmed. 2000; 28(5):38.

72. Schissel DJ, Godwin J. Effort-related chronic compartment syndrome of the lower extremity. Mil Med. 1999;164(11):830–832.

73. Edwards P, Myerson MS. Exertional compartment syndrome of the leg. Physician Sportsmed. 1996;24(4).

74. Swain R, Ross D. Lower extremity compartment syndrome. When to suspect acute or chronic pressure buildup. Postgrad Med. 1999;105(3):159–162, 165, 168.

75. Stuart MJ, Karaharju TK. Acute compartment syndrome. Physician Sportsmed. 1994;22(3).

76. Moyer RA, Boden BP, Marchetto PA, Kleinbart F, Kelly JD. Acute compartment syndrome of the lower extremity secondary to noncontact injury. Foot Ankle. 1993;14(9):534–537.

77. Fehlandt A, Jr., Micheli L. Acute exertional anterior compartment syndrome in an adolescent female. Med Sci Sports Exerc. 1995;27(1):3–7.

78. Tubb CC, Vermillion D. Chronic exertional compartment syndrome after minor injury to the lower extremity. Mil Med. 2001;166(4):366–368.

79. Hutchinson MR, Ireland ML. Common compartment syndromes in athletes. Treatment and rehabilitation. Sports Med. 1994;17(3):200–208.

80. Sebik A, Dogan A. A technique for arthroscopic fasciotomy for the chronic exertional tibialis anterior compartment syndrome. Knee Surg Sports Traumatol Arthrosc. 28 2007.

81. de Fijter WM, Scheltinga MR, Luiting MG. Minimally invasive fasciotomy in chronic exertional compartment syndrome and fascial hernias of the anterior lower leg: short- and long-term results. Mil Med. 2006;171(5): 399–403.

82. Blackman PG, Simmons LR, Crossley KM. Treatment of chronic exertional anterior compartment syndrome with massage: a pilot study. Clin J Sport Med. 1998;8(1): 14–17.

83. Gershuni DH, Yaru NC, Hargens AR, Lieber RL, O'Hara RC, Akeson WH. Ankle and knee position as a factor modifying intracompartmental pressure in the human leg. J Bone Joint Surg Am. 1984;66(9):1415–1420.

84. Batt ME. Shin splints – a review of terminology. Clin J Sport Med. 1995;5(1):53–57.

85. Cibulka MT, Sinacore DR, Mueller MJ. Shin splints and forefoot contact running: a case report. J Orthop Sports Phys Ther. 1994;20(2):98–102.

86. Michael RH, Holder LE. The soleus syndrome. A cause of medial tibial stress (shin splints). Am J Sports Med. 1985;13(2):87–94.

87. Beck BR, Osternig LR. Medial tibial stress syndrome. The location of muscles in the leg in relation to symptoms. J Bone Joint Surg Am. 1994;76(7):1057–1061.

88. Saxena A, O'Brien T, Bunce D. Anatomic dissection of the tibialis posterior muscle and its correlation to medial tibial stress syndrome. J Foot Surg. 1990;29(2):105–108.

89. Riddle DL. Foot and Ankle. In: Richardson JK, Iglarsh ZA, eds. Clinical Orthopaedic Physical Therapy. Philadelphia: W.B. Saunders; 1994.

90. Thomas S, Barrington, R. Hallux valgus. Current Orthopedics. 2003;17:299–307.

91. Lowe W. Orthopedic Assessment in Massage Therapy. Sisters, OR: Daviau-Scott; 2006.

92. Frank CJ, Robinson DE. Hallux Valgus. March 16; www.emedicine.com. Accessed March 25, 2005.

93. Frank CJ, Robinson DE. Hallux Valgus. e-Medicine; 2005.

94. Coughlin MJ, Grimes S. Proximal metatarsal osteotomy and distal soft tissue reconstruction as treatment for hallux valgus deformity. Keio J Med. 2005;54(2):60–65.

95. Roberts JM, Wilson K. Effect of stretching duration on active and passive range of motion in the lower extremity. Br J Sports Med. Aug 1999;33(4):259–263.

96. Ford P, McChesney J. Duration of maintained hamstring ROM following termination of three stretching protocols. J Sport Rehabil. 2007;16(1):18–27.

97. Travell J, Simons, D. Myofascial Pain and Dysfunction: The Trigger Point Manual. Vol 2. Baltimore: Williams & Wilkins; 1992.

98. Deland JT. The adult acquired flatfoot and spring ligament complex. Pathology and implications for treatment. Foot Ankle Clin. 2001;6(1):129–135, vii.

99. Turner NS. Pes Cavus. e-Medicine; 2007.

100. Burns J, Crosbie J, Hunt A, Ouvrier R. The effect of pes cavus on foot pain and plantar pressure. Clin Biomech (Bristol, Avon). 2005;20(9):877–882.

101. Alexander IJ, Johnson KA. Assessment and management of pes cavus in Charcot–Marie–Tooth disease. Clin Orthop Relat Res. 1989(246):273–281.

102. Sabir M, Lyttle D. Pathogenesis of pes cavus in Charcot–Marie–Tooth disease. Clin Orthop Relat Res. 1983(175): 173–178.

103. Turner N. Pes Cavus. March 18; www.emedicine.com. Accessed March 23, 2005.

104. Soderberg G. Kinesiology: Application to Pathological Motion. Baltimore: Williams & Wilkins; 1986.

105. Chaitow L, Delany J. Clinical Application of Neuromuscular Techniques. Vol 2. Edinburgh: Churchill Livingstone; 2002.

106. Stovitz SD, Coetzee C. Hyperpronation and foot pain. Physician Sportsmed. 2004;32(8).

Chapter 7

Knee and thigh

The knee is the largest joint in the body and is particularly susceptible to various types of injury or dysfunction due to its structural design. There are two articulations associated with the knee joint, the tibiofemoral and patellofemoral joints. The tibiofemoral is a true synovial joint where two long bones articulate with each other. It is the weight-bearing structure of the knee and as a result it plays an important role in shock absorption and locomotion. The patellofemoral articulation is neither a true synovial joint nor a weight-bearing articulation. The patellofemoral articulation is involved in numerous soft-tissue disorders at the knee because of the strong force loads associated with the quadriceps muscles during knee extension.

Knee injuries are rampant in sports activities, so the role of knee function in locomotion has been studied in great detail. Much attention has focused on joint trauma involving the internal knee structures, such as the cruciate ligaments, menisci, and articular surfaces. Yet soft-tissues acting on this joint are considerably important and massage plays an important role in management of numerous disorders in this area.

INJURY CONDITIONS

ANTERIOR CRUCIATE LIGAMENT SPRAIN

Description

The anterior cruciate ligament (ACL) is one of four primary stabilizing ligaments of the knee. The term *cruciate* means cross, and a lateral view of the knee shows how the anterior and posterior

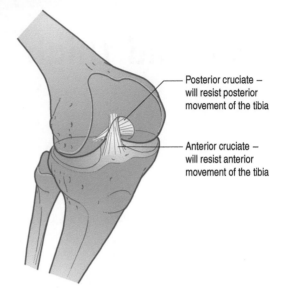

Figure 7.1   The knee joint showing where cruciate ligaments cross.

cruciate ligaments form a cross inside the knee joint (Fig. 7.1). The ACL attaches to the anterior aspect of the tibial plateau, and is designed to resist anterior translation of the tibia in relation to the femur. It also functions to limit hyperextension of the knee, and to resist medial rotation of the tibia in relation to the femur.

Sprains to the ACL are relatively common injuries. As more people become active in vigorous sports and recreational activities, these injuries are increasing even more. It has been estimated that ACL injuries occur at the rate of about 60 per 100,000 people per year.[1]

ACL sprains occur more often to women than to men. There are a number of different factors that may account for this statistic. The hormone estrogen can be a factor in causing relaxation in soft tissues, especially ligaments.[2,3] This greater degree of soft-tissue relaxation may account for an increase in ligamentous laxity and a greater number of ACL injuries. Women also have a larger Q angle than men. The *Q angle*, or Quadriceps angle, is determined by connecting a line between the tibial tuberosity and the midpoint of the patella. Another line is then drawn between the midpoint of the patella and the anterior superior

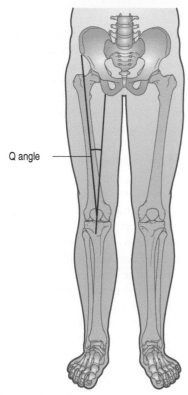

Q angle

Figure 7.2   The Q angle.

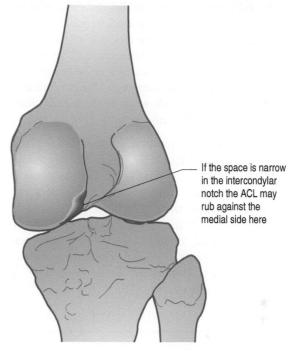

If the space is narrow in the intercondylar notch the ACL may rub against the medial side here

Figure 7.3   Posterior view of the right tibiofibular articulation showing the intercondylar notch.

iliac spine (ASIS). The angle formed between those two lines is the Q angle (Fig. 7.2).

Although sources vary on how much is too much for the Q angle, an angle of more than 15° in women and 10° in men is considered excessive.[4] Women have a larger Q angle because of the broader pelvis. There is some evidence that a larger Q angle may cause an increasing degree of pull by the quadriceps muscle group on the tibial tuberosity.[5]

The quadriceps group attaches to the tibial tuberosity. Due to its angle of pull, it pulls the tibia in an anterior direction. If there is a greater pull from the quadriceps on the tibial tuberosity, that increased quadriceps pull places a greater tensile load on the ACL and can contribute to ACL injury.

The quadriceps group pulls the tibia in an anterior direction. The ACL is designed to prevent excessive forward movement of the tibia. The hamstrings pull the tibia in a posterior direction. Consequently, they also prevent excessive forward tibial translation when contracting so their

contraction aids the role of the ACL. Hamstring function and strengthening becomes an important aspect of ACL rehabilitation because these muscles can aid the role of an injured ACL.

Narrowness of the intercondylar notch can also play a part in the onset of ACL injury. If the intercondylar notch is narrow, the ACL may rub against the medial side of the lateral femoral condyle (Fig. 7.3). Friction of the ligament against the side of the femoral condyle is likely to increase the incidence of ACL injury.[6]

Valgus stress to the knee increases tension on the ACL against the femoral condyles as well. Therefore, when attempting to identify the possible cause of ACL injury, it is important to analyze the mechanical factors that played a role in the initial injury.

ACL sprains are acute injuries that happen as a result of excessive loads placed on the ligament. These excessive loads commonly happen under certain circumstances:

1. Sharp deceleration or deceleration before a change in direction. When there is a sharp deceleration, one leg is placed in front of

the other to stop or slow the momentum of the body. There is a very strong anterior translation force of the tibia on the femur as the knee acts to absorb the body's momentum. The quadriceps muscles contract strongly to offer muscular resistance to the momentum. This combination of momentum and strong quadriceps force produces the ACL injury.

2. Landing from a jump is another activity that produces a sudden ACL sprain. The mechanics of this activity are much the same as those in the deceleration from running. There is a very strong anterior translation force placed on the knee when landing from a jump. The quadriceps contract strongly to resist gravity and absorb the body's weight. The strong quadriceps activity and body momentum lead to excessive loads on the ACL.

Treatment

Traditional approaches

If the sprain is not severe, it is usually treated with activity modification and the use of protective knee bracing. However, if the injury is more severe, surgical intervention is often required. Surgical techniques for treatment of ACL sprains have advanced significantly in recent years, and now these surgeries are performed with very good results and much shorter rehabilitation periods.

In instances, a total reconstruction of the ligament is the favored procedure.[7] This procedure involves taking the middle portion of the patellar tendon and using it to replace the damaged ACL. Small chunks of bone on each end of the tendon are also removed with the section of tendon that is used. The bone chunks on the end of the tendon are fixed to the femur and tibia, and eventually grow back into the bone creating a stronger attachment. Length of rehabilitation until the person can get back to full levels of activity for a complete ACL reconstruction is usually about 6 months.[4]

After the surgery physical therapy is very important during the rehabilitative phase. For example, strengthening of the hamstring muscles is important, as they are synergists for the ACL against anterior translation of the tibia.

Soft-tissue manipulation

General guidelines   Massage is not used for direct treatment of the ACL injury. Because the damaged ligament lies within the joint capsule deep inside the knee, it is inaccessible to palpation and massage treatment. However, massage still has a place in the rehabilitation of ACL sprains. Numerous secondary effects of the ACL sprain can benefit from massage treatment.

Spasm and/or tightness are/is common in the muscles surrounding the knee joint after an ACL sprain. Massage treatment to these muscles helps normalize biomechanical balance around the knee. Surgery is often performed for ACL injury and massage is advantageous for getting the individual back to optimum function following surgery. In the early stages after surgery, individuals may be prevented from moving their limbs through a full range of motion in order to protect the healing ligament. As a result, soft-tissue fibrosis may set in and cause longer delays in the healing process. Massage applications done during rehabilitation can enhance the healing process and prevent excessive fibrosis from developing. The various cross fiber and broadening techniques are most helpful in reducing the development of fibrosis.

The hamstrings are synergists with the ACL in stabilizing the knee against anterior tibial translation. As a result, they are prone to hypertonicity following ACL ligament injury. Massage applied to the hamstrings, helps them maintain proper neuromuscular tone. Reducing tension in the quadriceps with massage is also important because they pull the tibia in an anterior direction and place increased tensile stress on the ligament during healing.

Stretching of the quadriceps and hamstring muscles is advocated, but with some limitations. If the individual has had surgery for an ACL repair, it is crucial to consult with the client's physician and/or physical therapist to see what motions are being limited during the rehabilitation phase. During post-surgical rehabilitation certain motions are restricted to prevent excess stress on the ligament. Stretching must be performed within these motion limitations, and is usually not advised right after the surgical procedure. As the individual progresses through the post-surgical rehabilitation, more stretching is incorporated with the treatments, but should always be done within the functional limitations of the rehabilitation program.

Suggested techniques and methods

A. Sweeping cross fiber to quadriceps This technique applies superficial pressure to reduce tension in the quadriceps group. The stroke in the sweeping cross fiber technique travels diagonally across the fibers of the quadriceps muscle group with the sweeping motion of the hand and thumb (Fig. 7.4). Use successive sweeping strokes on the quadriceps until the entire muscle group has been covered.

B. Sweeping cross fiber to hamstrings A similar sweeping cross fiber technique is used to address superficial tension in the hamstrings, which might be hypertonic from the ligament sprain. Just as with the quadriceps technique, the stroke travels diagonally across the fibers of the muscle group (Fig. 7.5). Use successive sweeping strokes on the hamstrings until the entire muscle group has been covered.

C. Compression broadening to the quadriceps Increased pressure in this technique allows access to some of the deeper muscle fibers in this large muscle group. This broad cross fiber technique reduces hypertonicity. Use compression broadening strokes to work the entire length of the quadriceps muscle group. The application of each pressure stroke is directly transverse to the muscle fiber and primary circulatory flow (Fig. 7.6). Consequently, the muscle can be worked distal to proximal or proximal to distal.

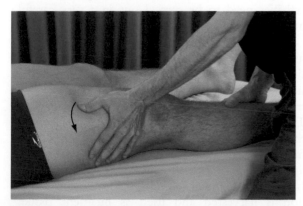

Figure 7.4 Sweeping cross fiber to quadriceps muscle group.

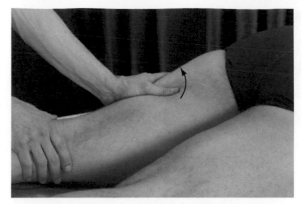

Figure 7.5 Sweeping cross fiber to hamstrings.

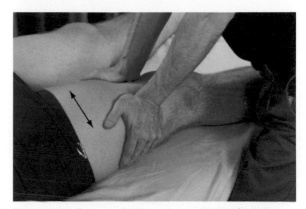

Figure 7.6 Compression broadening to quadriceps.

D. Compression broadening to the hamstrings Hypertonicity is further reduced with compression broadening. Apply the compression broadening techniques until the entire length of the muscle has been treated (Fig. 7.7). As with the quadriceps compression broadening technique, treatment can move distal to proximal or vice versa.

E. Deep longitudinal stripping to the quadriceps Elasticity and flexibility are enhanced with deep stripping applied to the quadriceps group. Deep stripping is used after broadening techniques and some of the more superficial applications are used to encourage adequate tissue fluid movement, warming, and superficial muscle pliability. Deep stripping can be performed first with a broad contact surface of pressure for more general muscle treatment and then with a small contact surface for deep specific muscle treatment (Fig. 7.8).

F. Deep longitudinal stripping to the hamstrings Stripping is used to treat the hamstrings for

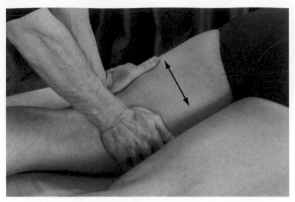

Figure 7.7 Compression broadening to hamstrings.

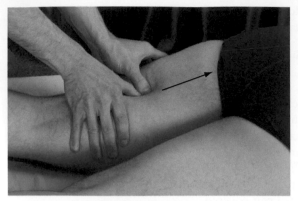

Figure 7.9 Deep stripping on hamstrings.

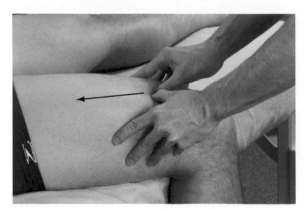

Figure 7.8 Deep stripping on quadriceps.

excessive muscle tension. Use the deep stripping techniques on the hamstrings in the same fashion as they are used with the quadriceps. Start with broad contact surface of pressure and then gradually perform the stripping techniques with a small contact surface (Fig. 7.9).

Rehabilitation protocol considerations

- The ACL is deep within the knee joint so no direct treatment of the damaged ligament is possible. The treatment techniques listed here are directed at secondary muscle spasm that results from the ligament injury or compensating biomechanical patterns.

- Consult with the physician or other supervising rehabilitation specialist about treatment approaches that would be most appropriate. Modifications to the suggested techniques mentioned above may be necessary for each unique client situation.

- The hamstrings serve an important synergistic function with the ACL in certain positions of the knee. It is not always advantageous to attempt complete flexibility and pliability of the hamstring muscle group. In severe ligament sprains hypertonicity in the hamstring group provides additional stabilizing support for the damaged ligament. Muscle tension can then be gradually reduced as the client progresses through the stages of rehabilitation.

Cautions and contraindications   Use caution with positioning if treatment is performed shortly after surgery. Protective braces are sometimes used to prevent the knee from going into full extension, which would stress the ACL. The practitioner must be careful not to put the knee in positions that compromise the ligament while it is healing. Range-of-motion activities need to be carried out in a very careful manner, so as not to further stress the ligament.

If surgery was performed for the ACL repair, use particular caution with treatment at the incision sites. It is wise to consult the orthopedic surgeon about the appropriateness of massage treatment in this region shortly after surgery. These sites can be susceptible to infection early in the healing process and all attempts should be made to keep them clean and free of massage lubricants that are being used during treatment. In some ACL repairs a section of the patellar tendon is harvested and used as ligament tissue. In this case use particular caution with massage treatment on or around the patellar tendon.

POSTERIOR CRUCIATE LIGAMENT SPRAIN

Description

The posterior cruciate ligament (PCL) connects the posterior aspect of the tibia to the anterior aspect of the femur. The primary function of the PCL is to prevent posterior movement of the tibia in relation to the femur (Fig. 7.1). PCL injuries are not as prevalent and cause far less functional instability than ACL injuries. However, PCL injuries may occur more often than they are actually reported.[8]

ACL injuries are most often the result of a non-contact injury where the momentum of the individual's body causes the injury. PCL injuries, however, occur more often from contact with an outside force. The mechanism of injury is usually a straight posterior force applied to the proximal tibia, driving it in a posterior direction. Common examples of PCL sprain include falling to the ground, where the proximal tibia hits the ground or another object first. This is especially likely to happen if the foot is dorsiflexed when the knee hits the ground, making the proximal tibia the initial point of impact.

Another example of PCL injury occurs to passengers in the front seat of a car in a head-on motor vehicle accident. If the force is sufficient, the passenger is thrown forward and the proximal end of the tibia hits the dashboard with a strong force. This force thrusts the proximal tibia posteriorly and causes a severe stretch or rupture to the PCL.

In addition to straight posterior stresses, the PCL may be injured from rotational stresses at the knee. Another role of the PCL is to prevent excessive rotation at the knee. Its orientation makes it a restraining ligament to lateral rotation of the knee.[9] Lateral rotation at the knee means the tibia is rotating laterally in relation to the femur. This motion occurs when an individual plants the foot and turns to the opposite side. This kind of sudden cutting motion happens a great deal in sporting activities, and is a common cause of ligamentous damage in the knee. Although its contribution to rotational stability is not great, there is still chance of ligament injury from excessive rotational stress. Biomechanical studies have also indicated that the PCL may play a stronger role in restraining rotational movements when the knee is in flexion compared to when it is in extension.

Isolated tears to the PCL can happen, but they are not very common. PCL injuries, especially those associated with rotational stresses at the knee, usually occur in conjunction with injuries to other soft tissues. The strong and powerful quadriceps, with their associated patellar tendon, lends additional resistance to direct posterior tibial translation. It is resisting rotational stress where the PCL and other soft tissues are under greater biomechanical demand.

Treatment

Traditional approaches

There are a number of different ways to treat PCL injuries. However, perhaps because isolated PCL injuries do not occur as often, treatment protocols for this problem remain undefined and controversial.[8]

Unlike ACL injuries, many PCL injuries are treated without surgery. If there is an isolated PCL injury and no other soft-tissue structure is significantly impaired, physical therapy is often sufficient to manage the condition.[10] Several authors have stated that non-operative procedures can be established for all grade 1 and 2 ligament injuries in the knee, as well as some grade 3 ligament tears that are isolated to the PCL only.[11]

Strengthening exercises are an important part of the rehabilitation process. Emphasis is placed on quadriceps strengthening because the quadriceps act as synergists to restrain posterior movement of the tibia on the femur.

Some PCL injuries are left untreated even if there is a significant tear to the ligament. If the client is not going to engage in activities that require a great deal of dynamic stability of the knee, the risks of surgery may outweigh the need for full knee stability. However, continued instability and excess movement in the knee are a potential risk factor leading to arthritic changes in the knee as the individual ages.

Soft-tissue manipulation

General guidelines   Massage approaches primarily play a supportive role in treating PCL injuries. Because the PCL is deep inside the knee joint, it is inaccessible to the palpating hand and therefore massage does not directly affect the ligament healing. However, massage may be used as an indirect adjunct to other treatments. As with treatment of ACL injuries varying levels of muscle spasm or biomechanical imbalance can occur around the knee joint. Massage reduces muscular hypertonicity and assists in restoring proper biomechanical function. As mentioned earlier, the quadriceps is a synergist with the PCL in preventing posterior translation of the tibia. As such, they may become hypertonic following an injury to the PCL. Massage treatment to the quadriceps is beneficial to make sure they maintain optimum biomechanical balance as the client regains knee function.

If surgery is performed for this condition, prevention of post-surgical fibrosis is a valuable contribution of massage. Various cross fiber and broadening techniques are most helpful in this process. During the rehabilitative phase, stretching helps restore proper biomechanical balance around the knee joint. Stretching that is aimed at maintaining a good length and flexibility balance between the quadriceps and hamstrings is the goal. Stretching methods should not put excessive stress on the healing ligament structure.

Suggested techniques and methods Treatment strategies for PCL sprains are indirect. The PCL is not accessible to palpation so no direct massage treatment is administered to the injured ligament. Massage approaches are all aimed at maintaining optimum biomechanical balance around the knee as the damaged ligament heals. See the suggested techniques and methods described above in the section on anterior cruciate ligament sprains. The same techniques, methods, and rehabilitation protocol considerations are applicable for PCL sprains.

Cautions and contraindications Because the PCL is not directly accessible to palpation, it is not likely that massage will damage the healing ligament. The main potential for harm in a healing PCL is excessive motion during joint movements or stretching procedures. As long as care is taken when performing those procedures and the client's tolerance for pain is considered, these treatments should be appropriate. Knowing the severity of injury will allow the practitioner to determine when to treat the condition and how much work

should be performed on the region. The more severe the injury, the greater must be the caution in applying soft-tissue interventions soon after the injury has occurred.

MEDIAL COLLATERAL LIGAMENT SPRAIN

Description

The medial (tibial) collateral ligament (MCL) is on the medial side of the knee and is the larger of the two collateral ligaments of the knee (Fig. 7.10). Its proximal attachment is on the medial condyle of the femur, and its distal attachment is on the medial side of the proximal tibia, just posterior to the pes anserine muscle group attachment. The pes anserine group includes the sartorius, semitendinosus, and gracilis. The angular direction of these muscles and their proximity to the MCL make them accessory stabilizers of the knee.[9] If there is a sprain injury to the MCL, these stabilizers can offer additional support.

The MCL is fibrously connected with the joint capsule of the knee. Injury to the MCL can also produce damage to the joint capsule. The medial meniscus also has a fibrous connection to the MCL. This fibrous connection is one of the main

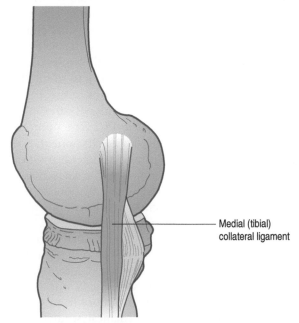

Medial (tibial) collateral ligament

Figure 7.10 Medial view of the right knee showing the medial collateral ligament.

reasons that MCL sprains often occur in conjunction with meniscal damage. When the MCL is exposed to high tensile forces, it can pull on the medial meniscus causing a tear in the cartilage.

The primary function of the MCL is to enhance medial stability of the knee. Specifically, it is designed to resist a valgus force to the knee. A valgus angulation at a joint is one in which the distal portion of the bony segment deviates in a lateral direction. At the knee a valgus force refers to the angulation of the tibia. Therefore, it would be a force directed in a medial direction that would cause the distal end of the tibia to deviate in a lateral direction (Fig. 7.11).

The ACL also provides some stabilization against valgus stresses at the knee. This may be one reason why ACL injuries often occur with extreme valgus stress on the knee. The ACL appears to play a stronger role in resisting valgus stress when the knee is in an extended position. It is for this reason that assessment procedures often put the knee in partial flexion when testing the MCL, so the role of the ACL in medio-lateral stability is minimized.

The MCL is part of a group of tissues called the *unhappy triad*. The unhappy triad includes the ACL, MCL, and medial meniscus.[12] The triad gets its name from the frequency with which these

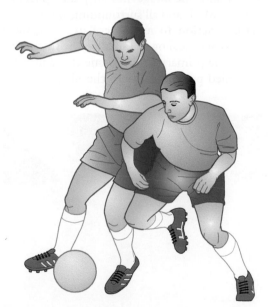

Figure 7.11 The player on the left is experiencing a valgus force to his left knee.

structures are injured together from a single incident. The injury commonly involves a strong valgus or rotary force to the knee. Injuries that involve the ACL and MCL together are quite common, even if they do not include damage to the medial meniscus. Several studies have indicated that the unhappy triad may really be a misnomer, because the authors had found more frequent injury to the lateral meniscus than the medial meniscus with combined ACL/MCL injuries.[12] What is important to keep in mind is that the MCL is often injured along with other structures in the knee, and they could all be part of a complex knee injury.

Treatment

Traditional approaches

MCL sprains are frequently treated without surgery. A number of sources have indicated that surgical repair of MCL injuries, rest, and immobilization are being de-emphasized in favor of early controlled motion and functional rehabilitation.[13–16]

In multiple ligament injuries, such as one where the MCL and ACL are both severely sprained, the ACL is often treated surgically, while the MCL is treated with conservative measures.[17,18]

There are several reasons why MCL injuries may fare better with conservative treatment than ACL injuries. The ACL has about half the expansibility of the MCL, and therefore it may be less resistant to tensile stress injuries.[16] Blood supply, which is essential for healing, may also play an important role. Blood supply to the collateral ligaments appears to be better than that to the cruciate ligaments. This is likely to have a negative impact on healing in the cruciate ligaments.[19]

Non-operative treatment includes the use of splints or hinged knee braces. The knee braces are adjustable to the severity of the knee ligament injury. Other forms of conservative treatment include protected weight bearing, inflammation control, range-of-motion and resistance exercises. The goal is to help provide support through accessory soft tissues while the primary ligamentous damage is healing. Following a ligamentous injury, muscles that cross the joint may play a greater role in joint stability, so strengthening of those muscles may be in order to create stabilization around the joint. The use of exercise measures such as resistance bands and balance boards may also be helpful, especially if the individual is trying to rehabilitate in preparation for a return to sporting activity.[20]

Soft-tissue manipulation

General guidelines   Unlike the cruciate ligaments, the MCL is easily accessible to treatment by soft-tissue manipulation. The client usually complains of a site of maximal tenderness in the ligament that corresponds to the primary site of tissue damage. Friction massage applied to the primary site of injury encourages fibroblast production and ligament healing.[21,22] In addition, the friction mobilizes the ligament against adjacent tissues and helps prevent fibrous adhesion with scar tissue during the healing process. Friction techniques used in treatment of a MCL sprain are most effective if they are performed perpendicular to the fiber direction of the ligament to prevent these adhesions.

In addition to the friction massage applications for the torn ligament fibers, massage can be applied to muscles that cross the joint to maintain their optimal tone and to decrease biomechanical imbalances that have been created in the process. It is likely that there is increased tension in the adductor muscles, as they will act as synergists for the medial collateral ligament. Following a sprain to this ligament, the adductor muscles can be hypertonic as they work to create stability around the knee. Stretching the adductor muscles is suggested if they have increased tightness following the injury. However, they may be contributing additional stability to the joint so over-zealous stretching can be counter productive.

Suggested techniques and methods

A. Sweeping cross fiber techniques to the medial knee Ligament, fascia, and muscle tissue is treated on the medial side of the knee with sweeping cross fiber techniques. There is an expanse of fascial connective tissue on the medial side of the knee. The sweeping cross fiber applications to the medial knee encourage mobility and pliability between the MCL and adjacent tissues. Start this technique with light pressure during the sweeping movements, then progress to gradually greater

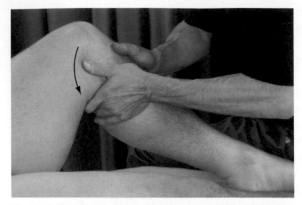

Figure 7.12   Sweeping cross fiber to medial side of the knee.

pressure. Use a sweeping motion with the thumb or fingers on the medial knee tissues with a mild to moderate amount of force (Fig. 7.12).

B. Multi-directional short stripping Deeper pressure is used with stripping applied to the medial aspect of the quadriceps retinaculum, distal pes anserine group, MCL, and all adjacent tissues. Use the thumb, finger, or pressure tool to apply deep short stripping strokes to all the tissues adjacent to the MCL (Fig. 7.13). The primary purpose of these strokes is to reduce tension in the surrounding tissues and encourage mobility and pliability between the MCL and all surrounding soft tissues.

C. Deep friction to medial collateral ligament Ligament tissue healing is enhanced with friction applied to the primary site of tissue damage. Friction is applied perpendicular to the fiber direction

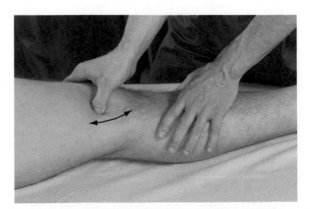

Figure 7.13   Multi-direction short stripping around medial collateral ligament and retinacular tissues.

of the MCL to encourage the greatest mobility between the healing ligament's scar tissue and adjacent soft tissues. Deep friction also encourages fibroblast proliferation that enhances the ligament healing. Perform the friction for several minutes and then follow with stretching and range-of-motion movements of the knee in multiple planes. Repeat the series of friction, movement, and stretching several times.

D. Sweeping cross fiber to the adductors Adductor tightness is likely to result from an MCL sprain. Sweeping cross fiber techniques are applied to the adductor muscle group to reduce excessive hypertonicity. The sweeping cross fiber movement has the thumb and hand moving with a diagonally curving motion across the adductor fibers (Fig. 7.14). It is also helpful to apply sweeping cross fiber techniques and effleurage to the thigh muscles to maintain optimum biomechanical balance.

Rehabilitation protocol considerations
- Direct treatment of an MCL sprain should only proceed if the injury is past the acute inflammatory stage.

- Properly assessing the degree of ligament damage guides the intensity and depth of deep stripping and deep friction techniques. The less severe is the injury, the earlier and more aggressive massage treatment can be. In a first-degree sprain, friction and deeper massage treatment can begin very soon, if not immediately. In a second- or third-degree sprain, superficial work in the area may begin right away, but direct work on the ligament injury should hold off at least several days after the acute inflammatory stage has ended. This waiting time gives the healing ligament a chance to have scar tissue spanning the torn and damaged fibers.

- Stretching and joint movement are an integral part of regaining optimum ligament function and should be immediately incorporated with the soft-tissue treatments administered in the clinic.

- Ice applications are sometimes used after more vigorous bouts of friction massage to reduce post-treatment inflammatory activity and decrease discomfort resulting from treatment.

Cautions and contraindications   The practitioner should accurately assess the condition to determine what level of friction massage is appropriate. Factors to consider include the severity of ligamentous injury (often determined with special orthopedic assessment tests), how recently the injury occurred, and visible signs of recent trauma in the area such as extreme redness, heat, or inflammation. If these signs or symptoms are present, it is better to delay massage treatment.

Stretching of the adductor muscles is advocated to reduce excess tension on surrounding thigh muscles that might be hypertonic after the injury. A number of the stretching positions for adductor muscles put increased valgus stress on the knee, so use caution in stretching the adductor muscle group.

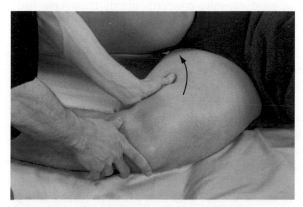

Figure 7.14   Sweeping cross fiber to adductors.

Box 7.1   Clinical Tip

One of the key factors when treating an MCL sprain is to make sure the healing ligament does not adhere to underlying tissues. Treatment with deep transverse friction is a valuable approach to address that concern. However, there is still the possibility of adhesion with underlying tissues, especially because the MCL may be fibrously attached to the meniscus. One way to enhance the mobility of the healing ligament is to perform deep friction treatments to the MCL while moving the knee in flexion and extension. Performing friction while moving the knee through a range of motion provides the greatest opportunity to have a strong ligament repair that is not adversely bound to adjacent tissues.

LATERAL COLLATERAL LIGAMENT SPRAIN

Description

The lateral (fibular) collateral ligament (LCL) attaches to the lateral condyle of the femur superiorly and the head of the fibula inferiorly (Fig. 7.15). The LCL is significantly smaller than its counterpart on the opposite side of the knee, the MCL. The LCL is not connected to the joint capsule of the knee or to the meniscus like the MCL is, so injuries to this ligament are rarely as severe as injuries to the MCL.

Sprains to the LCL usually occur from a pure varus load to the knee. A varus load to the knee would be one in which the knee was forced into a position with the proximal end of the tibia more lateral and the distal end more medial. This would occur, for example, with a direct blow to the medial side of the knee by a force that is moving from medial to lateral.

However, when a laterally directed force hits the medial side of the knee, an ankle sprain is more

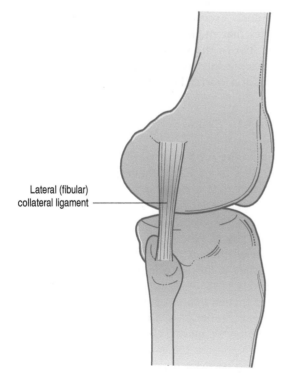

Figure 7.15 Lateral view of the right knee showing the lateral collateral ligament.

Lateral (fibular) collateral ligament

likely to result than an LCL sprain. The lateral ankle ligaments are a weaker point in the kinematic chain when excessive varus force is applied to the lower extremity so ankle sprains are more common than LCL sprains. Another reason the LCL is not injured as often is that it is protected by the opposite lower extremity. Consider a potential varus force hitting the left knee and coming from the person's right side. If an individual is hit from the right side, the right knee takes a valgus impact and protects the left knee from excessive varus force. The right knee would likely sustain the ligament sprain and protect the left knee from the varus force.

Treatment

Traditional approaches

Treatment for LCL sprains is similar to that for MCL sprains, and may include splints or hinged knee braces, protected weight bearing, inflammation control, range of motion and resistance exercises. The goal here is the same: to provide support through accessory soft tissues while the primary ligamentous damage is healing. However, since isolated tears of the LCL are not very common there is not a great deal of clinical evidence for effective treatments for this problem. The vast majority of these problems will be treated conservatively, with surgical treatment reserved for the most serious cases.

Soft-tissue manipulation

General guidelines   Deep friction massage is used to encourage fibroblast proliferation and the proper mobility of the healing ligament tissue. Because the LCL is not fibrously connected to the joint capsule, concerns about transverse friction applications being used to prevent adhesion to the capsule are not an issue. However, the concept of maintaining mobility with transverse friction massage plays a part with fibers of the iliotibial band that are directly on top of the ligament.

With LCL sprains there is rarely the same amount of correlating muscle hypertonicity that is present in MCL sprains. For one thing, there are fewer muscles producing abduction of the thigh than adduction. It is the abductors that work synergistically with the LCL. Primarily these are the tensor fasciae latae and gluteal muscles acting through the iliotibial band. While excess tension is not generally found in these muscles with an LCL sprain, there is benefit in addressing them as a part of the kinetic chain in knee stability.

Stretching will not play as much of a role in the rehabilitation process with LCL sprains, because there are not many tissues that can be adequately stretched across this area. The LCL has some synergistic help from the tensor fasciae latae through tension developed in the iliotibial band. However, hypertonicity in these muscles is not likely to develop in the same way it does, for example, with the adductors in an MCL sprain. Therefore, stretching plays a less significant role in the rehabilitation of this injury than it does with MCL sprains.

Suggested techniques and methods

A. Sweeping cross fiber techniques to lateral knee Superficial tissues are addressed and ligament adhesion reduced with cross fiber techniques applied to the lateral side of the knee (Fig. 7.16). This technique addresses the expanse of fascial connective tissues on the lateral side of the knee, just as they are treated on the medial knee in an MCL sprain. Start this technique with light pressure during the sweeping movements, then progress to gradually greater pressure.

B. Multi-directional short stripping Deeper and more specific pressure is applied with these short stripping techniques. The primary purpose of these strokes is to reduce tension in the surrounding tissues and encourage mobility and pliability between the LCL and all surrounding soft tissues. Short stripping is applied to the lateral aspect of the quadriceps retinaculum, iliotibial band,

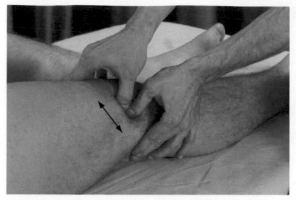

Figure 7.17 Multi-direction short stripping around lateral collateral ligament and retinacular tissues.

LCL, and all adjacent tissues. Use the thumb, finger, or pressure tool to apply deep short stripping strokes to all the tissues adjacent to the LCL (Fig. 7.17).

C. Deep friction to lateral collateral ligament Tissue healing is enhanced with deep friction applied to the site of fiber tearing in the LCL. The friction technique is applied perpendicular to the fiber direction of the LCL to encourage the greatest mobility between the healing ligament's scar tissue and adjacent soft tissues. Perform the friction for several minutes and then follow the friction treatment with stretching and range-of-motion movements of the knee in multiple planes. Repeat the series of friction, movement, and stretching several times.

D. Sweeping cross fiber to lateral thigh Iliotibial band and lateral thigh muscles are addressed with superficial sweeping cross fiber movements to reduce excessive hypertonicity (Fig. 7.18). Apply sweeping cross fiber techniques and effleurage to the thigh muscles to help maintain optimum biomechanical balance. Keep in mind when working on the lateral thigh region that the iliotibial band is a flat, sheet-like tendon and should never feel as pliable as the surrounding muscle tissue. Do not treat the iliotibial band aggressively in an effort to make it feel as soft and pliable as the surrounding muscle tissue.

Rehabilitation protocol considerations
● See the description of considerations under the MCL as they are virtually the same for this condition.

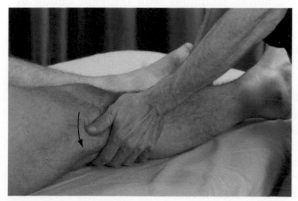

Figure 7.16 Sweeping cross fiber to lateral side of the knee.

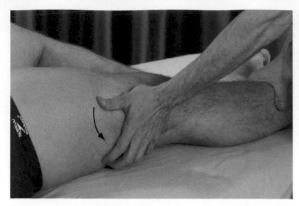

Figure 7.18 Sweeping cross fiber to iliotibial band and lateral thigh muscles.

- Surgery is performed far less often for LCL sprains, so there can be a greater reliance on soft-tissue treatment strategies to restore optimum function of the knee following an LCL sprain.

Cautions and contraindications The same cautions and contraindications exist as for treatment of MCL sprains except the cautions for stretching procedures are slightly different. Stretching procedures that focus on the thigh abductors are used most often to address tightness that may correspond with the ligament sprain. Use caution with thigh abductor stretches as some of the positions used to stretch this region put additional tensile stress on the LCL.

PATELLOFEMORAL PAIN SYNDROME

Description

Patellofemoral pain syndrome (PFPS) is not a specific condition with a clear cause or description. PFPS is a general term for anterior knee pain that may originate from a variety of causes. Some use the term incorrectly as a synonym for chondromalacia patellae. PFPS is characterized by anterior knee pain that is worse when using the extensors of the knee in activities such as ascending or descending stairs. The primary cause of the problem appears to be incorrect tracking of the patella during extension movements. Yet, it is not clear which tissues are the true source of pain in PFPS. Current literature indicates several possible sources of pain.

A basic comprehension of knee biomechanics is a prerequisite to understanding PFPS and patellar tracking disorders. To understand how a patellar tracking disorder occurs, it is important to understand some fundamental concepts of knee biomechanics. The patella is embedded in the quadriceps tendon, and its primary function is to improve the quadriceps' angle of pull on the proximal tibia. Because it is embedded in the quadriceps tendon, the patella is pulled superiorly along the quadriceps' line of pull. In most individuals, the quadriceps group does not pull in a straight superior direction, but along the line of the femur. The femur has a natural varus angulation (distal end of the femur deviating medially) so the quadriceps group pulls along this line. The degree to which this pull deviates from a straight vertical line can be visualized by evaluating the approximate Q angle for that individual and looking at the quadriceps line of pull (Fig. 7.19). See the description for how to determine the Q angle earlier in this chapter.

The distal portion of the vastus medialis muscle is called the VMO (vastus medialis obliquus), because its fibers run predominantly in an oblique (diagonal) direction. A primary function of the VMO is to offset the tendency of the other quadriceps muscles to pull the patella in a lateral direction. Strength imbalances between the VMO and the other quadriceps muscles are a main cause of tracking disorders and pain sensations associated with PFPS.[23]

Many anatomical structures around the knee joint, such as the quadriceps retinaculum and the fibrous joint capsule, are richly innervated. The medial and lateral sides of the patellar tendon have fibrous continuity with the joint capsule as well, and excessive stress on the tendinous fibers can pull on the capsule in turn. Consequently, it does not take a great deal of tensile force for the tissues to register pain.

Other tissues can also contribute to PFPS. The iliotibial band has fibrous connections with the lateral retinaculum of the quadriceps group. Excessive tightness in the iliotibial band could pull on the lateral retinaculum. Pain could result from the pull on the lateral side of the retinaculum, or from the tissues on the medial side of the knee that are also being pulled.

The client with PFPS complains of anterior knee pain that is aggravated by activities such as

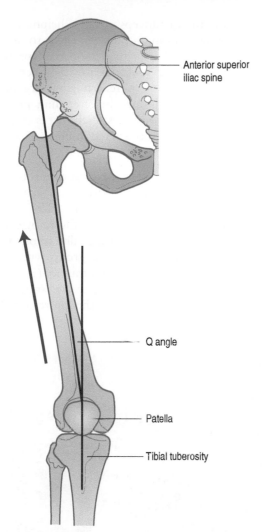

Anterior superior
iliac spine

Q angle

Patella

Tibial tuberosity

Figure 7.19 The quadriceps angle of pull depending on the Q angle (indicated by arrow).

ascending or descending stairs, squatting, or maintaining the knee in a flexed position for long periods. When the knee is maintained in a flexed position for long periods, many of the extensor tissues of the knee are pulled taut. The client may not feel anything until they change position. It is at this time that the pain sensations become most prominent. This experience is often called a *positive movie sign*, because it frequently happens in a theater when the individual stays seated in one position for about 2 hours. When they first get up and move around, there is a dramatic increase in pain sensations felt in the anterior knee region that gradually subsides after a few minutes.

Instability and feelings of giving way are also reported with PFPS. The instability is not necessarily from ligamentous damage or actual joint pathology. The cause of the sensation of instability and giving way comes primarily from reflex muscular inhibition. As there is a strong pain sensation in the knee extensors, the central nervous system essentially shuts off or decreases their contraction force. The individual experiences this sudden drop in quadriceps activity as the knee giving way and being unable to hold them up.

One of the clinical indicators that is often present in PFPS is atrophy of the quadriceps group. As a result of the knee pain, there is an inhibition of quadriceps activity. This can often lead to some degree of atrophy in the vastus medialis and lateralis muscles especially. This atrophy is evaluated by taking a circumferential measurement of the quadriceps group and comparing it to the unaffected side. A significant difference in circumferential measurement indicates some atrophy, and this can be a sign of extensor mechanism pathology. Atrophy is more apparent with quadriceps dysfunction than with some other muscle groups. That is because disuse atrophy affects anti-gravity muscles more than others. The quadriceps group is an anti-gravity muscle, and, therefore, more susceptible to this atrophy.[24]

Treatment

Traditional approaches

Conservative treatment is generally preferred for addressing PFPS. This is especially true if it is not clear which tissues are the source of pain. Conservative treatment comprises bracing, activity modification, and quadriceps strengthening exercises.[25]

There is some indication, although it is debated in the literature, that the VMO is most active in the last 20–30° of knee extension. Because one of its primary functions is to offset the tendency of lateral pull on the patella by the other quadriceps muscles, there is an emphasis on VMO strengthening.

Short arc quadriceps extension exercises against resistance are commonly used to strengthen the VMO. A short arc extension movement is performed in the last 20–30° of knee extension and repeated over and over. It is thought that strengthening the VMO in this range of the extension movement reduces the biomechanical imbalance around the joint.

Another intervention that has met with clinical success is patellar taping.[26–28] The client has restrictive tape placed on them similar to the way athletes do during sporting activities. The tape is thought to both encourage proper patellar tracking and influence proprioception in a way that leads to corrections in faulty biomechanical patterns.[29] Very often it is not one single treatment that is most effective, but a combination of various methods performed together.[30]

If conservative measures are not successful in alleviating the problem, surgical intervention may be used. One of the common surgical procedures for this problem is the lateral retinacular release. In this procedure the lateral retinaculum is cut in order to decrease the amount of lateral pull on the extensor mechanism. The effectiveness of lateral release surgery has been questioned recently.[31–33] One reason may be that the optimal biomechanical balance around the joint has been disturbed.

The problems from this procedure can also stem from the role of the lateral retinaculum. One study found that the lateral retinaculum helps stop the patella from moving laterally.[34] If this is actually true, surgically cutting the retinaculum can aggravate the problem.

Soft-tissue manipulation

General guidelines   Because a primary component of PFPS appears to be pain originating from the soft tissues around the knee, massage is valuable in treating this problem. Changes may not be immediate because the treatment is attempting to alter biomechanical patterns that have been established for some time. However, the client should feel some improvement in symptoms within three or four treatments. Massage treatment focuses on all of the quadriceps muscles as well as the patellar tendon and fascial retinacular tissues around the knee.

PFPS treatment addresses the soft-issue distress resulting from the patellar tracking disorder. In some cases there are other biomechanical issues, such as genu valgum or overpronation, which are exacerbating the tracking disorder. Some of these other biomechanical disorders may need correction in addition to the treatments that are focusing on the soft tissues around the patellofemoral articulation.

Stretching the quadriceps group is helpful both in the treatment room and for the client to do at home. It is a good idea to demonstrate proper quadriceps stretching methods for the client to make sure they are not overexerting or targeting the wrong muscles during the stretching procedure. An effective quadriceps stretch that is easy to perform at home is demonstrated in Figure 7.20.

Suggested techniques and methods

A. Sweeping cross fiber to quadriceps   Initial tension reduction in the quadriceps is achieved with sweeping cross fiber techniques. This technique also reduces excess pull on the retinacular tissues. The stroke travels diagonally across the fibers of the quadriceps muscle group with the sweeping motion of the hand and thumb. (See this picture in Fig. 7.4.) Use successive sweeping strokes on the quadriceps until the entire muscle group has been covered.

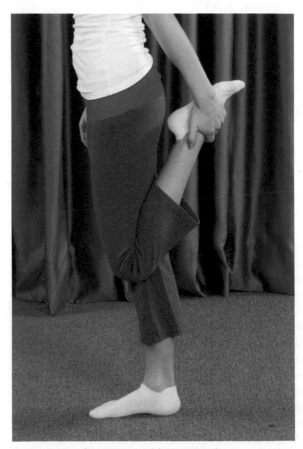

Figure 7.20   Common quadriceps stretch.

B. Compression broadening to the quadriceps Deeper pressure enhances muscle fiber spreading with compression broadening techniques. Use compression broadening strokes to work the entire length of the quadriceps muscle group. The application of each pressure stroke is directly transverse to the muscle fiber and primary circulatory flow. The muscle can be treated distal to proximal or proximal to distal. This technique is pictured in Figure 7.6.

C. Deep longitudinal stripping to the quadriceps Deep stripping is used after broadening techniques and some of the more superficial applications are used to encourage adequate tissue fluid movement, warming, and superficial muscle pliability. Deep stripping is performed first with a broad contact surface of pressure for more general muscle treatment and then followed with a small contact surface for deep specific muscle treatment. This technique is pictured in Figure 7.8.

D. Multi-directional short stripping on the retinaculum Short stripping strokes are applied to the medial and lateral aspects of the quadriceps retinaculum to reduce excess tension on the retinacular tissues. Use the thumb, finger, or pressure tool to apply deep short stripping strokes to the retinacular tissues around the patellofemoral joint. These techniques are illustrated in Figures 7.13 and 7.17. The primary purpose of these strokes is to encourage pliability and mobility in the fascial retinacular tissues.

E. Friction for patellar mobility Patellar mobility is enhanced with friction techniques applied around all sides of the patella. Grasp the patella between the thumb and fingers of both hands. Pull or push the patella as far to each side as possible and hold it in that position. When pushed medially, use short back and forth friction techniques along the medial side of the patella. When pushed laterally, use short back and forth friction techniques along the lateral border of the patella (Fig. 7.21).

F. Active engagement lengthening movements Increased pliability and flexibility are enhanced in the quadriceps with active engagement lengthening techniques. This technique also pulls on the retinacular tissues to encourage their pliability. The client can be positioned so the lower leg drops off the end or side of the table and is able to move through a full range of flexion and extension. Instruct the client to move the lower leg in full flexion and extension at a slow and steady pace.

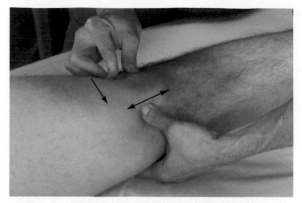

Figure 7.21   Patellar mobility friction treatment.

During the knee extension, perform a deep stripping technique to the quadriceps. Begin with a broad contact surface such as the fist or heel of the hand. Then gradually move to a more specific contact surface such as fingertips, thumbs, or a pressure tool (Fig. 7.22).

Rehabilitation protocol considerations

- While working on the soft tissues around the patellofemoral joint, pay particular attention to the tissues that reproduce the client's primary pain complaint when they are treated.

- After progress has been made with the techniques mentioned above and when the client is in the later stages of rehabilitation, additional resistance can be added to the active engagement methods with weights, resistance bands, or manual resistance offered by the therapist.

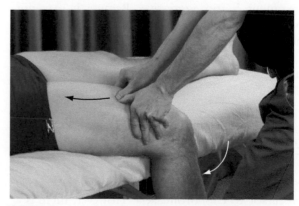

Figure 7.22   Active engagement lengthening for quadriceps.

- Pin and stretch techniques are also effective and can be used when active engagement methods are begun.

- In some cases fibrous adhesion has developed in the retinacular tissues. In these cases there can be significant pain when performing some of the deep friction or stripping techniques on the retinacular tissues, especially due to the rich innervation of these tissues. Work within the client's pain tolerance when addressing these fibrous restrictions. If the client is able to withstand a greater degree of discomfort, more progress can usually be made in tissue mobility enhancement.

- If the client is performing quadriceps strengthening as part of the treatment for patellar stability, achieving biomechanical balance of soft tissues around the knee with massage is an important adjunctive treatment.

- One of the common challenges in a problem like PFPS is overdoing activity once the condition begins to resolve. It is important to coach the client on a progressive and gradual return to activity that is not too fast. If the return to previous activity levels is too fast, the client is likely to stress the tissues that are attempting to return to normal function. This is likely to cause an aggravation of symptoms.

Cautions and contraindications   The practitioner should be careful pressure and intensity of certain treatments, especially the various deep stripping and friction treatments. The retinacular tissues are likely to be sore following treatment if the treatment is too aggressive. Because it may not be clear what the client's pain tolerance is and how his/her tissues react to the treatment, work a little less intensely in the first few treatments until the client's response can be evaluated.

CHONDROMALACIA PATELLAE

Description

Like PFPS, chondromalacia often starts with a patellar tracking problem. In fact, PFPS is a likely precursor to chondromalacia. However, there is a distinct difference between the two in that unlike PFPS, chondromalacia is a distinct clinical entity that can be verified through specific evaluation procedures. Chondromalacia literally means softening of the cartilage. The cartilage in this condition is not the meniscal fibrocartilage of the knee, but the hyaline cartilage on the underside of the patella.

If the patella is not tracking properly in the groove created by the two femoral condyles, there is an increased amount of friction on the underside of the patella. This increased friction eventually causes a softening and degeneration of the articular cartilage. The surface of the cartilage can become uneven and the client is likely to report crepitus (grating or grinding sensations) during flexion and extension of the knee.

For years it was assumed that the pain of chondromalacia was a result of the softening of the articular cartilage. Because the pain was happening in the same individuals who had crepitus and showed cartilage degeneration with arthroscopic examination, this only made sense. Yet, recent discoveries have indicated that the articular cartilage underneath the patella does not contain nerve endings so the cartilage degeneration is not causing the pain. However, the sub-chondral bone just below the surface of the cartilage is richly innervated and is the source of pain when the cartilage overlying it has degenerated.[35,36] Some clinicians state that chondromalacia should be used only as a descriptive term and not as a diagnosis of the pain since there is so little innervation of the articular cartilage.

Treatment

Traditional approaches

Because chondromalacia appears to develop from dysfunctions in patellar mechanics that are similar to PFPS, the treatment approaches are similar. This condition is initially managed conservatively with activity modification, bracing, stretching, and strengthening exercises. Strengthening exercises performed are generally the same as those for PFPS.

If the problem is not resolved through conservative treatment, surgical approaches can be used. Surgery for chondromalacia emphasizes smoothing the underside of the patella to prevent additional grinding of the articular surface resulting from the damaged and degenerated cartilage. This procedure is effective in alleviating symptoms for the majority of people who have it. Decreasing activities that place additional biomechanical stress on the knee is also important. Clients can also decrease biomechanical stress on the knee with compressive knee braces that encourage proper patellar tracking.

Soft-tissue manipulation

General guidelines   Massage treatment and rehabilitation protocol considerations for chondromalacia are the same as for PFPS. Because a large part of the problem is dysfunction in the extensor mechanism of the knee, treatment approaches focus attention in that area. The cartilage under the knee is inaccessible to massage and, therefore, no attempt is made to directly alter the course of the primary site of injury. In addition, because this problem involves roughening of the contact surface between two bones, massage would not have significant impact on changing the course of that problem.

Cautions and contraindications   One of the distinguishing characteristics that separate chondromalacia patellae from PFPS is the pain that is felt directly underneath the patella in chondromalacia. This pain is from friction and pressure on the subchondral bone. When performing massage or range-of-motion activities around the knee for chondromalacia, use caution not to exert undue pressure directly on the patella. It is likely to be painful and aggravate the existing condition.

Box 7.2   Clinical Tip

Chondromalacia and PFPS are two conditions that are closely related and the soft-tissue treatment for them is very similar. Stretching the fascial connective tissues of the quadriceps retinaculum is a valuable aspect of correcting patellar tracking problems that are creating these conditions. To stretch and fully mobilize the retinacular tissues, perform stripping techniques on the retinaculum itself while simultaneously moving the knee into flexion. These stripping techniques combined with lengthening the fascial retinacular fibers are very effective but can be uncomfortable for the client. Adjust the pressure and movement accordingly.

ILIOTIBIAL BAND FRICTION SYNDROME

Description

Iliotibial band (ITB) friction syndrome is an overuse condition that causes lateral knee pain. It occurs often in people who perform repetitive flexion and extension actions of the knee, such as runners and cyclists. Several predisposing factors make an individual more likely to develop this condition.

When the knee is in extension the iliotibial band lies anterior to the lateral epicondyle of the femur. As the knee moves into flexion the band moves in a posterior direction over the lateral epicondyle (Fig. 7.23). The posterior aspect of the band contacts the epicondyle first. Once the posterior fibers have made contact with the epicondyle the band drags across the epicondyle. Friction starts to occur between the band and the epicondyle at slightly less than 30° of flexion. This means the posterior edge of the band impinges against the lateral epicondyle just after foot strike in the gait cycle. Recurrent rubbing can produce irritation and subsequent inflammation, especially beneath the posterior fibers of the ITB. The posterior fibers can be tighter against the lateral femoral epicondyle than the anterior fibers.[37]

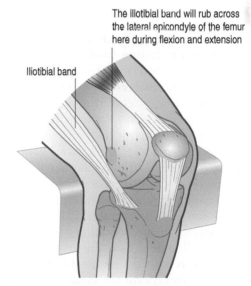

Figure 7.23   Movement of the iliotibial band in relation to the lateral epicondyle of the femur.

One of the primary functions of the iliotibial band is to enhance knee stability. There is a great deal of tension on the band to aid in this stability. However, excess tension can pull the band too tightly against the femoral epicondyle and this leads to the tissue irritation and inflammation of ITB friction syndrome.

In addition to tension on the band, anatomical variations in the knee, lower extremity, or ITB itself can contribute to this problem. A prominent lateral epicondyle can stick out further and cause excess friction. The postural distortion of genu varum (commonly referred to as 'bow legged') may cause increased tension on the band and subsequent pressure against the lateral knee. Activity that puts increasing varus stress on the lateral knee can also aggravate this problem. Running on the side of crowned roads can exacerbate this problem. The leg on the 'downhill' side of the slope is exposed to greater varus stress and therefore increased tension on the ITB.

One study found that individuals with ITB friction syndrome had a significantly thicker iliotibial band over the femoral epicondyle than a non-symptomatic control group.[38] Because it appears that the posterior fibers are primarily at fault, the thicker band makes it more difficult for the posterior fibers to roll over the lateral femoral epicondyle. It is not clear, however, if the thickened band is the cause of the condition or a result of continued friction.

Various sources have also described the pain of ITB friction as originating from a bursa that lies between the ITB and the femoral epicondyle. However, there is disagreement about the role played by this bursa, or even if it is an individual bursa. Nemeth and Sanders state the tissue under the ITB consists of a synovium that is a lateral extension and invagination of the actual knee joint capsule and not a separate bursa as often described in the literature.[39] In either event, there is a richly innervated cushioning tissue between the ITB and the femoral epicondyle that can also be the source of pain sensations in this condition.

While the literature on this condition has focused on the role of the iliotibial band and the synovial tissue underneath the band as the source of pain, there can be other possible causes for similar pain sensations. Restrictions in the local fascial tissue, and the development of myofascial trigger points in the vastus lateralis muscle can produce pain in a similar region and should be thoroughly investigated.[40]

Treatment

Traditional approaches

ITB friction syndrome is usually attributed to some repetitive activity that the client is performing. Therefore, activity modification is one of the primary methods of addressing the problem. If an individual is running, for example, the change can come through decreased distance or changing the location so they are not running on a sloped surface. Some authors advocate the use of orthotics to address lower-extremity biomechanical patterns that aggravate the ITB friction.[41,42]

Other methods of conservative treatment are employed as well. Anti-inflammatory medication can be used to decrease the inflammatory reaction of the ITB or the synovial tissue underneath it. Corticosteroid injection is one form of anti-inflammatory treatment that can be used in the region of the ITB friction. However, concerns over detrimental effects of corticosteroid injection have made this treatment method less desirable.[43]

Surgery is performed on ITB friction syndrome if conservative treatment is unsuccessful. However, surgery should generally only be recommended if attempts at conservative treatment have failed.[44] In the surgical procedure for this problem a small section of the posterior aspect of the ITB is cut away, so the band may more easily glide over the lateral epicondyle of the femur.

Soft-tissue manipulation

General guidelines   Massage can be an important part of the treatment arsenal for ITB friction syndrome. However, there are some important considerations in how and where massage techniques should be applied. As mentioned earlier, it is likely that myofascial trigger points, especially in the vastus lateralis muscle, may be contributing to pain sensations in the area. Investigate the possibility of these trigger points being the source of lateral knee pain. If the tissues are tight and sensitive but produce no characteristic referral sensations, myofascial treatments can still be effective.[45]

Bear in mind that, when working on the vastus lateralis muscle, pressure is being applied directly through the ITB. It is tempting to think that the ITB is loosening or 'releasing' through this type of work. However, the ITB is tendinous tissue and is not shortened or contracted itself. The tightness in the ITB, if it is excessive, is originating with the muscles that insert into the band up near the hip – the tensor fasciae latae and the gluteus maximus. Because these muscles are likely contributing to ITB friction, they should be a primary focus of treatment.

Suggested techniques and methods

A. Sweeping cross fiber to lateral and anterior thigh region This technique is moderately superficial in its pressure level and is designed primarily to enhance flexibility and tissue pliability in the soft tissues of the lateral thigh. Use the sweeping cross fiber motion that glides diagonally across the anterior and lateral thigh muscles (Fig. 7.24). There is initially a light to moderate pressure in this technique which can be increased as further treatment progresses.

B. Deep stripping techniques to lateral thigh muscles Stripping techniques should start with a broad contact surface such as the palm or back side of the hand first, and then gradually move into a small contact surface, such as the finger, thumb, or pressure tool (Fig. 7.25). Use caution with pressure when performing stripping techniques on the lateral thigh, especially directly over the iliotibial band. This region is likely to be very tender.

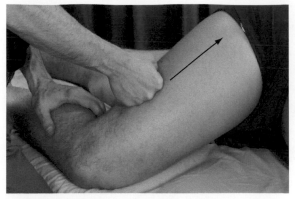

Figure 7.25 Stripping with broad contact surface on the lateral thigh.

C. Static compression Trigger points in the vastus lateralis, gluteus maximus, or tensor fasciae latae can contribute to ITB tension. Use the stripping techniques mentioned in B above to identify myofascial trigger points and encourage tissue elongation. Once trigger points or particular areas of heightened neuromuscular tension have been identified, static compression is applied to decrease neuromuscular activity (Fig. 7.26).

D. Pin and stretch to tensor fasciae latae Tension on the ITB is reduced by treating the tensor fasciae latae. The client is in a side-lying position on the table. The lower extremity is brought into a position of extension and abduction to shorten the tensor fasciae latae. Once in that position, apply pressure to the tensor fasciae latae muscle. It is a good idea to use a broader contact surface first and then gradually incorporate a small contact

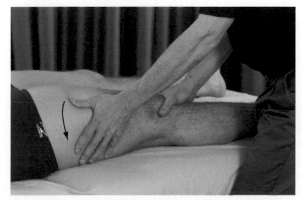

Figure 7.24 Sweeping cross fiber to lateral thigh muscles.

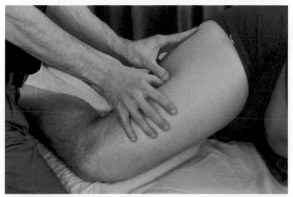

Figure 7.26 Static compression to lateral thigh region to treat trigger points.

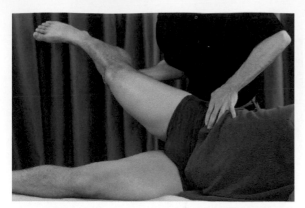

Figure 7.27   Pin and stretch on tensor fasciae latae. The muscle's shortened position is pictured (prior to moving the lower extremity into the muscle's stretch position).

surface as the technique is repeated several times. While maintaining pressure on the muscle, gradually lower the client's leg off the back side of the table until the tensor fasciae latae is fully stretched (Fig. 7.27). In later stages of treatment or to get an even greater effect of the pressure applied, have the client slowly drop their own leg, so the tensor fasciae latae is working eccentrically during the pin and stretch.

E. Deep friction to the iliotibial band Apply deep friction to the fibers of the iliotibial band (ITB) to stimulate fibroblast proliferation and encourage a positive healing response for the damaged tissue (Fig. 7.28). Depending on where the primary site of irritation is in the ITB, friction can aggravate the inflamed synovial tissue underneath the band. To avoid working directly over the epicondyle and irritating the synovial tissue, place the knee in different positions as the friction treatment is applied. To

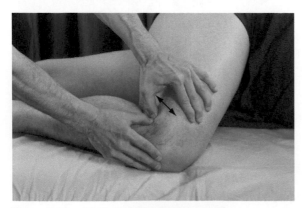

Figure 7.28   Friction to the iliotibial band.

work the anterior edge of the band, keep the knee in extension. To work the posterior edge of the band, keep the client's knee in full flexion. Try several different knee positions to see which produce the least discomfort to work the middle fibers of the band.

Rehabilitation protocol considerations

- If the condition is in an advanced stage, it may be too tender for friction or direct pressure techniques directly over the lateral epicondyle. Evaluate the severity of the condition to determine if these techniques should be used initially or held for later stages of rehabilitation.

- Presence of a tight ITB does not necessarily mean ITB friction syndrome will result. Consequently, a client can have an ITB that feels tight due to the tension on the tendinous fibers. It should not be a treatment goal to make the ITB as pliable and flexible as surrounding tissue.

- Biomechanical compensations in the lower extremity can play a role in the onset of ITB friction syndrome. Address soft-tissue tension in muscles throughout the lower extremity, especially the quadriceps group as they can contribute to ITB tension.

- Heat applications applied to the lateral thigh tissues may enhance stretching and massage treatment approaches through increased connective tissue pliability.

Cautions and contraindications   When performing friction techniques over the distal end of the ITB, use caution if the client reports a pain sensation with this treatment that mimics the pain they were experiencing during activity. This could indicate pressure from the technique is aggravating the ITB, and further compressing the inflamed synovial tissue underneath the band.

MENISCAL INJURY

Description

Inside the knee are two fibrocartilage structures that separate the tibia and femur – the lateral and medial meniscus (Fig. 7.29). Their primary function is to absorb shock and provide a greater degree of contact surface between the femur and the tibia. The shock absorbency of the meniscus

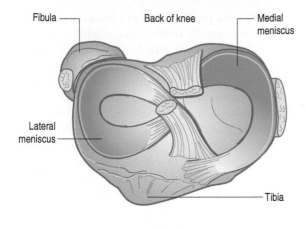

Figure 7.29   Superior view of the right knee showing the medial and lateral meniscus.

is crucial for long-term knee joint health. Each meniscus also provides a protective function to prevent the femur from rolling off the top of the tibial plateau. If the meniscus is severely damaged or removed from the knee, joint degeneration with arthritis is likely to follow.

The meniscus can be damaged from either compressive or tensile forces. Compressive forces can cause the meniscus to break, chip or tear. It is easy to see the amount of compressive force focused on the articulation between the femur and the tibia due to body weight. Tensile forces can also cause meniscal injury because the medial collateral ligament is connected to the medial meniscus. If there is an acute valgus force to the knee that pulls the MCL, it may be enough to pull or tear a portion of the meniscus as well.

Pieces of the meniscus can become separated from the intact meniscus and float around in the knee joint cavity. These loose bodies of cartilage can interfere with proper knee mechanics and often cause a locking or disruption of smooth knee movement.[46] Commonly, the knee will lock during one motion, but not lock when that motion is immediately repeated. This periodic locking occurs because the loose body of cartilage has moved slightly and is not in the same position to cause a joint restriction. Because this loose body of cartilage is often moving around in the joint and can so easily appear and then disappear it is sometimes referred to as a *joint mouse*.

Treatment

Traditional approaches

If the meniscal damage is not severe, physical therapy is usually successful in the gradual management and healing of the meniscal damage. Tears that occur in the outer edge of the meniscus, which has a greater vascular supply, have a good potential for healing. Tears on the inner portion of the meniscus where there is less blood supply do not have a good prognosis for healing on their own and may need to be treated surgically.[47]

While there have been a number of innovative surgical procedures for addressing meniscal damage, it does not appear imperative that meniscal tears always be treated surgically. Clinical evidence shows that people often get along fine with non-surgical treatment of meniscal problems. In fact, the risks of removing a meniscus can far outweigh those of leaving a tear in a portion of it.[48] Yet there are some concerns with non-operative treatment as well. Loose fragments can detach and a potentially repairable tear can pulverize and become too damaged for repair.

Soft-tissue manipulation

General guidelines   In this condition, the structures of concern are deep within the knee joint and out of reach for treatment with massage. There is little, if anything, that massage can do to address torn cartilage itself. As with ACL and PCL injuries, massage treatment and rehabilitation protocol considerations for meniscal damage focus on restoring proper biomechanical balance around the joint. Various muscles in the lower extremity can be hypertonic in an effort to compensate for altered knee mechanics resulting from the meniscal injury. Soft-tissue manipulation is a helpful adjunct to other measures used to treat the meniscal injury. To address meniscal damage with massage use the techniques and recommendations listed under ACL sprain at the beginning of the chapter.

Cautions and contraindications   When performing soft-tissue treatments around the knee, use caution with techniques that put pressure on the lateral or medial side of the knee near the joint line. If there is a meniscal injury that is near the periphery of the meniscus, pressure in this area could cause additional discomfort for the client. The pressure is unlikely to aggravate the injury, but could cause additional discomfort for the client.

PATELLAR TENDINOSIS

Description

This condition is frequently referred to as patellar tendinitis. The suffix -itis indicates an inflammatory condition. However, many are moving away from this term because a majority of overuse tendon disorders result from collagen degeneration in the tendon and not inflammatory activity.[49] Patellar tendinosis is also called jumper's knee because of the frequency with which it occurs in people who perform jumping activities like basketball or volleyball. However, the problem is by no means limited to people who do jumping activities. Pain is felt at the onset of activity and it is common for pain to subside during activity, only to return later when activity ceases.

The patellar tendon is the distal attachment tendon for the quadriceps muscle group. The patella is imbedded within the patellar tendon dividing the tendon into an upper and lower section (Fig. 7.30). The upper section is called the suprapatellar tendon and the lower section, the infrapatellar tendon. The lower section is sometimes erroneously

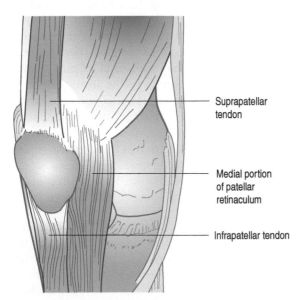

Figure 7.30 Suprapatellar and infrapatellar portions of the patellar tendon.

Suprapatellar tendon

Medial portion of patellar retinaculum

Infrapatellar tendon

identified as the patellar ligament because the fibers pass from the patella to the tibia, connecting bone to bone. However, the patella is imbedded within the tendon, making it structurally, functionally, and physiologically tendon tissue. The proper name for this structure is the infrapatellar tendon.[50]

Tendinosis occurs in either the suprapatellar or infrapatellar tendons. The condition appears in order of frequency at the infrapatellar tendon's insertion into the patella (65% of cases), the attachment of the suprapatellar tendon into the patella (25% of cases), and the patellar tendon insertion into the tibial tuberosity (10% of cases).[51,52] Dysfunction with the infrapatellar portion of the tendon accounts for 75% of all cases. If the tendinosis is not properly managed a complete rupture of the tendon can result.[53]

If left untreated, it can progress to a chronic state of degeneration and necrosis in the tendon.[54] Healing of collagen degeneration in tendinosis can take months instead of weeks because of the slow metabolic rate in tendon tissue.[55] As with a number of other conditions affecting the extensor mechanism of the knee, pathology with the patellar tendon can cause quadriceps atrophy. This may be detectable on visual comparison of the affected and unaffected sides, but can be confirmed by comparing circumferential measurements of the distal quadriceps on each side.

Treatment

Traditional approaches

Various anti-inflammatory medications have been used for treatment, but since this is not truly an inflammatory problem their benefit is highly questionable and generally ineffective.[49,56] When the problem is viewed as one that is not an inflammatory reaction in the tendon, the entire treatment paradigm shifts. While cryotherapy is traditionally considered as a modality aimed at reducing the inflammatory process, it may still be a beneficial part of tendinosis treatment. Cryotherapy is a vasoconstrictor and one of the keystones of this problem is abnormal development of vascularity in the injury site.[57] Cryotherapy is also beneficial for pain management during treatment.

Strength training has been used effectively in the treatment of tendinosis. It is employed early in the development of the condition as a means of conditioning the tendon for increased demands. However, if the tendinosis has progressed too far, strength training can be detrimental and aggravate the problem. In a measured amount it appears beneficial. One reason it may be effective is the stimulation of collagen production during tensile load on the tendon. As long as tendon load during strength training is not excessive and repetitive, it can assist the healing process.

Soft-tissue manipulation

General guidelines Because a primary part of the problem in tendinosis results from excess tensile load on the quadriceps group, soft-tissue manipulation should focus attention on reducing tension in these muscles. Numerous techniques used on the quadriceps group are effective for that purpose. Friction treatments are aimed at the site of primary discomfort in the tendon (usually infrapatellar tendon) in order to encourage fibroblast proliferation and tendon healing. Friction massage applied to tendinosis can be uncomfortable so cryotherapy is sometimes used prior to or immediately after friction treatment to reduce the discomfort.

Activity modification is an important part of addressing tendinosis conditions. The collagen degeneration in tendinosis takes a long time to heal, so reducing offending activities decreases the load on the tendon and gives the body time to mend the damaged collagen fibers. Along with activity modification, regular stretching of the quadriceps group is an important component of treatment.

Suggested techniques and methods All of the treatment techniques A–F that are described in the section on PFPS are valuable in the treatment of patellar tendinosis. In addition, deep friction applied directly to the site of primary tendon dysfunction is important.

A. Deep friction Friction treatment can be performed transversely or longitudinally (along the tendon's fiber direction). Deep friction treatment is generally more effective if the tendon being treated is on a slight stretch, so keep the knee in partial flexion during the treatment (Fig. 7.31). Stretching and range-of-motion movements should be incorporated along with the friction treatments.

Rehabilitation protocol considerations

- Treatment of tendinosis is likely to have limited benefit if the client is not able to decrease or eliminate certain offending activities, especially

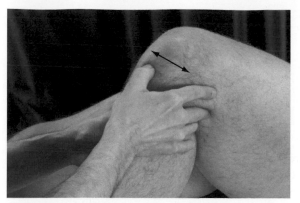

Figure 7.31 Deep transverse friction to the infrapatellar tendon with the knee flexed and the tendon on stretch.

during the course of treatment. The tendency for those recovering from tendinosis is to return to activities once the pain recedes in the affected tendon. However, tendon healing is much slower than other tissues and an early return to activity can easily re-aggravate the condition, making for a prolonged and chronic condition. It is better to be conservative in returning to activities that are likely to irritate the condition.

- The primary treatment goals of addressing any tendinosis condition involve decreasing tension on the offending muscle group and stimulating fibroblast proliferation. These objectives should be addressed simultaneously.

- If the condition is not severe, massage treatment can employ more intense forms of treatment such as pin and stretch or active engagement methods relatively soon. If the tendinosis is more advanced, it is best to gradually build up to the use of those treatment techniques. Use sweeping cross fiber, compression broadening, and passive stripping techniques first.

- The length of time necessary for positive outcomes with tendinosis varies significantly. If the tendinosis is of recent onset, the likelihood for a quicker resolution is greater. If the condition has been around a long time, there is likely damage to the collagen matrix of the tendon and healing time will be greater.

- Strength training is routinely used to condition tendons for the increased loads that are placed on them. However, if strength training begins too soon, it could further stress the damaged tendon fibers. It is best to wait until the rehabilitation process is well underway before engaging in significant strength training. Pain can be a guide. There should not be tendon pain associated with strengthening activities. If there is pain, long-term tendon damage could result.

Cautions and contraindications In some cases tendon damage is not the result of excessive activity. Certain systemic disorders or medications, such as fluoroquinolone antibiotics, could cause collagen degeneration in the tendon.[58–60] Massage that is too aggressive in these cases could potentially produce further tendon damage. If there is no overuse activity or recent change in activity levels that would indicate the onset of tendinosis, consider a systemic, metabolic, or medication-induced tendon injury as a possibility. Treatments should be tempered to a decreased intensity level in those conditions. Tendon pathologies caused by a systemic disorder could be continually aggravated, even despite the complete cessation of activity.

HAMSTRING STRAINS

Description

Hamstring strains involve a tear in the muscle-tendon unit of the hamstring muscles; biceps femoris, semitendinosus, or semimembranosus. These strains, as with all other muscle strains, are graded as first degree (mild), second degree (moderate), or third degree (severe). Strains can occur anywhere along the muscle, but frequently occur at or near the musculotendinous junction. This is a common location for tears to occur, because it is a place where the contraction force is transmitted from a yielding tissue type (muscle) to a non-yielding tissue type (tendon). This tissue interface becomes a focal point of stress and, consequently, a common site for muscle tearing. Third-degree muscle strains in the hamstrings also commonly occur at the interface where the tendon meets the bone at the ischial tuberosity.[61]

Muscle strains can happen to any muscle in the body, but are more common in the hamstrings than in other muscles. There are several reasons for this injury frequency. Strength imbalances between the hamstrings and quadriceps are a primary cause of hamstring strains. The structure and biomechanical demands placed on the hamstrings can be another reason. The hamstrings are multi-articulate muscles because with the exception of the short head of the biceps femoris they all cross more than one joint.

Multi-articulate muscles are more susceptible to muscle strain because they are acting across more than one joint at a time. The relationship of muscle length to the amount of tension generated in the muscle, referred to as the length/tension relationship, is such that great demands are placed on the hamstring muscles when they are not in a position to handle the mechanical load of their length/tension relationship. These high loads overwhelm the contractile unit and connective tissues within the muscle and cause a strain or tear in the fibers. It is interesting, however, that despite the short head of the biceps femoris only crossing the knee joint, the greatest number of hamstring strains occur in the biceps femoris.[62]

Various factors including lack of flexibility, muscle fatigue, insufficient warm-up, and strength imbalances play a role in the onset of hamstring strains.[63] Hamstring strains are usually an acute injury, but small levels of stress can accumulate and cause chronic low-grade tearing as well. Along with acute strains it is common to have a large amount of bruising. Bruising can extend down the posterior lower extremity over the days following the injury, making the problem look much more widespread than it really is.

Hamstring strains are characterized by sharp pain that occurs at the initial time of injury. The client frequently describes hearing a loud pop or snap when the injury occurred. Pain is strong locally, and the three hallmarks of musculotendinous injury are present – pain with palpation, pain with manual resistance, and pain with stretching. Symptoms may persist for long periods and re-injury is common.

Adverse neural tension can also play a part in the onset of hamstring strains.[64] The increase in neural tension causes an elevated level of tonus in the muscle, which in turn makes the muscle more susceptible to mechanical strain. This can become a vicious cycle because adverse neural tension can occur as a result of hamstring strain as well.[65] Fibrous adhesions or scar tissue in the hamstring muscles from a strain can restrict mobility of the sciatic nerve. Then a situation of adverse neural tension develops leading to the likelihood of frequent recurrence of the strain.

Treatment

Traditional approaches

The principle mode of treatment starts with PRICE (Protection, Rest, Ice, Compression, Elevation). A physician may prescribe anti-inflammatory medication, although long-term use of anti-inflammatory medication is generally not advised for this condition.[66]

Functional treatment involving stretching and strength training to build the muscle back to its original level of strength is a mainstay of this conservative approach. Treatment that includes movement and strength training can become more active after the sub-acute phase when the initial swelling has subsided.[67] Conservative treatment emphasizing a reduction in offending activities is usually enough to let the body's healing processes take care of the strain if it is not severe.

If there is a grade three strain, or one that includes a tendon avulsion (tearing away of the tendon from its attachment to the bone), surgery may be indicated, although not all avulsions need surgery. If there is suspicion of a severe muscle strain, it should be properly evaluated to determine if there is a tendon avulsion or avulsion fracture. An avulsion fracture occurs when the tendon pulls a small chunk of bone with it as it pulls away from the attachment site.

Soft-tissue manipulation

General guidelines   The primary function of massage treatment for hamstring strains is to reduce reactive muscle tightness and address the primary site of the fiber tearing. Reduction of muscle tightness is accomplished with effleurage, compression broadening techniques, sweeping cross fiber, and longitudinal stripping techniques performed on the hamstrings.

In addition to these passive techniques, various forms of massage with active engagement are effective as well. These methods enhance functional restoration to the hamstring group by emphasizing soft-tissue manipulation during movement. Both shortening and lengthening movements are used for this purpose. Additional muscular effort can be recruited to enhance the effectiveness of elongating deeper fascial tissues. Use a piece of resistance band or the hand to produce additional eccentric load for the hamstrings during the elongation.

It is also important to address the primary site of tissue damage. Massage is an effective way to stimulate collagen production at the site of tissue damage. Deep transverse friction (DTF) helps create a healthy and mobile scar. Identification of the actual strain is accomplished by finding a site of maximum tenderness that reproduces the primary complaint the client initially had. If the strain is of sufficient intensity, a palpable defect is likely to be felt in the muscle.

Apply friction to the site of the strain for several minutes. The friction massage should be alternated with other forms of tissue mobilization including effleurage, sweeping cross fiber, and stretching. That series of techniques should then be repeated several more times.

As the injury site is beginning to heal, stretching is an important aspect of treatment. Stretching has benefits not only in elongating the myofascial tissues in the leg, but also in reducing adverse neural tension that can contribute to perpetuation of the problem.[64]

Suggested techniques and methods   Numerous techniques and methods will be valuable in addressing hamstring strains. The following techniques that have been described in prior sections of this chapter are used to address hamstring strains.

A. Sweeping cross fiber to hamstrings   This stroke reduces initial muscle tension throughout the muscle group. The stroke travels diagonally across the fibers of the muscle group (Fig. 7.5). Use successive sweeping strokes on the hamstrings until the entire muscle group has been covered.

B. Compression broadening to the hamstrings   Further fiber broadening and muscle pliability is enhanced with compression broadening techniques. Apply the compression broadening techniques until the entire length of the muscle has been treated. Compression broadening techniques can move distal to proximal or vice versa (Fig. 7.7).

C. Deep longitudinal stripping   Tissue elasticity is enhanced with deep stripping techniques. Start with a broad contact surface of pressure and then eventually perform the stripping techniques with a small contact surface (Fig. 7.9). Use caution in stripping techniques near the site of muscle strain, especially if the strain is more severe.

D. Deep transverse friction   Friction is applied to the primary site of tissue damage. In most cases this

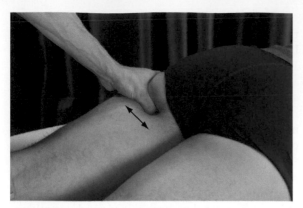

Figure 7.32 Deep transverse friction to proximal musculotendinous junction of hamstring muscles.

will be at the musculotendinous junction, but use proper assessment to identify the injury site specifically. Friction is applied transverse to the fiber direction of the hamstrings to help proper alignment of scar tissue as the damaged tendon fibers are healing (Fig. 7.32).

Rehabilitation protocol considerations

* The degree or intensity of work is directly related to the severity of the strain. For example, vigorous stripping is not used early in the rehabilitation process, especially in the case of a second- or third-degree strain. In the case of a more severe strain, use lighter work such as effleurage and sweeping cross fiber until a greater degree of tissue repair has occurred at the primary injury site. Accurate assessment is crucial for identifying the severity of injury and appropriate treatment at different stages of the injury management.

* When working with athletes or others in active lifestyles, deeper and more penetrating methods such as active engagement shortening or lengthening techniques can also be incorporated. These techniques are used in the latter stages of rehabilitation when a significant degree of tissue remodeling has already been accomplished. There should be sufficient strength and resiliency rebuilt in the hamstring muscle before attempting these procedures.

* Stretching should be a fundamental component of the treatment from the outset. Stretching enhances tissue mobility and will aid in developing an optimally functioning tissue repair site.

Cautions and contraindications The primary cautions and contraindications with massage treatment of hamstring strains are related to working aggressively on the injury too soon after its occurrence. If the strain is severe and affects the attachment site instead of the musculotendinous junction, there could be a tendon avulsion. If an avulsion is suspected refer the client for orthopedic evaluation in case surgical reattachment of the tendon is deemed necessary.

ADDUCTOR STRAINS

Description

Strains to the adductor muscle group are relatively common, especially for people engaged in various sporting and recreational activities. They are also called, *groin strain* or *groin pull*. Regardless of the name, the pathology is a strain to one of the adductor muscles of the thigh. The adductor group is composed of five different muscles: adductor longus, adductor brevis, adductor magnus, pectineus, and gracilis (Fig. 7.33). Of these five, the adductor longus is the muscle most often strained.[68] However, the fibers of these different muscles often blend together near their attachment

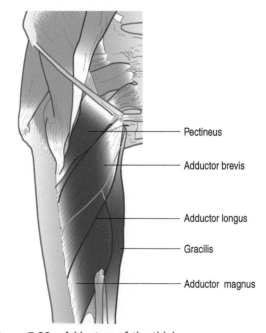

Pectineus

Adductor brevis

Adductor longus

Gracilis

Adductor magnus

Figure 7.33 Adductors of the thigh.

sites, so it is difficult to distinguish among them at the musculotendinous junction.

As with other muscles, an adductor strain is graded as either mild (first degree), moderate (second degree), or severe (third degree). A third-degree strain usually indicates a complete rupture of the muscle tendon unit or an avulsion of the tendon from its attachment site on the bone. The classification for grading strains is somewhat subjective, so there can be slight variations in determining the category of this injury.

There are several common causes of adductor strain. A forced abduction of the thigh that goes beyond the individual's flexibility limit is a common cause. An example of this is when a person slips on the ice and one leg suddenly goes out to the side. Another example is during a blocked kick in soccer. A sudden eccentric load is put on the adductors when the individual is kicking the ball with the instep of the foot and they are blocked in mid stride of the kick. The sudden stopping of the kick can be enough to produce a strain on one of the adductor muscles. The same type of sudden loading to the adductors can occur when an individual suddenly changes direction while running, turning to the side opposite that of the planted foot.

Strength deficits are a factor in the development of adductor strains. For example, ice-skating is an activity that uses a tremendous amount of adductor muscle activity, both to maintain balance and create forward propulsion on the skates. One study with hockey players found that the players were 17 times more likely to sustain an adductor muscle strain if the adductor muscle strength was less than 80% of the abductor muscle strength.[69]

Clients who have sustained an adductor strain generally complain of pain localized near the attachment of the adductor muscles on the pubic bone. The majority of adductor strains occur near the proximal attachment of the muscles. Swelling or ecchymosis may be present, but their absence does not rule out an adductor strain. Look for the classic musculotendinous injury triad, which includes pain with palpation, pain with stretching, and pain with manual resistance.

Treatment

Traditional approaches

The usual treatment of PRICE (Protection, Rest, Ice, Compression, Elevation) is the first line of treatment for an individual who has sustained an adductor strain. A physician may prescribe anti-inflammatory medication, although long-term use of anti-inflammatory medication is generally not advised for this condition.[66]

Functional treatment involving stretching and strength training later in the course of rehabilitation is used to build the muscle back to its original level of strength. Treatment that includes movement and strength training can become more active after the sub-acute phase when the initial swelling has subsided.[67] Conservative treatment emphasizing a reduction in offending activity is usually enough to let the body's healing processes take care of the strain if it is not severe.

Strength training is used as a preventive strategy for individuals who are at risk of developing adductor strains. The strength increase allows the muscles to develop greater resistance to the forces that produce muscle strain.[70] Strength training can be used following a strain, but should not be performed aggressively because the increased demands on the tissue could produce further damage.

Soft-tissue manipulation

General guidelines   As with other muscle strains, the primary function of treating them with massage will be to reduce reactive muscle hypertonicity and address the site of tissue tearing. Reduction of muscle hypertonicity can be accomplished primarily with effleurage, compression broadening techniques, sweeping cross fiber, and longitudinal stripping techniques.

Deep friction massage is applied to the site of the strain in the muscle. Identify the primary site of tissue injury in the strain by finding a site of maximum tenderness that reproduces the client's complaint. If the strain is of sufficient intensity, a palpable defect may also be felt in the muscle. The triad of signs for musculotendinous injury should be present: pain with palpation, pain with manual resistance, and pain with stretching. In each of these three situations, it is likely that the primary site of pain is going to be the location of tissue tearing.

Deep transverse friction is applied to the site of the strain to help develop a functional, flexible, and pliable injury repair site. The friction massage should be alternated with other forms of tissue mobilization including effleurage, sweeping cross fiber, and stretching. That series of techniques should then be repeated several more times.

In addition to the soft-tissue treatment methods advocated, stretching is an important part of the rehabilitation process. Stretching methods can be performed in the clinic at the same time that other soft-tissue treatments are being administered. The client can also be instructed in stretching procedures which can be performed at home.

Suggested techniques and methods

A. Sweeping cross fiber to adductors Superficial relaxation and fiber broadening occurs with sweeping cross fiber methods. The stroke travels diagonally across the fibers of the muscle group (Fig. 7.34). Use successive sweeping strokes on the adductor group until the entire region has been covered.

B. Compression broadening to the adductors Deeper compression broadening techniques reduce hypertonicity as well as encourage muscle fiber repair and development of a functional scar. Apply the compression broadening techniques until the entire length of the muscle has been treated. Compression broadening techniques can move distal to proximal or vice versa (Fig. 7.35).

C. Deep longitudinal stripping Stripping techniques emphasize muscle elasticity and pliability. Start with a broad contact surface of pressure and then gradually perform the stripping techniques with a small contact surface (Fig. 7.36). Use caution in stripping techniques near the site of muscle strain, especially if the strain is more severe.

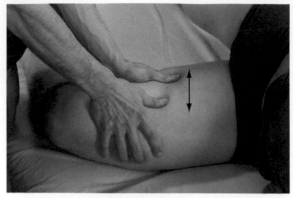

Figure 7.35 Compression broadening to adductors.

D. Deep transverse friction Friction is applied to the primary site of tissue damage, which is usually at the musculotendinous junction. Use proper assessment to identify the injury site specifically. See the discussion of deep friction treatments in Chapter 4 for guidelines about length of friction treatments and incorporating friction with movement and stretching of the affected tissues. Friction is applied transverse to the fiber direction of the hamstrings to encourage proper alignment of scar tissue as the damaged tendon fibers are healing (Fig. 7.37).

A common site of strain to the hamstrings is at the proximal musculotendinous junction. This poses challenges in treatment because of the proximity to the groin. Soft-tissue work in the groin area can be uncomfortable both physically and psychologically for the client. Consequently, a great sense of presence and care is needed when performing treatments. Special attention to draping and hand position assures

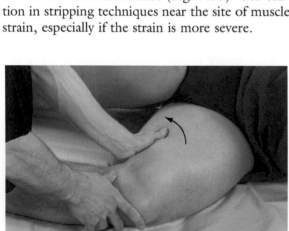

Figure 7.34 Sweeping cross fiber to adductors.

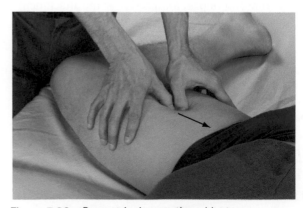

Figure 7.36 Deep stripping on the adductors.

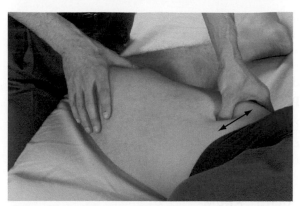

Figure 7.37 Deep friction to the adductors.

the client will feel a greater sense of comfort and confidence with the treatment. One way to address this issue is to have the client place a hand over the top of the drape to hold it in place over the groin while working this region. This reduces the possibility of unintentional contact with the genital region. Pay close attention to hand and finger position when performing friction or stripping techniques in this region. Keeping the fingers curled into the palm when treating this region also decreases the chance of unintentional contact by the practitioner's finger tips.

Rehabilitation protocol considerations   See the description of rehabilitation protocol considerations for hamstring strains in the previous section. These considerations will be the same for treating adductor strains.

Cautions and contraindications   Bear in mind that there are vascular structures traveling through the femoral triangle in the region of the adductor muscles. The femoral artery and vein, as well as the femoral nerve, can be compressed during manual treatment of the adductors. Keep in close communication with the client in order to recognize signs or symptoms of compressing these structures.

POSTURAL DISORDERS

The next section includes a number of structural and postural disorders of the knee and thigh. These disorders are not considered injury conditions, as are the prior conditions in this chapter. However, they can produce considerable stress on other tissues or structures and contribute to their dysfunction. Massage is generally not used to correct these postural deviations, but can be a therapeutic approach to restoring appropriate biomechanical balance around the joint.

GENU VALGUM

Description

This is the condition that is known in layman's terms as *knock-knees*. It is a structural deviation of the lower extremity that is defined by a varus angulation of the femur and a valgus angulation of the tibia (Fig. 7.38). It is unclear exactly what causes this problem. In some cases it seems to be a congenital postural distortion, while in others it seems to be more of an acquired condition. Children often have genu valgum during the growth years, and eventually grow out of the problem as their skeletal and muscular structures mature.

There are a number of problems that can result from genu valgum, which often involve biomechanical dysfunction of the lower extremity, especially around the knee. The femur already has a natural varus angulation so it does not drop straight down onto the tibial plateau. Yet, weight

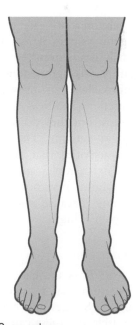

Figure 7.38 Genu valgum.

is transmitted from the femur to the lower leg. It would be best if this weight could be transmitted as evenly as possible. When the angulation is increased as it is in genu valgum, there is an increasing amount of compressive force on the lateral meniscus and the lateral aspect of the tibial plateau. There is also, consequently, a greater degree of tensile stress on some of the soft-tissue structures on the medal side of the knee that are spanning the joint, such as the joint capsule or the medial collateral ligament. The increased tensile stress causes these structures to be more vulnerable to injury.

A more significant concern with genu valgum is the effect it has on patellar tracking. The patella must glide in a superior and inferior direction in relation to the femoral condyles during flexion and extension of the knee. With an individual that has genu valgum, there is a tendency for the patella to track in a more lateral direction as it moves superiorly during knee extension. This alteration in patellar tracking can lead to a number of soft-tissue pain complaints in and around the knee, such as patellofemoral pain syndrome or chondromalacia patellae.

Treatment

Traditional approaches

Changing genu valgum is not easy. If there appears to be a severe genu valgum it may be addressed surgically, especially in children. However, changing lower-extremity misalignment in adults with non-surgical approaches has proved difficult.[71] Orthotics are used to address lower-extremity alignment problems, but they do not appear very effective with genu valgum. The client can be advised to avoid activities that could make the problem worse. For example, an individual with significant genu valgum may not be cut out for recreational running because the likelihood of developing knee pain is high.

Soft-tissue manipulation

General guidelines   It is unclear if there is any soft-tissue intervention that is successful in correcting genu valgum. Suggestions have been made that adductor muscle tightness can play a role in genu valgum, but how much of a role it plays is unclear. There are other factors of bony alignment that do not appear to be significantly affected by soft-tissue tightness. However, massage treatment of all the thigh musculature can aid in developing optimal biomechanical balance and postural correction.

Cautions and contraindications   Other than general precautions there are no major contraindications for working on a client with genu valgum.

GENU VARUM

Description

This postural distortion is just the opposite of genu valgum. It is the condition commonly referred to as *bow-legged*. In this problem there is a valgus angulation of the femur and a varus angulation of the tibia (Fig. 7.39). Both genu valgum and genu varum take their name from the angulation of the tibia, and not of the femur. Genu varum can occur frequently in children as their bones are growing. It is quite common for children to have genu varum in the first years of life and then grow out of it and have genu valgum for several years after that before finally achieving a more normal degree of knee alignment.

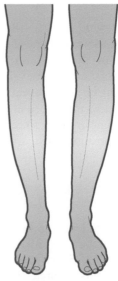

Figure 7.39   Genu varum.

Like genu valgum, this postural distortion can aggravate other lower-extremity problems. In genu varum there is greater compressive stress on the medial meniscus, and greater tensile stress on the lateral knee structures such as the lateral collateral ligament or the iliotibial band. Greater tensile stress on the iliotibial band from genu varum is a common contributing factor to iliotibial band friction syndrome.

In most cases, genu varum is associated with structural changes that cause the misalignment, and not soft-tissue changes that can be improved with massage. Genu varum has a reputation of occurring in certain activities like riding horses for long periods. It is unlikely that soft-tissue treatment can actually reverse this process without significant postural retraining. However, soft-tissue treatment of conditions like iliotibial band friction syndrome that result from genu varum may be addressed with massage treatment.

Treatment

Traditional approaches

Genu varum is addressed in the same way as genu varum. Orthotics are sometimes used to address the ramifications of this postural disorder. If genu varum appears that it is going to be a problem in children, corrective braces or surgery are sometimes used to address the postural distortion.

Soft-tissue manipulation

General guidelines   Massage treatment for genu varum is only an adjunctive procedure that focuses on restoring optimal biomechanical balance in the muscles and fascia of the thigh region.

Cautions and contraindications   Other than general precautions there are no major contraindications for working on a client with genu varum.

Box 7.3   Case Study

Background

Marie is a 46-year-old advertising executive who travels a great deal. In order to reduce stress and stay in shape she has recently begun a recreational running program. She really likes running and does not want to give it up. Unfortunately, she has been experiencing anterior knee pain on her left knee and she believes it is associated with her running as she first noticed it about a month after starting her running program. The pain comes on while she is running and does not seem to bother her as much on the days when she does not run. She also notices the pain when she squats down to pick something up off the floor. She has tried to increase stretching prior to and after her activities, but said she also feels the knee pain somewhat when she attempts quadriceps stretching.

Observation of Marie's posture from an anterior position indicates a slight genu valgum posture in her lower extremity. Viewed from the lateral direction there is also a slight degree of anterior pelvic tilt apparent. When palpating the soft tissues around her knee there is tenderness in the fascial, retinacular, and tendinous tissues around the medial and inferior side of her patella.

Questions to consider

- What are three different tissues around the knee that could be responsible for Marie's pain?
- While we don't have enough information from a thorough evaluation, does Marie's knee pain initially sound like something that would be treatable with massage? Why or why not?
- Marie travels a great deal and long trips on an airplane sometimes cause an increase in her symptoms. Why might sitting for long periods cause an increase in pain?
- Do you think that she might have an internal joint disorder, such as a meniscal injury or ligament sprain? Why or why not?
- How might other postural conditions, such as overpronation or pelvic tilt, contribute to Marie's knee pain?
- Is there anything Marie might be able to do at home that will help this condition?

References

1. Arnold T, Shelbourne KD. A perioperative rehabilitation program for anterior cruciate ligament surgery. Physician Sportsmed. 2000;28(1):283–293.

2. Arendt E, Dick R. Knee injury patterns among men and women in collegiate basketball and soccer. NCAA data and review of literature. Am J Sports Med. 1995;23(6):694–701.

3. Boden BP, Griffin LY, Garrett WE, Jr. Etiology and prevention of noncontact ACL injury. Physician Sportsmed. 2000;28(4):53–60.

4. Torg J, Shephard R. Current Therapy In Sports Medicine. 3rd ed. St. Louis: Mosby; 1995.

5. Nisell R. Mechanics of the knee. A study of joint and muscle load with clinical applications. Acta Orthop Scand Suppl. 1985;216:1–42.

6. Harner CD, Paulos LE, Greenwald AE, Rosenberg TD, Cooley VC. Detailed analysis of patients with bilateral anterior cruciate ligament injuries. Am J Sports Med. 1994;22(1):37–43.

7. Delay BS, Smolinski RJ, Wind WM, Bowman DS. Current practices and opinions in ACL reconstruction and rehabilitation: results of a survey of the American Orthopaedic Society for Sports Medicine. Am J Knee Surg. 2001;14(2):85–91.

8. Morgan EA, Wroble RR. Diagnosing posterior cruciate ligament injuries. Physician Sportsmed. 1997;25(11):224–232.

9. Kapandji IA. The Physiology of the Joints: Volume 2 – Lower Limb. Vol 2. 5th ed. Edinburgh: Churchill Livingstone; 1987.

10. Parolie JM, Bergfeld JA. Long-term results of nonoperative treatment of isolated posterior cruciate ligament injuries in the athlete. Am J Sports Med. 1986;14(1):35–38.

11. Kannus P, Jarvinen M. Nonoperative treatment of acute knee ligament injuries. A review with special reference to indications and methods. Sports Med. 1990;9(4):244–260.

12. Shelbourne KD, Nitz PA. The O'Donoghue triad revisited. Combined knee injuries involving anterior cruciate and medial collateral ligament tears. Am J Sports Med. 1991;19(5):474–477.

13. Azar FM. Evaluation and treatment of chronic medial collateral ligament injuries of the knee. Sports Med Arthrosc. 2006;14(2):84–90.

14. Edson CJ. Conservative and postoperative rehabilitation of isolated and combined injuries of the medial collateral ligament. Sports Med Arthrosc. 2006;14(2):105–110.

15. Deckey JE, Gibbons JM, Hershon SJ. Rehabilitation of collateral ligament injury. Sport Med Arthroscopy. 1996;4(1):59–68.

16. Meislin RJ. Managing collateral ligament tears of the knee [Electronic Version]. Physician Sportsmed. 24. Retreived 3-24-08.

17. Reider B. Medial collateral ligament injuries in athletes. Sports Med. 1996;21(2):147–156.

18. Shelbourne KD, Porter DA. Anterior cruciate ligament-medial collateral ligament injury: nonoperative management of medial collateral ligament tears with anterior cruciate ligament reconstruction. A preliminary report. Am J Sports Med. 1992;20(3):283–286.

19. Fu F, Stone D. Sports Injuries: Mechanisms, Prevention, Treatment. Baltimore: Williams & Wilkins; 1994.

20. Morris PJ, Hoffman DF. Injuries in cross-country skiing. Trail markers for diagnosis and treatment. Postgrad Med. 1999;105(1):89–91, 95–88, 101.

21. Davidson CJ, Ganion LR, Gehlsen GM, Verhoestra B, Roepke JE, Sevier TL. Rat tendon morphologic and functional changes resulting from soft-tissue mobilization. Med Sci Sport Exercise. 1997;29(3):313–319.

22. Hammer WI. Functional Soft-Tissue Examination and Treatment by Manual Methods. 3rd ed. Boston: Jones and Bartlett; 2007.

23. Thomee R, Augustsson J, Karlsson J. Patellofemoral pain syndrome: a review of current issues. Sports Med. 1999;28(4):245–262.

24. McComas A. Skeletal Muscle: Form and Function. Champaign: Human Kinetics; 1996.

25. Tria AJ, Jr., Palumbo RC, Alicea JA. Conservative care for patellofemoral pain. Orthop Clin North Am. 1992;23(4):545–554.

26. Callaghan MJ, Selfe J, McHenry A, Oldham JA. Effects of patellar taping on knee joint proprioception in patients with patellofemoral pain syndrome. Man Ther. 2007:19–24.

27. Herrington L. The effect of corrective taping of the patella on patella position as defined by MRI. Res Sports Med. 2006;14(3):215–223.

28. Aminaka N, Gribble PA. A systematic review of the effects of therapeutic taping on patellofemoral pain syndrome. J Athl Train. 2005;40(4):341–351.

29. Crossley K, Cowan SM, Bennell KL, McConnell J. Patellar taping: is clinical success supported by scientific evidence? Man Ther. 2000;5(3):142–150.

30. Crossley K, Bennell K, Green S, McConnell J. A systematic review of physical interventions for patellofemoral pain syndrome. Clin J Sport Med. 2001;11(2):103–110.

31. Kolowich PA, Paulos LE, Rosenberg TD, Farnsworth S. Lateral release of the patella: indications and contraindications. Am J Sports Med. 1990;18(4):359–365.

32. Christoforakis J, Bull AM, Strachan RK, Shymkiw R, Senavongse W, Amis AA. Effects of lateral retinacular release on the lateral stability of the patella. Knee Surg Sports Traumatol Arthrosc. 2006;14(3):273–277.

33. Panni AS, Tartarone M, Patricola A, Paxton EW, Fithian DC. Long-term results of lateral retinacular release. Arthroscopy. 2005;21(5):526–531.

34. Desio SM, Burks RT, Bachus KN. Soft tissue restraints to lateral patellar translation in the human knee. Am J Sports Med. 1998;26(1):59–65.

35. Niskanen RO, Paavilainen PJ, Jaakkola M, Korkala OL. Poor correlation of clinical signs with patellar cartilaginous changes. Arthroscopy. 2001;17(3):307–310.

36. Radin EL. A rational approach to the treatment of patellofemoral pain. Clin Orthop. 1979(144):107–109.

37. Nishimura G, Yamato M, Tamai K, Takahashi J, Uetani M. MR findings in iliotibial band syndrome. Skeletal Radiol. 1997;26(9):533–537.

38. Ekman EF, Pope T, Martin DF, Curl WW. Magnetic resonance imaging of iliotibial band syndrome. Am J Sports Med. 1994;22(6):851–854.

39. Nemeth WC, Sanders BL. The lateral synovial recess of the knee: anatomy and role in chronic iliotibial band friction syndrome. Arthroscopy. 1996;12(5):574–580.

40. Travell J, Simons, D. Myofascial Pain and Dysfunction: The Trigger Point Manual. Vol 2. Baltimore: Williams & Wilkins; 1992.

41. Barber FA, Sutker AN. Iliotibial band syndrome. Sports Med. 1992;14(2):144–148.

42. McNicol K, Taunton JE, Clement DB. Iliotibial tract friction syndrome in athletes. Can J Appl Sport Sci. 1981; 6(2):76–80.

43. Fadale PD, Wiggins ME. Corticosteroid injections: their use and abuse. J Am Acad Orthop Surg. 1994;2(3):133–140.

44. Martens M. Iliotibial band friction syndrome. In: Torg JS, Shephard RJ, eds. Current Therapy in Sports Medicine. St. Louis: Mosby; 1995:322–324.

45. Fredericson M, Guillet M, DeBenedictis L. Quick solutions for iliotibial band syndrome. Physician Sportsmed. 2000;28(2).

46. Bernstein J. Meniscal tears of the knee. Physician Sportsmed. 2000;28(3):83–90.

47. Weiss CB, Lundberg M, Hamberg P, DeHaven KE, Gillquist J. Non-operative treatment of meniscal tears. J Bone Joint Surg Am. 1989;71(6):811–822.

48. Noble J, Erat K. In defence of the meniscus. A prospective study of 200 meniscectomy patients. J Bone Joint Surg Br. 1980;62–B(1):7–11.

49. Torstensen ET, Bray RC, Wiley JP. Patellar tendinitis: a review of current concepts and treatment. Clin J Sport Med. 1994;4(2):77–82.

50. Lowe W. Orthopedic Assessment in Massage Therapy. Sisters, OR: Daviau-Scott; 2006.

51. Fredberg U, Bolvig L. Jumper's knee. Review of the literature. Scand J Med Sci Sports. 1999;9(2):66–73.

52. Ferretti A. Epidemiology of jumper's knee. Sports Med. 1986;3(4):289–295.

53. Depalma MJ, Perkins RH. Patellar tendinosis. Physician Sportsmed. 2004;32(5):41–45.

54. Pellecchia GL, Hamel H, Behnke P. Treatment of infrapatellar tendinitis – a combination of modalities and transverse friction massage versus iontophoresis. J Sport Rehabil. 1994;3(2):135–145.

55. Khan KM, Cook JL, Bonar F, Harcourt P, Astrom M. Histopathology of common tendinopathies – update and implications for clinical management. Sport Med. 1999; 27(6):393–408.

56. Almekinders LC, Temple JD. Etiology, diagnosis, and treatment of tendinitis – an analysis of the literature. Med Sci Sport Exercise. 1998;30(8):1183–1190.

57. Khan KM, Cook JL, Maffulli N, Kannus P. Where is the pain coming from in tendinopathy? It may be biochemical, not only structural, in origin. Br J Sports Med. 2000; 34(2):81–83.

58. Williams RJ, III, Attia E, Wickiewicz TL, Hannafin JA. The effect of ciprofloxacin on tendon, paratenon, and capsular fibroblast metabolism. Am J Sports Med. 2000;28(3): 364–369.

59. Casparian JM, Luchi M, Moffat RE, Hinthorn D. Quinolones and tendon ruptures. South Med J. 2000; 93(5):488–491.

60. Khaliq Y, Zhanel GG. Musculoskeletal injury associated with fluoroquinolone antibiotics. Clin Plast Surg. 2005; 32(4):495–502, vi.

61. Kujala UM, Orava S, Jarvinen M. Hamstring injuries. Current trends in treatment and prevention. Sports Med. 1997;23(6):397–404.

62. Garrett WE, Jr., Rich FR, Nikolaou PK, Vogler JB, 3rd. Computed tomography of hamstring muscle strains. Med Sci Sports Exerc. 1989;21(5):506–514.

63. Worrell TW. Factors associated with hamstring injuries. An approach to treatment and preventative measures. Sports Med. 1994;17(5):338–345.

64. Kornberg CaL, P. The effect of stretching neural structures on grade one hamstring injuries. Journal of Orthopaedic and Sports Physical Therapy. 1989;10(12):481–487.

65. Turl SE, George KP. Adverse neural tension – a factor in repetitive hamstring strain. J Orthop Sport Phys Therapy. 1998;27(1):16–21.

66. Mishra DK, Friden J, Schmitz MC, Lieber RL. Anti-inflammatory medication after muscle injury. A treatment resulting in short-term improvement but subsequent loss of muscle function. J Bone Joint Surg Am. 1995; 77(10):1510–1519.

67. Kisner C, Colby LA. Therapeutic Exercise: Foundations and Techniques. 2nd ed. Philadelphia: F.A. Davis; 1985.

68. Renstrom PA. Tendon and muscle injuries in the groin area. Clin Sports Med. 1992;11(4):815–831.

69. Tyler TF, Nicholas SJ, Campbell RJ, McHugh MP. The association of hip strength and flexibility with the incidence of adductor muscle strains in professional ice hockey players. Am J Sports Med. 2001;29(2):124–128.

70. Garrett WE, Jr., Safran MR, Seaber AV, Glisson RR, Ribbeck BM. Biomechanical comparison of stimulated and nonstimulated skeletal muscle pulled to failure. Am J Sports Med. 1987;15(5):448–454.

71. Krivickas LS. Anatomical factors associated with overuse sports injuries. Sports Med. 1997;24(2):132–146.

Chapter 8

Hip and pelvis

The hip and pelvis region make up the structural core of the body and contain its center of gravity. The functional relationships between the pelvis, hip, lumbar spine, and lower extremity are crucial for proper gait, movement, and function. The interaction between this region and other areas of the body are also crucially important. Muscular, fascial, and neurological connections between the pelvic region, upper extremity, and cranium create a symbiotic relationship necessary for human movement in the vertical gravity plane.

The hip and pelvis region have two major articulations on each side of the body: the sacroiliac (SI) joint and the iliofemoral (hip) joint. Iliofemoral and sacroiliac joint mechanics are closely related and understanding the numerous pathologies in this region requires familiarity with both. The SI joint is an articulation designed for stability and is often viewed as a *keystone* in the architecture of the pelvis. Body weight is transmitted from the upper body across the SI joint to the lower extremities. The joint is held tightly in place by a complex webbing of ligaments on the anterior and posterior sides to manage the high force loads of the region.

The hip is a far more mobile joint. It is the body's largest ball and socket joint, and permits movement in several planes. Although muscles acting across the hip joint can generate large force loads, hip joint pathologies generally result from chronic compressive stress. This region also houses the largest diameter nerves in the body. As a result of being so large, these nerves are susceptible to compression by adjacent bone and soft tissues in a number of locations. This is such a biomechanically complex region that entire textbooks have been written on lumbo-pelvic mechanics. Yet, soft-tissue pathology plays an important role in numerous disorders in this region and the orthopedic massage practitioner can make valuable contributions to relieving pain and injury complaints.

INJURY CONDITIONS

PIRIFORMIS SYNDROME

Description

Piriformis syndrome is frequently described as an entrapment of the sciatic nerve by the piriformis muscle. However, there are other nerves in the region that the piriformis can compress; these nerve compression pathologies may be called piriformis syndrome as well. By far the most common problem involves compression of one or both divisions of the sciatic nerve by the piriformis muscle in the gluteal region.

The normal path of the sciatic nerve courses from the anterior region of the sacrum through the greater sciatic notch in the ilium. The nerve then passes inferior to the piriformis and over the top of the other five deep hip rotator muscles (Fig. 8.1). The sacrospinous ligament is just inferior to the piriformis muscle. The sciatic nerve courses between the inferior border of the piriformis muscle and the superior border of the sacrospinous ligament. Because the sacrospinous ligament is a dense and taut structure, nerve damage can occur from compression against the sacrospinous ligament. The sciatic nerve is susceptible to damage even from light levels of pressure.[1]

The superior gluteal nerve also exits through the greater sciatic notch, but travels superior to the piriformis muscle on its way to innervate the gluteal muscles (Fig. 8.1). Tightness or tendinous fibers in the superior portion of the piriformis can trap the superior gluteal nerve against the greater sciatic notch. If this occurs, the client describes aching

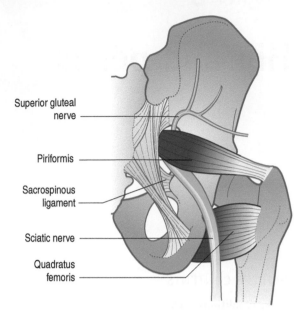

Figure 8.1   Posterior view of the right pelvis showing sciatic nerve and superior gluteal nerve in relation to the piriformis muscle.

buttock pain and usually demonstrates weakness in the hip abductors.

Pain sensations similar to those in piriformis syndrome can also come from myofascial trigger points in the piriformis muscle. Sacroiliac joint dysfunction can also produce pain in the hip and pelvis region, although it is not as likely to cause radiating pain down the posterior lower extremity.[2] Myofascial trigger points in this region should be treated even if it appears that nerve compression is the primary problem. Trigger points are often the root of the problem by causing greater tightness in the piriformis and deep hip rotator muscles.

Anatomical variations in the gluteal region create a number of different ways that nerve compression can occur. The sciatic nerve often separates into the tibial and peroneal divisions as it passes through the greater sciatic notch and passes the piriformis muscle. Cadaver dissections have indicated that about 10% of the population has one division of the nerve going through the muscle and the other division going below it. Another 2–3% has one division of the nerve above and one division below. A remaining 1% of the population has both divisions going right through the middle of the muscle.[2] Figure 8.2 shows these different variations.

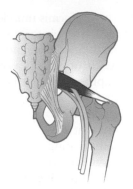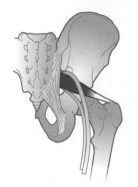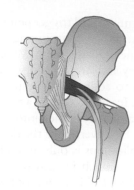

Figure 8.2   Variations on sciatic nerve and piriformis arrangement.

When looking at these different anatomical variations, it seems likely that an individual with the sciatic nerve perforating the piriformis muscle would be in serious discomfort all the time. However, this does not always occur. There are numerous locations where a nerve goes through a muscle without adverse symptoms. For example, the musculocutaneous nerve perforates the coracobrachialis muscle in the arm, and few people ever have a problem.

In the common arrangement of the sciatic nerve, it lies just inferior to the piriformis muscle and superior to the sacrospinous ligament. The ligament is a very dense and unyielding structure, and therefore when the nerve is pressed against it, symptoms are likely. On the other hand, muscle tissue is relatively soft and pliable. Therefore, it provides a greater cushion around the nerve even if the nerve travels directly through the middle of the muscle.

A client with piriformis syndrome usually reports pain and/or paresthesia in the gluteal region that is also felt down the posterior lower extremity, sometimes all the way to the foot. Low back pain is common with this problem as well. The concurrent presence of low back pain makes identification of this problem even more crucial. The symptoms of piriformis syndrome are similar to those arising from problems with the lumbar nerve roots. Making the assumption that the client's pain comes from nerve roots rather than the piriformis, unless this is the case, could delay healing or prevent it entirely as the cause of the pain may not be addressed.

Symptoms of piriformis syndrome are aggravated from sitting for long periods, as this places compression on the nerve and causes local tissue ischemia as well. Sitting with a wallet in the back pocket is another common aggravator of nerve compression.

While piriformis syndrome is most common as a chronic compression injury, it is also possible to occur as an acute injury resulting from a direct blow or fall on the buttock region.[3]

Treatment

Traditional approaches

One of the more important factors in addressing piriformis syndrome is to establish the primary cause of compression. If there are any activities that exacerbate the problem, such as sitting on a large wallet, they need to be modified or terminated first. In many cases, changing this pattern is all that is needed to resolve the condition.

Stretching and range-of-motion activities are used to address tightness in the piriformis muscle that leads to nerve compression. Stretching can be performed in the clinic as well and the client can be instructed to do these stretches at home. Anti-inflammatory medications have been used to treat this problem, but their use for this problem is questionable.[4]

Surgery may be performed for piriformis syndrome if conservative treatment is ineffective. Physicians use diagnostic tests such as MRI and CT scans to determine anatomical variations of the piriformis muscle and sciatic nerve.[5] If the nerve is perforating the piriformis muscle, the nerve can be surgically repositioned. However, surgery for this condition is controversial, because it is believed that surgery is not warranted in many cases. For example, if the person has not been symptomatic with the nerve in this position and it suddenly becomes a problem, there is a question as whether the muscle needs to be cut and the nerve repositioned, or if conservative treatments are a better option.

Because myofascial trigger points in the piriformis muscle can be a contributing factor, treatment focuses on neutralizing them. Myofascial treatments, such as spray and stretch or dry needling, are sometimes used to address trigger point dysfunction in this region. Ice is also used as a treatment to decrease neurological activity in the piriformis muscle prior to stretching. However, since the depth of penetration of cold applications is only around 1 cm, it is questionable how much ice can really do to affect the piriformis muscle.[6] Injection of the trigger points is sometimes performed to reduce their activity and treat the muscular components of the problem.

Soft-tissue manipulation

General guidelines There are a number of massage and soft-tissue treatment approaches for piriformis syndrome. Myofascial trigger points in the piriformis muscle can be treated with static compression techniques. This may be done with either a broad contact surface or a small contact surface like the thumb, elbow, or pressure tool.

The piriformis may be difficult to palpate, due to the thickness of the overlying gluteus maximus. However, anatomical landmarks can help identify its location. Find the upper and lower borders of the sacrum and then locate a point about half way between those two landmarks. Connect a line from that point to the greater trochanter of the femur. This will be the approximate path and location of the piriformis muscle (Fig. 8.3).

It is important to know the location of the piriformis muscle, because this condition involves nerve compression by the piriformis muscle. Treatment involves pressure to the piriformis, so it is important that the practitioner does not exacerbate the problem. If the client reports a reproduction of the primary symptoms, then it is apparent that the area where pressure is being applied is aggravating the nerve compression, and pressure should be removed from that area.

One way to avoid complicating the nerve compression is to apply treatments to the ends of the piriformis muscle and avoid putting further direct compression on the site of nerve entrapment. The muscle will still get a strong soft-tissue treatment intervention, and a reduction of muscle tension will result.

Another way to effectively treat hypertonicity in the piriformis muscle without putting direct pressure on the compression site is through active-assisted stretching procedures. Passive or active stretching techniques effectively address the piriformis but do not put additional compression on the sciatic nerve.[7] However, similar to massage, stretching the hypertonic muscle can increase compression on the nerve by tightening the tissues around the nerve. Practitioners should pay close attention to any symptom changes reported by the client during therapy.

Suggested techniques and methods

A. Sweeping cross fiber Superficial sweeping cross fiber techniques are applied to the gluteal muscles to reduce hypertonicity and make it easier to treat the piriformis. Use a sweeping motion of the hand and thumb to deliver broad cross fiber sweeping techniques to the gluteal muscles (Fig. 8.4).

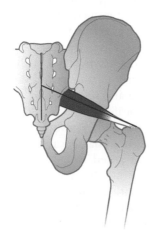

Figure 8.3 Locating the piriformis muscle for treatment.

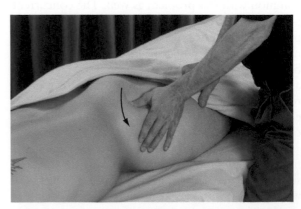

Figure 8.4 Sweeping cross fiber to gluteal muscles.

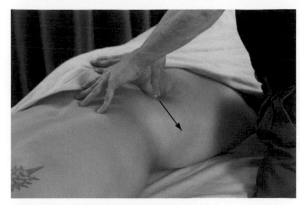

Figure 8.5 Stripping on the piriformis.

B. Longitudinal stripping on piriformis Use the thumb, finger tips, pressure tool, or other small contact surface to perform a stripping technique on the piriformis muscle (Fig. 8.5). The stripping technique can be performed from either the proximal to distal attachment of the piriformis or vice versa. There is no clear physiological preference of one direction over the other.

C. Pin and stretch for piriformis The client is in a prone position with the knee flexed. Grasp the ankle with one hand and move the client's thigh into full lateral rotation; this places the piriformis in its shortest position. Apply pressure to the piriformis with the other hand using a thumb, finger, pressure tool, or other small contact surface. With pressure maintained on the muscle, pull the client's leg laterally (notice that the thigh moves in medial rotation), fully stretching the piriformis (Fig. 8.6). Repeat this technique several times for the maximal benefit.

D. Active engagement lengthening to piriformis More specific treatment of the piriformis is accomplished with active engagement methods. This technique can feel intense for the client, but it is highly effective for reducing tension in the muscle. The client is in a prone position with the knee flexed. Instruct the client to engage an initial (non-maximal) isometric contraction by holding the leg in the starting position while the practitioner attempts to pull the leg in a lateral direction, which rotates the thigh medially. The client is instructed to slowly release the contraction while the practitioner continues to pull the leg. Simultaneously, the practitioner performs a longitudinal stripping technique on the piriformis (Fig. 8.7). The piriformis is engaged eccentrically during this treatment.

E. MET (active-assisted stretching) to piriformis This technique is effective if there is concern about putting additional compression on the region of nerve entrapment near the piriformis. The client is in a prone position with the knee flexed. Instruct the client to hold the leg stationary as the practitioner attempts to pull the leg laterally (moving the thigh in medial rotation). This resisted movement engages an isometric contraction. The client holds the contraction for about 5–8 seconds and then releases the contraction. Upon release, the practitioner pulls the leg laterally (thigh moving in medial rotation) thereby stretching the piriformis.

Rehabilitation protocol considerations

- The gluteal musculature is thick in this region and soft-tissue applications must go through this tissue to reach the piriformis. Appropriate time should be spent working to relax these

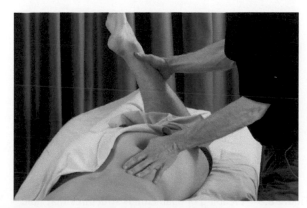

Figure 8.6 Pin and stretch on piriformis.

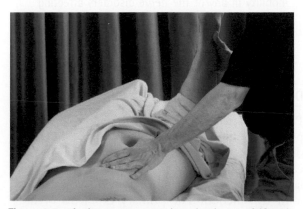

Figure 8.7 Active engagement lengthening to piriformis.

more superficial tissues prior to commencing deep work on the piriformis. If appropriate attention is not paid to treating the muscles first, the treatment can feel invasive to the client.

- After treating all of the muscles in this region, stretching is valuable to enhance muscle pliability and reduce compression on the affected nerve(s).

- Relevant activity modifications should be included with treatment strategies to decrease aggravating factors.

Cautions and contraindications A number of other conditions can produce symptoms similar to entrapment of the sciatic nerve by the piriformis muscle. Use comprehensive assessment procedures to identify the particular nerve and compression location as accurately as possible. If any treatment aggravates the neurological sensations it should be terminated. An increase in sensory irritation by further compressing the nerve is likely to make the muscle even tighter.

Box 8.1   Clinical Tip

Piriformis syndrome is routinely misdiagnosed as a problem resulting from lumbar disc pathology. However, even though it is a nerve compression in the gluteal region, there can be muscular tightness in the low back region and other regions of the lower extremity that should be addressed. Treat the tissues adjacent to the entire length of the sciatic nerve and its branches from the lumbar nerve roots to the distal fibers of the plantar nerves in the foot. This can encourage full neural mobility in any of the nerve disorders affecting extremity nerves.

SACROILIAC JOINT DYSFUNCTION

Description

Pain that is felt in the sacroiliac region, low back, pelvis, or thigh, may be the result of sacroiliac dysfunction. There are a number of problems that can occur at this joint, all of which may have similar symptoms, and can be classified as sacroiliac joint dysfunction. The primary problems occurring at the sacroiliac joint include ligament sprains,

friction between the articular surfaces, and joint misalignment.

The sacrum acts as a wedge between the two halves of the pelvis, holding the weight of the upper body. As such, there are large compressive forces on the joint that force the sacrum in an inferior direction. The sacrum is held firmly into this joint by a tight webbing of ligamentous structures (Fig. 8.8).

Because of the need for stability, there is very little motion possible at the SI joint. There is a slight degree of motion in the sagittal plane. The forward tipping of the superior surface of the sacrum is called *nutation* and the backward tipping is called *counternutation*; the range for both is only 7–8°. This motion is essential for proper mechanics during walking, bending over, and other motions because each innominate (half of the pelvis) must rotate independently. Motion at a joint is usually controlled by muscles that span directly between the two bones of the joint. At the SI joint no muscles span directly from the sacrum to the ilium. Instead joint motion is controlled by a collection of muscles, ligaments, and fascia in the lumbosacral region.[8,9]

Movement must be equal at the sacroiliac joints on both sides of the body. If movement is not equal, joint dysfunction occurs and pain

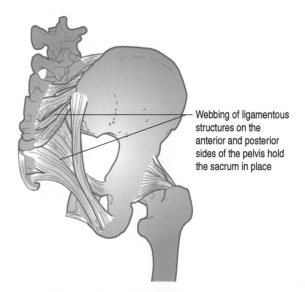

Webbing of ligamentous structures on the anterior and posterior sides of the pelvis hold the sacrum in place

Figure 8.8   Webbing of ligamentous structures that hold the sacroiliac joint.

production from that dysfunction is likely. Despite the fact that the sacroiliac joints on each side of the body are symmetrical in design and close to each other, they operate somewhat independently in relation to the pelvis. Many sacroiliac dysfunctions are unilateral.[10]

Even though there is slight motion at the joint, it is held close to stationary by a complex structure of ligaments. Ligaments that contribute to stability in the region include the anterior sacroiliac, posterior sacroiliac, iliolumbar, sacrotuberous, and sacrospinous ligaments. Because there are no muscles that go directly from the sacrum to the ilium, the importance of these ligaments in maintaining stability at the joint is increased.

With ligaments as the primary joint stabilizers, the likelihood of joint dysfunction and sprain is heightened during pregnancy, when relaxin is released in the body. The effect of the hormone relaxin is to increase the pliability of ligament tissue, especially in the ligaments around the pelvis. Therefore, during pregnancy, more motion may be permitted at the sacroiliac articulation with less resultant stability.

Ligaments stabilizing this joint are influenced by muscle activity that is distant from the joint. After examining fascial connections in numerous cadaver studies, Vleeming and his colleagues made some interesting discoveries about lumbopelvic biomechanics.[11] They found that (1) gluteus maximus tissue is connected to the sacrotuberous ligament, (2) there is fascial continuity between part of the biceps femoris long head and the sacrotuberous ligament, and (3) there is fascial continuity from the posterior aspect of the piriformis to the posterior sacroiliac ligament. As a result, contractions from these muscles can affect tension levels on the ligament structures, which in turn affect the biomechanics of the sacroiliac joint. Similar concepts have been described by Tom Myers, with his discussion of *Anatomy Trains.*[12]

Other regions of muscular activity can also be influential. There is evidence that the thoracolumbar fascia transmits tensile force through the connective tissue to the contralateral gluteus maximus. Because the gluteus maximus has fascial connections with the sacrotuberous ligament, muscular activity in the latissimus could conceivably affect

mechanics at the sacroiliac joint. Muscle tightness that affects bony alignment through tension on the related ligaments is what researchers refer to as a *force closure* of the joint, as opposed to a *form closure* that results from bony displacement.[13]

Unlike other joints in the body, the articulation between the bony surfaces of the sacrum and ilium are not smooth. The two joint surfaces are moderately rough and irregular because the joints are not designed for free gliding motion. The rough surface between the two bones helps produce stability in the joint. However, the irregular surface can become problematic if the joint surfaces become misaligned. It has been suggested due to the misalignment of the ridges and depressions that the joint can become 'locked' this is one explanation for the sensation of joint locking that client's report. This would be an example of *form closure* mentioned above. It may also be an explanation for the effectiveness of some high velocity joint manipulations that are used to treat sacroiliac joint problems. The sudden movement allows the irregular contact surfaces of the joint to be realigned once again.

Dysfunction of the sacroiliac joint can result from either acute injury, such as an automobile accident, or from chronic dysfunctional biomechanics, such as gait alterations. A good example of dysfunctional biomechanics affecting the SI joint is a structural leg-length discrepancy. If one leg is longer than the other, an unequal amount of force is placed on the two sacroiliac joints. The unequal force causes altered biomechanical function and pain. The patient with sacroiliac joint dysfunction often complains of diffuse pain in the lumbar or sacral region, which can be mistaken for lumbar disc pathology.[14] Pain can also refer into other areas such as the groin or posterior leg.

Treatment

Traditional approaches

There are a number of approaches for treating sacroiliac dysfunction, but no ideal treatment protocol has been established. Joint mobilization and manipulation are used with success in many cases. The exact mechanism by which these approaches work is not clear. Manipulation could be altering joint position, but there is not full agreement on this theory. Some suggest manipulation does not alter the position of the sacroiliac joint, yet manipulation does reduce pain in many cases.[15] Various physical therapy modalities such as ultrasound with or without phonophoresis (cortisone or other medications driven through the skin with ultrasound) are sometimes used.[16]

Strength training and exercise programs function to gain stability in the sacroiliac joint. Bracing or lumbar corsets may be worn to decrease dysfunctional biomechanics. Another method that has been used with some success involves proliferant injections. In this procedure, a substance is injected into the joint region that aids in the proliferation of fibrous tissue, subsequently making the joint more stable.

Soft-tissue manipulation

General guidelines No muscles span directly from the sacrum to the ilium and govern SI joint mechanics. However, myofascial connections span the SI joint indirectly and aid in controlling movement at the joint. Muscles with a strong influence on SI joint mechanics include the gluteus maximus, biceps femoris, and latissimus dorsi. It is important to address these muscles along with others in the region, as they all have effects on SI joint mechanics.

While strength training is used to regain stability in the joint, an argument could be made that reducing hypertonicity in the muscles that have produced the force closure of the sacroiliac joint may be more helpful. The problem around the joint, after all, is usually not a strength deficiency, but an imbalance in the forces acting on the joint. Massage can function to bring the body back to homeostasis by reducing tension in the hypertonic muscles rather than increasing strength (tension) in other muscles. The end result of reducing muscle tension is a more biomechanically balanced joint.

Other muscles that are important for sacroiliac mechanics should be addressed with massage as well. In particular, treatment should focus on the lumbar, gluteal, and hamstring muscles. Stretching of the muscles in this region after soft-tissue treatment is an important adjunct. Stretching procedures should be performed with care so as not to put excess tensile load on tissues contributing to the biomechanical imbalance.

Suggested techniques and methods

A. Sweeping cross fiber Superficial hypertonicity in the gluteal muscles is reduced with sweeping cross fiber techniques. Use a sweeping motion of the hand and thumb to deliver broad cross fiber sweeping techniques to the gluteal muscles (Fig. 8.4).

B. Deep stripping to gluteus maximus Gluteus maximus crosses the SI joint and has facial connections with ligaments in the region, so excess tension in this muscle can adversely affect SI joint mechanics. Apply stripping techniques to the gluteus maximus along the direction of the fibers. Use a broad contact surface, such as the backside of the fist initially, then follow with stripping techniques using a small contact surface, such as finger tips, thumbs, or pressure tool (Fig. 8.9).

C. Static compression to gluteal muscles Myofascial trigger points play an important role in altering SI joint mechanics. Static compression techniques are an effective way to neutralize trigger points' adverse effects. Begin the static compression with a broad contact surface first and follow with small contact surface compression such as the elbow, thumb, finger, or pressure tool (Fig. 8.10).

D. Sweeping cross fiber to lumbar muscles The superficial lumbar muscles are treated to reduce tension on the myofascial tissues spanning the SI joint. Use the thumb, backside of the fingers, base of the hand, or other broad contact surface to perform longitudinal and sweeping cross fiber applications (Fig. 8.11). Pay particular attention to the lumbodorsal fascia, quadratus lumborum,

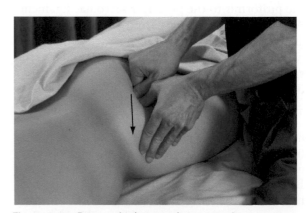

Figure 8.9   Deep stripping on gluteus maximus.

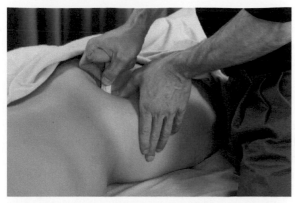

Figure 8.10   Static compression to gluteal muscles.

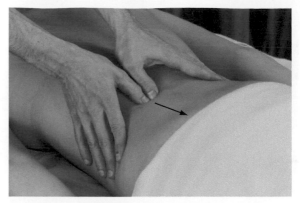

Figure 8.12   Deep longitudinal stripping on lumbar muscles.

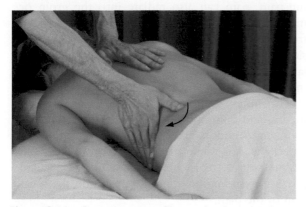

Figure 8.11   Sweeping cross fiber to lumbar muscles.

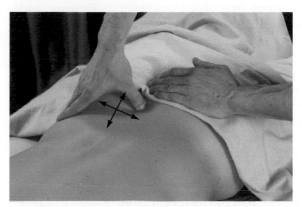

Figure 8.13   Friction to posterior sacroiliac ligaments.

and erector spinae due to the fascial continuities from these muscles that act on the SI joint.

E. Deep longitudinal stripping on the lumbar muscles Deep stripping techniques are applied to the same muscles addressed in D above. Encourage elongation in the specific myofascial fibers with small contact surface pressure such as the finger tips, thumb, or pressure tool (Fig. 8.12).

F. Friction to posterior sacroiliac ligaments In some cases there is fiber stretching or tearing to the posterior sacroiliac ligaments. Perform short back and forth friction directly on the sacroiliac ligaments, paying particular attention to any actions that reproduce the client's discomfort (Fig. 8.13).

G. Deep longitudinal stripping on hamstrings Hamstring tension can play a prominent role in SI joint dysfunction. Deep stripping is used to treat the hamstrings for excessive muscle tension that may contribute to dysfunctional SI joint mechanics. Start with a broad contact surface of

pressure and then eventually perform the stripping techniques with a small contact surface (Fig. 8.14).

Rehabilitation protocol considerations

- The techniques presented above may not be necessary for each client or for every session. Accurate assessment is crucial to determine the primary factors that will guide the clinical decision of which techniques to employ.

- Strength training is sometimes used for SI joint dysfunction, but it is best reserved for the later stages of rehabilitation. It can be used when the symptoms have significantly decreased, joint mechanics appear more normalized, and soft-tissue hypertonicity has been resolved. Strengthening activities performed too early in the rehabilitative process may adversely alter joint mechanics.

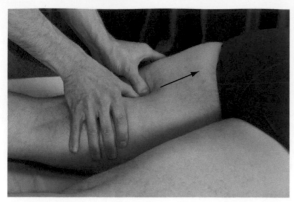

Figure 8.14   Deep longitudinal stripping on hamstrings.

Cautions and contraindications Patients with sacroiliac joint dysfunction may have difficulty lying in certain positions on the treatment table. It is a good idea to have several options for positioning when determining which treatment methods to perform. Use caution when applying pressure around the SI joint region, especially with techniques such as that of F described above. Pressure applied directly on the sacrum during friction treatment can be painful if they aggravate misaligned joints or overstretch ligament tissue.

Encourage clients to move slowly when getting up from the treatment table or changing positions after soft-tissue treatment for SI joint pathology. Proprioception and joint position can change substantially when in a non-weight-bearing position after treatment. When the client gets up and weight is once again transmitted through the SI joint, the relaxed tissues of the joint may allow greater joint movement, which could be painful.

TROCHANTERIC BURSITIS

Description

The trochanteric bursa lies directly over (superficial to) the greater trochanter of the femur. Its primary purpose is to reduce friction between the greater trochanter of the femur and the iliotibial band, which is superficial to it. This bursa can become irritated and inflamed from an acute blow to the lateral hip region, such as falling directly on the hip.

Chronic compression or repetitive friction from the iliotibial band (ITB) can also cause inflammation of the bursa. Trochanteric bursitis is more common in the middle age to older population.[17, 18] Chronic trochanteric bursitis from iliotibial band friction is more common than the acute type.

Symptoms from trochanteric bursitis include aching pain over the lateral hip region. Pain is usually aggravated by additional pressure directly over the greater trochanter. Clients complain that it hurts to lie on the affected side. Repeated activities of hip flexion such as stair climbing or running are also likely to aggravate the symptoms.

Although the most common symptom is lateral hip pain, pain can also radiate into the groin or into the lateral thigh region.[19] Because friction from the iliotibial band is a causative factor, tension in the gluteus maximus and tensor fasciae latae that attach to the iliotibial band play a role in the onset of the problem as well.

The other gluteal muscles, especially gluteus medius and minimus should not be ignored in this problem. Tendon pathology in these muscles, especially near their distal attachment sites, can masquerade as trochanteric bursitis.[20] A detailed physical examination should help clarify the location of the pain.

Treatment

Traditional approaches

The primary goal of any bursitis treatment is to reduce inflammation in the affected bursa. This can be done with a number of different conservative methods such as rest, ice, stretching of the muscles attached to the ITB, and non-steroidal anti-inflammatory drugs (NSAIDs).[17] Strength training of hip musculature is also used, although it should be avoided if it aggravates the problem.

If conservative treatment is not successful, corticosteroid injections are used to reduce inflammation in the bursa. Steroid injections are usually effective and yield prolonged results.[19] In the event that steroid injections are not successful, surgery might be performed for trochanteric bursitis. This is not a common procedure, but excision (removal) of the irritated bursa can be performed if all other treatment options have been unsuccessful.[21]

Soft–tissue manipulation

General guidelines Soft-tissue manipulation for treatment of trochanteric bursitis takes an indirect approach. There is no benefit from applying direct massage to an inflamed bursa and, in fact, this approach is contraindicated because of further compression and irritation to the bursa. However, if the bursa is being irritated by tightness in structures, such as the tensor fasciae latae acting through the iliotibial band, then soft-tissue manipulation can reduce tension in those structures.

Hypertonicity in the gluteal muscles can be effectively reduced with deep longitudinal stripping techniques. Stripping methods should also focus on the gluteus medius and minimus because tension in these muscles can further aggravate bursa compression. Myofascial trigger point pain referral patterns in these muscles can also mimic trochanteric bursitis.

Treatment should also focus on the tensor fasciae latae muscle, as it is one of the primary causes of excess tension on the iliotibial band. Static compression and deep longitudinal stripping are some of the best techniques for addressing tension in this muscle. These procedures are more effectively performed with the client in a side-lying position.

Suggested techniques and methods

A. Sweeping cross fiber to gluteal muscles Sweeping cross fiber techniques are applied to the gluteal muscles to reduce superficial hypertonicity. Use a sweeping motion of the hand and thumb to deliver broad cross fiber sweeping techniques to the gluteal muscles (Fig. 8.4). Similar techniques should be applied to the tensor fasciae latae prior to deeper techniques such as stripping or pin and stretch.

B. Deep stripping to gluteus maximus The gluteus maximus pulls on the iliotibial band and when tight can contribute to the band rubbing over the trochanteric bursa. Apply stripping techniques to the gluteus maximus along the direction of the fibers. Use a broad contact surface, such as the back-side of the fist first and eventually follow with stripping techniques using a small contact surface, such as finger tips, thumbs, or pressure tool (Fig. 8.9).

C. Static compression to the tensor fasciae latae The client is in a side-lying position. Use a small

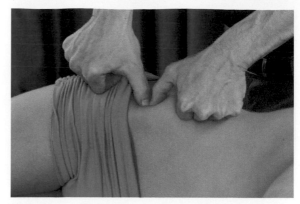

Figure 8.15 Static compression on tensor fasciae latae.

contact surface such as the thumb, finger, elbow, or pressure tool to apply compression to the areas of tightness in the TFL muscle (Fig. 8.15). In particular, search for active myofascial trigger points that reproduce lateral hip or high pain.

D. Deep stripping to the tensor fasciae latae The client is in a side lying position. Perform a series of effleurage and sweeping cross fiber techniques on the TFL first to begin reducing tension in the muscle prior to deep stripping. Use a small contact surface such as a finger, thumb, or pressure tool to apply longitudinally stripping techniques to the TFL from the proximal attachment all the way through its insertion into fibers of the ITB (Fig. 8.16).

E. Pin and stretch for the tensor fasciae latae This technique uses the pin and stretch concept along with eccentric activity in the TFL to encourage lengthening of the muscle and lessen tension on the ITB. The client is in a side-lying position.

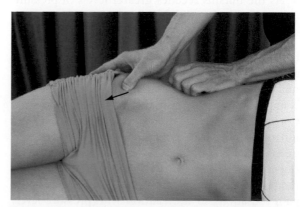

Figure 8.16 Deep stripping on the tensor fasciae latae.

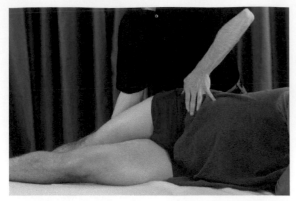

Figure 8.17 Pin and stretch on tensor fasciae latae. Photo shows the final position at the end of the stretch.

Bring the client's thigh into a position of abduction to shorten the TFL muscle. Ask the client to hold their leg in that position. Apply static compression to the muscle while the client holds the leg in the abducted position. Then instruct the client to slowly drop the leg off the back-side of the table (Fig. 8.17). This can feel intense for the client so gauge the pressure carefully with this technique. A variation on this technique can be used by applying a stripping technique during the client's eccentric adduction of the thigh instead of static compression; this is even more effective in reducing tension in the TFL muscle.

Rehabilitation protocol considerations
- Greater caution should be observed if the bursitis is in a more aggravated condition. Use caution with techniques that increase pressure on the bursa.

- As the bursitis recedes greater levels of pressure can be used and rehabilitative exercise can be combined with the soft-tissue treatment

Cautions and contraindications Because the aggravated and inflamed bursa is close to where treatment is being performed on the lateral hip muscles, it is important to make sure that additional pressure is not applied to the irritated bursa. The area over the inflamed bursa will be tender, so the client will describe local tenderness in the region. Trochanteric bursitis may be managed with anti-inflammatory medications. These medications can alter the client's pain sensations so use caution with pressure levels if the client is using these medications.

POSTURAL DISORDERS

The next section includes a number of structural and postural disorders of the hip and pelvis. These disorders are not considered injury conditions, as are the prior conditions in this chapter. However, they can produce considerable stress on other tissues or structures and contribute to their dysfunction. Massage is not always used to correct these postural deviations, but it may be a helpful approach to restoring appropriate biomechanical balance in the region.

ANTERIOR PELVIC TILT

Description

In an anterior pelvic tilt, both innominates (halves of the pelvis) are rotated in an anterior direction (Fig. 8.18). The increased anterior pelvic tilt also causes an exaggeration of the lumbar lordosis. It is valuable to measure the innominates separately as sometimes one may rotate more than the other.[22] Several factors may contribute to an anterior pelvic tilt, but typically it is from an imbalance of muscles pulling on the pelvis and/or lumbar region.

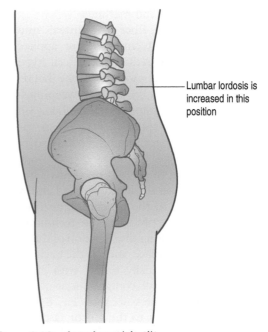

Lumbar lordosis is increased in this position

Figure 8.18 Anterior pelvic tilt.

An anterior pelvic tilt is part of a postural distortion pattern affecting the low back and pelvic muscles called the lower crossed syndrome.[23,24] The lower crossed syndrome got its name from the pattern of tension in the muscles when the body is viewed from the side (Fig. 8.19). There are two types of muscles in the body that play a central role in the lower crossed syndrome. The postural muscles are important for maintaining erect posture during locomotion. When fatigued, the postural muscles have a tendency to become hypertonic.

The phasic muscles play a greater role in creating movement. Containing a higher concentration of fast-twitch muscle fibers, the phasic muscles have a tendency to fatigue more easily and become weakened when overstressed.[25] The tendency for the phasic muscles to weaken is exaggerated by the law of reciprocal inhibition. The law of reciprocal inhibition that when one muscle gets a stimulus to contract, its oppo site – or antagonist – muscle is neurologically inhibited to contract. If the postural muscles are hypertonic, they naturally inhibit the phasic muscles. A look at these two groups of muscles illustrates this point.

Primary postural muscles that tend toward hypertonicity in the low back and pelvic region include the iliopsoas, erector spinae, rectus femoris,

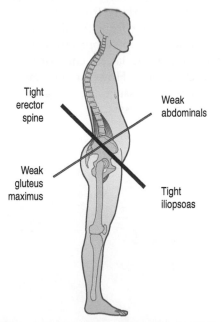

Tight erector spine

Weak abdominals

Weak gluteus maximus

Tight iliopsoas

Figure 8.19   Lower crossed syndrome (from Chaitow L, DeLany J. Clinical Application of Neuromuscular Techniques. Vol 1. Edinburgh: Churchill Livingstone; 2000).

and quadratus lumborum. When hypertonic, these muscles exaggerate the lumbar lordosis and create an anterior pelvic tilt. In addition, the postural muscles are susceptible to the development of myofascial trigger points as they become hypertonic.[26] In the graphic above (Fig. 8.19) the line connecting the regions where these muscles are located demonstrates one side of the cross.

Opposing this group are the phasic muscles of the abdomen and pelvis. The phasic muscles in this region include the gluteus maximus, gluteus medius, and rectus abdominis. The line connecting between the phasic muscles establishes the other side of the cross. Our current sedentary lifestyle encourages overuse of the postural muscles at the expense of the phasic muscles. The phasic muscles can become weak from disuse.

Treatment

Traditional approaches

The treatment protocol suggested is usually for the individual to strengthen the abdominal muscles, often through sit-ups or crunches. However, these exercises can recruit the iliopsoas as a flexor of the trunk if the legs or feet are held on the floor in the sit-up. This is counter-productive if the desire is to reduce hypertonicity in the iliopsoas.

While strengthening of the abdominal musculature can be beneficial, these muscles are often weak primarily because they are phasic muscles and the hypertonic postural muscles are inhibiting them. Clinical experience has shown that an effective resolution is to reduce hypertonicity in the postural muscles, and not necessarily attempt to increase strength in the inhibited phasic ones.[27] It is also important for the client to engage in postural re-education to deal with established biomechanical patterns.

Soft-tissue manipulation

General guidelines   Soft-tissue treatment for anterior pelvic tilt focuses on the hypertonic muscles creating the distortion. Emphasis is on reducing tightness in spinal extensor muscles, quadratus lumborum, iliopsoas, and rectus femoris. A variety of techniques including sweeping cross fiber, deep longitudinal stripping, pin and stretch, and active-assisted stretching are used to treat these muscles.

Direct massage is used to address the muscles responsible for creating the anterior pelvic tilt. Treatment of the iliopsoas is more challenging. Soft-tissue practitioners often treat this muscle with techniques that apply pressure through the abdomen to get to the muscle. Because the iliopsoas attaches to the anterior aspect of the lumbar vertebral bodies, it is very deep in the abdomen. It is contacted with finger pressure by pressing on the lateral side of the abdomen in a posterior and medial direction.

However, there are potentially dangerous contraindications to performing palpatory treatment of the iliopsoas in this region. This muscle lies directly adjacent to the external iliac artery (Fig. 8.20). Pressure on the external iliac artery can cause a back flow of pressure in the vascular structures, and could eventually cause the rupture of an aortic aneurysm. For that reason, performing the deep abdominal approach described above is not advised and it is beneficial to have alternative methods for treating the iliopsoas muscle. The MET procedure described in D below is effective in reducing muscle tightness, but does not put

pressure directly on the iliopsoas and so concerns of vascular pressure are eliminated.

Suggested techniques and methods

A. Effleurage and sweeping cross fiber to lumbar muscles Superficial muscle tension is reduced in the lumbar muscles with long gliding effleurage and sweeping cross fiber techniques are applied to the lumbar muscles. These techniques are performed prior to deep stripping applications. Use the thumb, back-side of the fingers, base of the hand, or other broad contact surface (Fig. 8.11).

B. Deep longitudinal stripping on the spinal extensors Deep stripping techniques are applied to the erector spinae and other lumbar extensor muscles close to the spine. Encourage elongation in the specific myofascial fibers with small contact surface pressure such as the finger tips, thumb, or pressure tool (Fig. 8.12).

C. Deep stripping for quadratus lumborum The client is in a prone position. Use the thumb or fingertips to perform a longitudinal stripping technique on the quadratus lumborum (Fig. 8.21). Use stripping motions from the iliac crest to the transverse processes, iliac crest to twelfth rib, and transverse processes to twelfth rib as the quadratus lumborum has fibers running in all these directions. When working from lateral to medial on the fibers running from the iliac crest to the transverse processes, apply pressure deep enough to treat up under the lateral edge of the erector spinae muscle group. However, use caution not to apply too much pressure directly against the tips of the transverse processes.

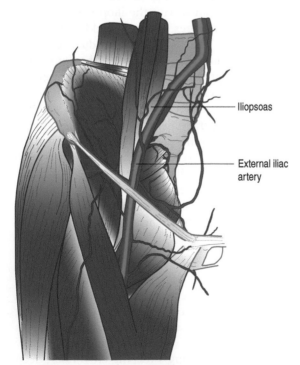

Iliopsoas

External iliac artery

Figure 8.20 Relationship of the iliopsoas to the external iliac artery.

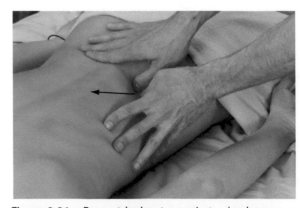

Figure 8.21 Deep stripping to quadratus lumborum.

D. MET for iliopsoas The client is in a supine position with one thigh hanging off the side of the table. The client holds the opposite thigh in a fully flexed and bent knee position. The client attempts hip flexion of the hanging thigh, while the practitioner offers resistance. The client holds the contraction for about 5–8 seconds, and then releases the contraction. As the client releases the contraction, the practitioner pushes the thigh into extension to stretch the iliopsoas muscle (Fig. 8.22). If the client experiences discomfort, instruct the client to further flex the opposite hip, which will increase rotation of the pelvis, straighten the spine, and reduce facet joint compression.

Rehabilitation protocol considerations

- Perform soft-tissue treatment methods several times before engaging in strength training for muscles in this region. The body needs to re-adjust to different proprioceptive and neuro-muscular patterns.

- Strength training methods are routinely used to address the postural distortion of anterior pelvic tilt. Studies on the use of strength training have indicated that if hypertonic muscles are not properly addressed, dysfunctional compensation and recruitment patterns develop. That is why strength training should not be the first inter-vention, but should come at a point after soft-tissue treatment interventions.

- Many postural disorders such as anterior pelvic tilt persist because neuromuscular patterns of

tension are continually reinforced. Despite soft-tissue treatment or strengthening activities, correction of many anterior pelvic tilts will not have a lasting change unless the client engages in some form of postural re-training which reinforces corrected biomechanical patterns.

Cautions and contraindications

Use great caution with any iliopsoas treatment technique that uses direct pressure through the abdomen. As mentioned above, there is a risk of adverse vascular responses. When performing MET for the iliopsoas above, be aware that some clients experience back discomfort with this technique due to compression of the lumbar facet joints.

POSTERIOR PELVIC TILT

Description

A posterior rotation of the two innominates that make up the pelvis is a posterior pelvic tilt. This postural distortion gives the individual an appearance of a very flat back and buttocks that appear tucked under (Fig. 8.23). The posterior

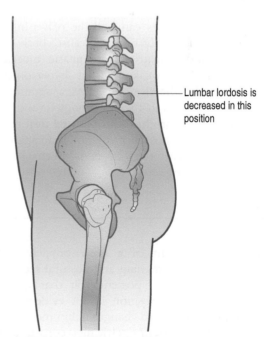

Lumbar lordosis is decreased in this position

Figure 8.23 Posterior pelvic tilt.

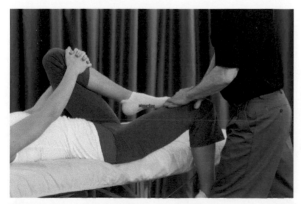

Figure 8.22 MET for iliopsoas from Thomas test position with the leg off the side of the table.

tilt is less common than the anterior tilt. There are detrimental ramifications to the posterior tilt.

There is only slight movement at the sacroiliac joints, so when the pelvis moves it also brings the sacrum and lumbar spine along with it. A posterior rotation decreases the lumbar lordosis and causes the vertebrae to be stacked vertically on top of one another. A primary function of the lumbar lordosis is to decrease compressive forces in the spine and to allow for proper shock absorption. The more vertical arrangement of the vertebral bodies on top of each other increases the compressive forces on the intervertebral discs and can play a role in lumbar disc pathology.[28]

Several factors contribute to posterior pelvic rotations; many of these stem from chronic postural misuse such as sitting in a slouched position. Because the posterior pelvic rotation may be exacerbated by a continual reinforcement of poor biomechanics, like slouching, short-term interventions may not be effective unless accompanied by repeated postural re-education and a reconditioning of proper body mechanics.

The muscular and soft-tissue factors that contribute to posterior pelvic rotation are opposite those that create the anterior pelvic rotation. Tightness in the abdominal muscles and/or tightness in the hamstrings can pull the pelvis into a posterior rotation. However, because both the abdominals and hamstrings are phasic muscles, they tend toward weakness, not hypertonicity when fatigued. Therefore, it takes a significant amount of tightness in the hamstrings or abdominals combined to produce this postural distortion alone. More often, posterior rotation is an adapted pattern that is reinforced by poor mechanics in sitting and standing.

Treatment

Traditional approaches

Traditional treatment of a posterior pelvic tilt focuses on strength training and postural reeducation. In many cases a posterior tilt that appears evident in a sitting position is not evident in a standing position due to changes in hip mechanics. Treatment of the posterior pelvic tilt is consequently not emphasized as greatly.

Soft-tissue manipulation

General guidelines   Treatment of posterior pelvic rotations should address hypertonicity evident in the abdominal and hamstring muscle groups. Investigate these muscles for presence of myofascial trigger points as well. Unlike the anterior pelvic tilt, muscular hypertonicity is not as much of a factor in creating a posterior pelvic tilt. The postural distortion is more related to chronic postural positions in either standing or sitting. Consequently, postural re-education is an essential component of treating the posterior pelvic tilt. Soft-tissue manipulation alone, without some form of postural retraining is unlikely to achieve a lasting effect.

Suggested techniques and methods

A. Sweeping cross fiber for rectus abdominis The rectus abdominis pulls its attachments on the pubis in a superior direction. Sweeping cross fiber techniques reduce muscle tightness that contributes to the postural distortion. Sweep diagonally across the fibers of the rectus abdominis with the thumb (Fig. 8.24). Treat the whole length of the rectus abdominis from the rib cage to the inferior attachments near the pubis.

B. Sweeping cross fiber to hamstrings The hamstrings can pull inferiorly on the pelvis causing the posterior rotation. Reducing tension in this muscle group helps decrease their downward pull on the pelvis. The stroke travels diagonally across the fibers of the muscle group (Fig. 8.25). Use successive sweeping strokes on the hamstrings until the entire muscle group has been covered.

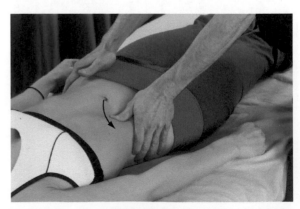

Figure 8.24   Sweeping cross fiber to rectus abdominis.

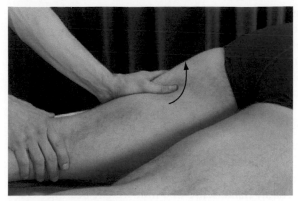

Figure 8.25   Sweeping cross fiber to hamstrings.

C. Deep longitudinal stripping Hamstring tension is further reduced with deep stripping techniques. Use the deep stripping techniques on the hamstrings after some of the more superficial techniques such as the sweeping cross fiber. Start with broad contact surface of pressure and then gradually perform the stripping techniques with a small contact surface (Fig. 8.26).

Rehabilitation protocol considerations

- Massage treatment can help reduce hypertonicity that may be contributing to the problem. However, postural change should be encouraged early on in the treatment process and reinforced on a regular basis.

- Stretching methods are valuable after soft-tissue treatment to encourage flexibility of the involved tissues. It is helpful if stretching is performed prior to regular postural retraining exercises.

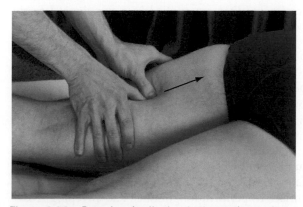

Figure 8.26   Deep longitudinal stripping to hamstrings.

Cautions and contraindications   Other than general precautions and working within the client's pain and comfort tolerance, there are no major contraindications or cautions for addressing a posterior pelvic tilt with massage.

LATERAL PELVIC TILT

Description

When one side of the pelvis is higher than the other side, the individual has a lateral pelvic tilt (Fig. 8.27). The tilt is named for the side toward which the pelvis tilts. If the right side is higher, it is considered a left lateral tilt because the pelvis is tilting to the left. Think of the pelvis as a bowl and the side to which the water would spill is the side the tilt is named for.

The lateral pelvic tilt can result from muscular dysfunction, in which case it is considered a functional disorder. When it is caused by irregular bone size or alignment issues in the lumbar spine or lower extremity, it is considered a structural disorder. Failure to discriminate between structural and

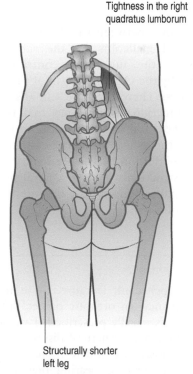

Tightness in the right
quadratus lumborum

Structurally shorter
left leg

Figure 8.27   Lateral pelvic tilt.

functional causes of a lateral pelvic tilt can cause clinical confusion and inappropriate treatment. Two of the most common causes of lateral pelvic tilt are functional changes from lumbar muscle tightness, and structural problems resulting from a true leg-length discrepancy.

The pelvis can tilt in a lateral direction if there is hypertonicity or spasm in the low back muscles, especially if the tightness is exaggerated on one side. This is particularly apparent with hypertonicity of the quadratus lumborum (QL), because it is a primary lateral flexor of the lumbar spine. The QL muscle is particularly susceptible to hypertonicity because it is a postural muscle of the trunk. If tightness in the QL is markedly greater on one side than the other, it can pull the pelvis higher on the side that is tighter. The tightness may be the result of an acute episode of back pain, or it may occur from improper habitual postural patterns that have been adopted over time.

If the client has a true, structural leg-length discrepancy, it causes a lateral pelvic tilt. A true, structural leg-length discrepancy is accurately evaluated with a full lower-extremity X-ray. However, that is not practical in many cases and a comparable test can be achieved by using a tape measure to measure the distance between the ASIS on one side to the medial malleolus on the same side.[29] Regardless of the functional contribution to pelvic tilting by the QL, the length of these bones never changes. Therefore, one can discriminate between a functional shortening that is caused by QL tightness and one that is caused by a true difference in the length of the bones of the lower extremity. In addition to the leg-length discrepancy, other structural causes of lateral pelvic tilt include a smaller innominate on one side and structural scoliosis.

Treatment

Traditional approaches

If the lateral pelvic tilt is caused by a true leg-length discrepancy, an orthotic or heel lift under the short side is usually prescribed. Lateral pelvic tilts caused by major structural disorders, such as structural scoliosis, are much more difficult to treat. They may involve wearing braces, corsets,

or, in more extreme cases, surgical treatment to correct the spinal deformity. Traditional treatment of lateral pelvic tilts that are functional disorders and caused by muscular tightness usually involves physical therapy, stretching, and in some cases muscle relaxants.

Soft-tissue manipulation

General guidelines   It is suggested that the hamstrings contribute to lateral pelvic tilt by pulling down on the low side of the pelvis.[30] This would certainly make sense in a non-weight bearing position. However, with the weight of the upper body resting on the femoral heads, it is unclear how the pelvis could be pulled any further inferiorly. Hypertonicity in the hamstrings would more likely pull the pelvis into a posterior rotation, as their angle of pull has a greater tendency to act on the pelvis in the sagittal plane.

If the apparent leg-length difference is primarily functional and caused by hypertonicity in the QL, then treatment of the hypertonic QL is the most effective approach. There are a variety of techniques to address tightness in the quadratus lumborum including static compression, deep longitudinal stripping, pin and stretch, and active-assisted stretching.

If the cause of the lateral pelvic tilt is a structural disorder, massage has limited effectiveness in making a postural correction. However, various detrimental ramifications can result from the structural dysfunction and these can be addressed by massage. For example, if a structural scoliosis has caused the lateral pelvic tilt, muscles on the concave side of the scoliotic curve are likely to be hypertonic. They benefit from the same muscular treatments that are applied in a functional lateral pelvic tilt.

Suggested techniques and methods   It is valuable to treat the lumbar muscles bilaterally in a lateral pelvic tilt. However, place greater emphasis on the high side of the lateral tilt because these muscles need the most therapy to reduce hypertonicity.

A. Effleurage and sweeping cross fiber to lumbar muscles Use the thumb, back-side of the fingers, base of the hand, or other broad contact surface to perform longitudinal and sweeping cross fiber applications to the lumbar muscles (Fig. 8.11). If the lateral pelvic tilt is resulting from an acute spasm, use caution with the amount of pressure in this technique because deep pressure moving rapidly across the muscle fibers can cause reactive muscle splinting.

B. Static compression to hypertonic lumbar muscles Apply static compression to the lumbar muscles with a broad contact surface such as the fist or palm. After achieving some initial relaxation in the lumbar tissues, use a more specific contact surface, such as the fingertip, thumb, or pressure tool (Fig. 8.28). Be cautious about the depth of pressure with these more specific pressure applications, especially if the QL is in spasm.

C. Deep stripping to quadratus lumborum After achieving some relaxation in the superficial back muscles and initial tension reduction in the QL, apply deep longitudinal stripping to the QL muscle. Use the thumb or fingertips to perform a longitudinal stripping technique on the quadratus lumborum (Fig. 8.21). Use stripping motions from the iliac crest to the transverse processes, iliac crest to twelfth rib, and transverse processes to twelfth rib as the quadratus lumborum has fibers running in all these directions. When working from lateral to medial on the fibers running from the iliac crest to the transverse processes, apply pressure deep enough to treat under the lateral edge of the erector spinae muscle group. However, use caution not to apply too much pressure directly against the tips of the transverse processes.

D. Pin and stretch for quadratus lumborum This technique uses the pin and stretch concept along with eccentric activity in the QL to encourage reduction of hypertonicity. The client is in a side-lying position. Bring the client's thigh into a position of abduction to shorten the QL muscle. Abducting the thigh shortens the QL because when the thigh is abducted the pelvis lifts a little higher on the same side. Ask the client to hold their leg in that position (as long as this does not produce further muscle pain in a client with muscle spasm). Apply static compression to the QL with the thumb while the client holds the leg in an abducted position. Instruct the client to slowly drop the leg down off the back-side of the table; continue to hold the static compression position as the client lowers the leg (Fig. 8.29). This treatment can feel intense for the client so gauge the pressure carefully. A variation on this technique can be used by applying a stripping technique during the client's eccentric adduction of the thigh instead of static compression. This variation is even more effective in reducing tension in the quadratus lumborum.

Rehabilitation protocol considerations

- Unlike the posterior and anterior pelvic tilts, which appear to be postural aberrations reinforced from chronic misuse over time, muscular (functional) lateral pelvic tilts are often caused by recent dysfunctional muscular activity. Consequently, massage and soft-tissue treatment interventions are more effective in this condition.

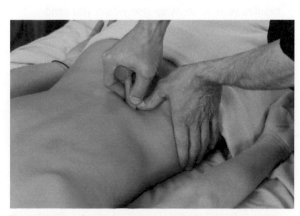

Figure 8.28   Static compression to lumbar muscles.

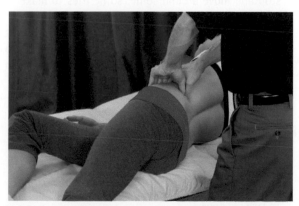

Figure 8.29   Pin and stretch to quadratus lumborum. Photo shows the final position at the end of the stretch.

- Massage and soft-tissue treatments should be engaged immediately. Stretching procedures are most effective when performed after massage treatment has made the lumbar muscles more pliable.

- Self-massage or stretching procedures that the client can perform at home will assist in maintaining optimum tissue flexibility and restoring proper balance to the pelvic musculature.

Cautions and contraindications Other than general precautions and working within the client's pain and comfort tolerance, there are no major contraindications or cautions for addressing a lateral pelvic tilt with massage.

Box 8.2   Case Study

Background

Daniel is a 42-year-old insurance specialist who spends a great deal of time traveling in his car. He is also moderately active at home, as he likes to keep in shape. He has not been able to do as much physical activity recently due to an accident he had several weeks ago. While getting out of his car he slipped on the ice in the parking lot and fell against the curb, landing on his right gluteal region. It was painful at the time, and has continued to give him problems ever since. The pain he reports is mostly a dull aching pain felt in his gluteal region and right lower extremity. He went to the doctor after the accident and had X-rays performed. The doctor mentioned that he did not have any broken bones or serious injuries. The doctor suggested he rest for a while and come back if the condition did not get better or got worse.

His pain is aggravated from long hours in his car, which unfortunately he must keep doing for his work. He says it usually feels better when he can stop and move around some, so he tries to make more frequent stops when he is driving to decrease the discomfort. Sometimes the pain wakes him up at night, and he will take aspirin so he can go back to sleep. He thinks massage might be able to help him reduce his pain and get back to his active regimen.

Questions to consider

- The doctors have ruled out any fractures with an X-ray, but based on the information we have, what might be the cause of Daniel's injury?
- A sudden fall like his could have caused an injury to ligaments such as the iliolumbar, posterior sacroiliac, or sacrotuberous ligaments. Would you choose to treat these problems with massage? If so, how would you go about it?
- Daniel is reporting pain down his lower extremity so it is possible that he has a nerve injury. If he suffered a compression injury to one or more of the nerves in the gluteal region, would you choose to treat him with massage?
- Do you think thermal modalities would be advantageous for Daniel to use at home? If so, which ones would you recommend and why?
- A multi-disciplinary approach is often valuable in treatment. Based on what we know from Daniel's condition, do you think he might benefit from seeing another health professional besides you? If so, who else would you send him to?
- What are some of the major cautions and possible contraindications you want to be aware of in addressing Daniel's condition.

References

1. Rask MR. Superior gluteal nerve entrapment syndrome. Muscle Nerve. 1980;3(4):304–307.
2. Travell J, Simons, D. Myofascial Pain and Dysfunction: The Trigger Point Manual. Vol 2. Baltimore: Williams & Wilkins; 1992.
3. Benson ER, Schutzer SF. Posttraumatic piriformis syndrome: Diagnosis and results of operative treatment. J Bone Joint Surg Am 1999;81A(7):941–949.
4. Almekinders LC. Anti-inflammatory treatment of muscular injuries in sport – An update of recent studies. Sport Med. 1999;28(6):383–388.
5. Jankiewicz JJ, Hennrikus WL, Houkom JA. The appearance of the piriformis muscle syndrome in computed tomography and magnetic resonance imaging. A case report and review of the literature. Clin Orthop. 1991;262:205–209.

6. Prentice W. Rehabilitation Techniques in Sports Medicine. St. Louis: Mosby; 1990.

7. Chaitow L. Modern Neuromuscular Techniques. New York: Churchill Livingstone; 1996.

8. Lowe W. Orthopedic Assessment in Massage Therapy. Sisters, OR: Daviau-Scott; 2006.

9. Voorn R. Case report: can sacroiliac joint dysfunction cause chronic Achilles tendinitis? J Orthop Sports Phys Ther. 1998;27(6):436–443.

10. Basmajian J, Nyberg R. Rational Manual Therapies. Baltimore: Williams & Wilkins; 1993.

11. Vleeming A, J.P. VW, Snijders CJ, et al. Load application of the sacrotuberous ligament: influences on sacroiliac joint mechanics. Clinical Biomechanics. 1989;4:203–205.

12. Myers TW. Anatomy Trains. Edinburgh: Churchill Livingstone; 2001.

13. Snijders C, Vleeming A, Stoeckart R, Mens J, Kleinrensink G. Biomechanics of the interface between spine and pelvis in different postures. In: Vleeming A, Mooney V, Dorman T, Snijders C, Stoeckart R, eds. Movement, Stability, & Low Back Pain. New York: Churchill Livingstone; 1999.

14. Weksler N, Velan GJ, Semionov M, et al. The role of sacroiliac joint dysfunction in the genesis of low back pain: the obvious is not always right. Arch Orthop Trauma Surg. Dec 2007;127(10):885–888.

15. Tullberg T, Blomberg S, Branth B, Johnsson R. Manipulation does not alter the position of the sacroiliac joint. A roentgen stereophotogrammetric analysis. Spine. 1998;23(10):1124–1128; discussion 1129.

16. Gotlin R. Sacroiliac joint injury. e-Medicine; 2006.

17. Browning KH. Hip and pelvis injuries in runners. Physician Sportsmed. 2001;29(1):23–26.

18. Mehta A. Common Musculoskeletal Problems. Philadelphia: Hanley & Belfus; 1997.

19. Shbeeb MI, Matteson EL. Trochanteric bursitis (greater trochanter pain syndrome). Mayo Clin Proc. 1996;71(6):565–569.

20. Kingzett–Taylor A, Tirman PF, Feller J, et al. Tendinosis and tears of gluteus medius and minimus muscles as a cause of hip pain: MR imaging findings. AJR Am J Roentgenol. 1999;173(4):1123–1126.

21. Slawski DP, Howard RF. Surgical management of refractory trochanteric bursitis. Am J Sports Med. 1997; 25(1):86–89.

22. Vleeming A, Mooney V, Dorman T, Snijders C, Stoeckart R. Movement, Stability, & Low Back Pain. New York: Churchill Livingstone; 1999.

23. Chaitow L. Muscle Energy Techniques. New York: Churchill Livingstone; 1996.

24. Janda V. Muscles as a pathogenic factor in back pain. Paper presented at: IFOMT, 1980; New Zealand.

25. Liebenson Ce. Rehabilitation of the Spine. Baltimore: Williams & Wilkins; 1996.

26. Chaitow L, DeLany J. Clinical Application of Neuromuscular Techniques. Vol 1. Edinburgh: Churchill Livingstone; 2000.

27. Janda V. Rational therapeutic approach of chronic back pain syndromes. Paper presented at: Chronic back pain, rehabilitation, and self-help, 1985; Turku, Finland.

28. Soderberg G. Kinesiology: Application to Pathological Motion. Baltimore: Williams & Wilkins; 1986.

29. Magee D. Orthopedic Physical Assessment. 3rd ed. Philadelphia: W.B. Saunders; 1997.

30. Phaigh R. The Treatment of Pain. Eugene: Onsen Techniques; 1991.

Chapter 9

Lumbar and thoracic spine

Back pain is a persistent and costly problem for society today. It is estimated that approximately 70% of Americans will have back pain at some point in their life.[1] For many people these conditions will occur more than once. The direct and indirect medical costs of low-back pain (LBP) are staggering. In 1991 it was reported that these costs equaled somewhere between $50 and $100 billion per year in the United States, with more recent studies showing these costs increasing.[2,3–5] Attempts have been made to identify which treatments are most cost effective in dealing with this pervasive musculoskeletal disorder, but studies have yet to come away with a clear determination.[6,7] Other countries also report a high incidence of LBP indicating this disorder places a high economic burden on the health care system worldwide.[8–12]

The causes of LBP are poorly understood and treatment for the condition can be inadequate. For many years LBP was thought to result primarily from structural disorders, such as herniated discs.[1] While herniations do exist in some cases, many LBP complaints do not involve disc pathology. For numerous cases there is no easily identifiable structural or organic cause for the pain.

It is becoming increasingly clear that LBP problems are multi-dimensional, involving anatomy, biomechanics, and important psychosocial factors.[1] In fact, a back pain diagnosis is often dependent on the theoretical perspective of the health care practitioner treating the condition. In general, the type of health care specialist chosen mainly determines an individual's treatment options.[13] In LBP, these options run the gamut from surgery to soft-tissue therapy.

Despite the fact that a large percentage of the population develops back pain, the ability to effectively treat this problem has lagged. A large percentage of patients report dissatisfaction with the quality of care they receive for back pain.[14,15] This is one of the primary reasons that individuals seek help from various alternative therapies, such as massage. Non-specific back pain often has a muscular origin, resulting from hypertonicity or myofascial trigger points.[16,17] Massage is an ideal therapeutic intervention in many of these cases.[18-23]

INJURY CONDITIONS

NEUROMUSCULAR LOW BACK PAIN

Description

Muscular dysfunction is one of the most common sources of LBP and can lead to altered movement patterns as well as postural stress in both standing and sitting positions. The postural distortions that occur in the spine have led clinicians to focus on the bones of the spine as the root of the problem, with an associated emphasis on joint pathology.[24] In a large number of cases, however, the problem is muscular in nature, with postural changes a result not the cause.

Myofascial trigger points in muscles such as the quadratus lumborum, erector spinae, multifidi, and other short intrinsic muscles of the spine cause pain referral patterns in the back. A sudden and awkward loading movement or trauma often activates trigger points. Perpetual trigger points can become a chronic source of back pain if they are not properly neutralized.[25-27]

In some cases, a seemingly benign activity, like reaching down to pick up a pencil, can cause acute muscular back pain and the development of subsequent trigger points. In these cases, lumbar musculature is close to a level of fatigue, and all it takes is a little bit of additional stress to cause overload and subsequent dysfunction. This kind of injury often results from the combined motions of lateral flexion and rotation, which put the lumbar spine in a mechanically disadvantaged position.[28] Recent studies in spinal biomechanics indicate that neuromuscular pain and acute back injury often start with dysfunctional coordination between muscle recruitment and fascial tension in the lumbar spine.[29,30]

Constant neuromuscular tension can produce a number of postural distortions. These postural distortions, conversely, can produce excess neuromuscular activity and create muscular imbalance. For example, the quadratus lumborum can be the cause of an apparent leg length difference because the muscle pulls superiorly on the pelvis. The difference in leg length can then cause neuromuscular dysfunction in the lumbar muscles, especially the quadratus lumborum. A cycle of pain and discomfort is the result.

Due to the nature of motor learning, movement and dysfunctional postural distortions follow a pattern that, once set, tend to be repeated.[31] Patterns of pain or dysfunction occur in the same location repeatedly, especially in the stabilizing postural muscles of the spine. Individuals with back pain regularly describe an area to which the pain always returns whenever their problem flares up.

Biomechanical ramifications of muscular dysfunction, while sometimes subtle, can have far-reaching effects. Movement of the spine is an integrated process of motion between each of the different functional segments. Restricted motion at one vertebral segment (from either joint pathology or soft-tissue dysfunction) can increase or decrease motion at another segment. The subsequent lack of proper coordination leads to mechanical overload and neuromuscular dysfunction of the numerous thoracic and lumbar muscles.[32]

Treatment

Traditional approaches

For many years bed rest was a treatment suggestion for muscular LBP. That idea has changed as evidence now suggests that bed rest is more detrimental than helpful.[1,33] Prolonged immobilization appears to cause further muscle splinting and limitations to improved range of motion, despite the initial pain relief that may be felt during the rest. A complication of prolonged bed rest for back pain is the development of deep vein thrombosis in the lower extremity.[34]

Non-steroidal anti-inflammatory drugs (NSAIDs) are used with great frequency for neuromuscular back pain. In many cases there is no muscular inflammation, even though muscle is the primary pain-producing tissue in the condition. The rationale for use of anti-inflammatory medications is then questionable. The detrimental effects of prolonged NSAID are a factor in reconsidering this approach. Corticosteroid injections are also used for their anti-inflammatory and pain management properties.[35,36]

Physical medicine approaches, including exercise, stretching, or educational programs, have met with clinical success.[37,38] Physical intervention along with the active involvement of the patient are important components of this approach. Manipulation and joint mobilization also achieve favorable results in many cases.

Soft-tissue manipulation

General guidelines While there is a limited research base for clinical massage, LBP is one area that is studied more than others. At this point the evidence is strong that massage is very helpful in neuromuscular LBP problems.[18,19,21,39] Myofascial techniques are a great way to start treatment of neuromuscular back pain. They are generally performed before lubricant is applied and produce an initial soothing sensation for the client. In addition, neurological responses in the fascia encourage reductions in muscular tension.[40] Myofascial techniques can be followed up with effleurage and sweeping cross fiber treatments to the back muscles. These techniques are effective at reducing superficial muscle tension, increasing tissue circulation, and enhancing pliability in the subcutaneous fascia. As treatment progresses pressure levels can increase to access the deeper muscles. Increasing pressure levels enhances the neurological and mechanical effects that help reduce tension throughout the spinal muscles.

Various deep and specific massage techniques are an excellent method for treating the muscular tension that is at the root of neuromuscular LBP. Static compression, deep longitudinal stripping, pin and stretch, and active-assisted massage techniques are all effective methods for addressing neuromuscular back pain. Each of these techniques can be modified with different positions or methods to address specific muscles.

Suggested techniques and methods The suggested treatments section is expanded here to provide more attention to the different techniques that can be used to address the muscles in this area. Yet, this selection is only a small fraction of the many approaches and variations that are used to treat LBP.

A. Myofascial approaches These techniques can be performed in many areas of the lumbar or thoracic regions. The primary goal is to place a moderately light tangential (tensile) force on the subcutaneous fascia. Pulling the fascia in multiple directions enhances its pliability. Place the hands lightly on the client's back in the region where the myofascial stretch is to be applied. Pull the hands apart to take the slack out of the tissue and apply a light degree of tensile (pulling) force between the hands (Fig. 9.1). Once there is a slight degree of pull between the hands, hold this position until a subtle sensation of tissue release is felt between the hands.

B. Effleurage and sweeping cross fiber These techniques are some of the most effective methods for achieving relaxation of the superficial back muscles. They also produce extensibility in the superficial fascia. Effleurage is performed with long gliding strokes parallel to the muscle fiber

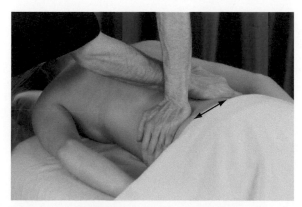

Figure 9.1 Myofascial techniques on lumbar area.

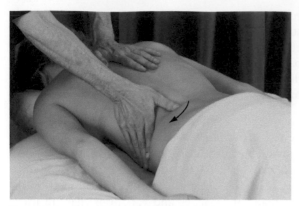

Figure 9.2   Sweeping cross fiber to lumbar muscles.

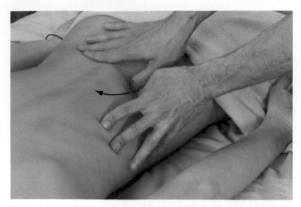

Figure 9.4   Deep stripping on quadratus lumborum.

direction. The cross fiber techniques sweep diagonally across the primary fiber direction of the muscles. Perform both throughout the low back (Fig. 9.2). Increasing levels of pressure are used to access deeper muscles.

C. Deep longitudinal stripping to spinal extensors Deep stripping techniques are applied to the erector spinae and spinal extensor muscles. Use a broad contact surface of pressure at the outset, especially if there is a greater degree of tension in these muscles. After relaxation of superficial tissues and to work more specifically on particular regions of the muscle, apply the stripping techniques with a small contact surface pressure, such as the finger tips, thumb, or pressure tool (Fig. 9.3).

D. Deep longitudinal stripping on quadratus lumborum The client is in a prone or side-lying position. Use the thumb or fingertips to perform a longitudinal stripping technique on the quadratus lumborum (Fig. 9.4). Use stripping motions

from the iliac crest to the transverse processes, iliac crest to twelfth rib, and transverse processes to twelfth rib as the quadratus lumborum has fibers running in all these directions. When working from lateral to medial on the fibers running from the iliac crest to the transverse processes, apply pressure deep enough to treat up under the lateral edge of the erector spinae muscle group. However, use caution not to apply too much pressure directly against the tips of the transverse processes.

E. Static compression To reduce muscular hypertonicity in a specific location, use static compression methods. With greater muscle tension, use a broad contact surface first such as the back side of the hand, palm, or fist. To treat more localized areas of tension or specific myofascial trigger points, use static compression with a small contact surface directly on those areas of increased tension (Fig. 9.5). Pressure maintained for 8–10 seconds is usually sufficient to achieve a reduction of muscle tension.

F. Deep stripping in lamina groove Numerous intrinsic muscles of the spine are difficult to treat unless deep specific work with a small contact surface is applied. Use the thumb, finger tip, or pressure tool to apply deep longitudinal stripping techniques to these muscles in the lamina groove. A hand position that uses two thumbs is the most effective way to perform this technique. This technique can be performed moving in a superior or inferior direction. The thumbs are positioned at right angles to each other. One thumb applies pressure against the spinous processes, while the other is applying pressure forward in the direction

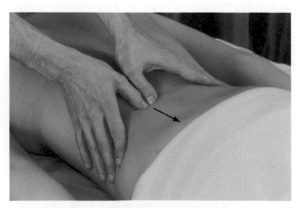

Figure 9.3   Deep stripping on erector spinae.

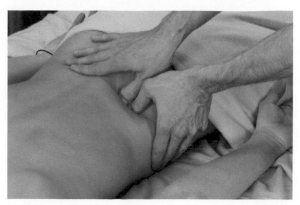

Figure 9.5 Static compression (small contact surface) on lumbar mucles.

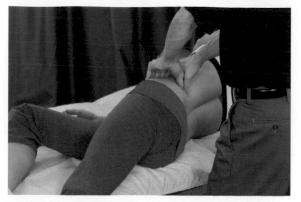

Figure 9.7 Pin and stretch to quadratus lumborum. Photo shows position at the end of the stretch procedure.

that the hands are moving (Fig. 9.6). Pause and repeat short stripping movements on any areas where increased muscle tension is palpated or the client reports greater tenderness.

G. Pin and stretch for quadratus lumborum This technique uses the pin and stretch concept along with eccentric activity in the quadratus lumborum (QL) to reduce hypertonicity. The client is in a side-lying position. Bring the client's thigh into a position of abduction to shorten the QL muscle. Abducting the thigh shortens the QL because when the thigh is abducted the pelvis lifts a little higher on the same side. Ask the client to hold their leg in that position (as long as this does not produce further muscle pain in a client with muscle spasm). Apply static compression to the QL with the thumb while the client is holding the leg in the abducted position. Continue to

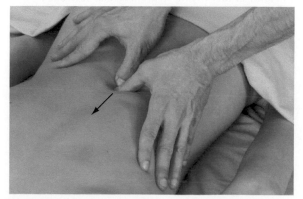

Figure 9.6 Deep stripping to the lamina groove.

apply the compression as the client slowly lowers the leg off the back-side of the table (Fig. 9.7).

This can feel intense for the client so gauge the pressure carefully as the technique is applied. A variation on this technique can be used by applying a stripping technique during the client's eccentric adduction of the thigh instead of static compression. This is even more effective in reducing tension in the QL.

H. Active assisted stretching for quadratus The client is in a side-lying position. Have the client reach up overhead and grasp the opposite end of the treatment table to both stabilize the torso and further stretch the lateral trunk muscles. Bring the client's thigh into a position of abduction to shorten the QL muscle just as in G above. Ask the client to hold the thigh in this position for 5–8 seconds, producing an isometric contraction in the QL. Have the client release the contraction and help them lower the abducted thigh off the back side of the table. As the thigh gets near the end range of motion press down on the thigh with one hand while the other hand pushes the client's pelvis in an inferior direction, creating a stretch (Fig. 9.8).

Rehabilitation protocol considerations

- Prior to constructing a treatment program for neuromuscular back pain, complete a thorough assessment to rule out more serious pathologies that need referral to another health professional.

- Facilitated patterns of postural distortion are an impediment to lasting change for

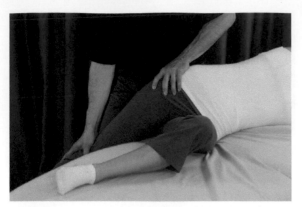

Figure 9.8 Active assisted stretching for quadratus lumborum. Photo shows position at the end of the stretch procedure.

neuromuscular back pain. Even after an effective massage treatment that provides relief, the neuromuscular pain pattern can immediately recur when long-established dysfunctional movement or postural patterns are repeated. It is important to encourage changes in these movement or postural patterns early in the treatment process as muscle tension is addressed through massage treatment.

- Strengthening techniques are often suggested by physical therapists or exercise specialists as a means of addressing neuromuscular back pain. If the strengthening activities are engaged too early in the rehabilitative process, they can reinforce dysfunctional patterns of muscle tension or posture. Massage can help reinforce gains made with strengthening or conditioning activities as long as it is later in the rehabilitation stage. Stretching and flexibility enhancement are essential components of treating neuromuscular back pain. Stretching is most effective when it performed after the soft-tissue manipulation so the benefits of enhanced tissue pliability can be maximized. If strength training is used in the rehabilitation program, stretching should be an integral aspect of the treatment process. Stretching is beneficial after the exercises to reduce any lingering muscle tension.

Cautions and contraindications Pay close attention to the pain reported by the client when working in this area. The quality of pain the client

reports helps determine the primary tissues at fault. There can be other causes of LBP, such as systemic disorders, tumor, or infectious processes, and many of these conditions can mimic muscular pain problems. The general guideline of common sense should apply here. If there is doubt about the nature of the client's condition, refer that person to another more qualified practitioner for further evaluation.

Sometimes neuromuscular back pain appears to resolve while the client is on the treatment table, only to return when the client stands or performs some slightly awkward movement, such as getting dressed after the treatment. Decreasing pain-producing tension on the muscular soft tissues in the lumbar and thoracic region can dramatically alter muscular proprioception. When the individual moves around after treatment there are very different muscular recruitment patterns being used and these new patterns can overtax certain tissues that have not appropriately developed to accommodate for the new neuromuscular patterns. The body's reaction to the sudden overload is muscle spasm. The best way to avoid that occurring is to remind the client to move slowly and carefully when first getting up from the massage treatment and for a short time afterward.

Box 9.1   Clinical Tip

Despite the advances in high-tech diagnostic tools such as X-ray or MRI, these tools are not very helpful in identifying neuromuscular low back pain. One of the most valuable tools for identifying muscular back pain is the trained palpation of practitioners specializing in soft-tissue manipulation. Knowledge of anatomy combined with specialized palpatory skills enhances the practitioner's ability to accurately identify tissues responsible for neuromuscular pain complaints. The ability to identify the source of neuromuscular soft-tissue pain and then immediately treat it with manual therapy is a distinct advantage for the massage practitioner in addressing numerous cases of low back pain.

HERNIATED NUCLEUS PULPOSUS

Description

The herniated nucleus pulposus (HNP) is routinely considered a primary cause of LBP, especially if that pain involves neurological symptoms. This problem is also known as a herniated disc, or inappropriately in laymen's terms, as a *slipped disc*. The diagnosis of disc herniation as a cause of back pain has become so extensive in the medical field that it has been referred to as the *dynasty of the disc*.[1]

One of the first articles to appear in the scientific literature indicating the intervertebral disc as a cause of back pain was the paper published by Mixter and Barr in 1934.[41] After their original article, there were numerous other studies published in medical journals that set out to prove the intervertebral disc as being at fault in many, if not most, LBP cases. The Mixter and Barr article appeared at a time when there were significant developments occurring in surgical techniques that made back surgery more feasible. Because discs could be observed protruding near nerve roots, it was a logical conclusion to assume that they were the cause of much back pain. However, as it turns out, this concept contained a jump in logic that has not proven accurate now that more sophisticated evaluation techniques have been developed.

Herniation technically means a pushing through. The primary problem in this condition is that degeneration of the annulus fibrosis allows the nucleus to push through it (Fig. 9.9). As the nucleus continues to press into the annulus, it causes the annulus to change shape. Eventually, if not halted, the nucleus can push all the way through the annulus. Degeneration of the annulus can be the result of numerous factors, including poor disc nutrition, loss of viable cells, loss of water content, and others.[42] These problems typically originate from chronic excessive compressive loads on the spinal structures.

There are several names given to disc herniations, and these reflect the level of severity of the disc damage. These names are not always consistent in the literature, but they do give a greater degree of specificity as to the severity of the herniation.[43] Figure 9.10 illustrates the different types of disc herniation. In a disc protrusion (also called

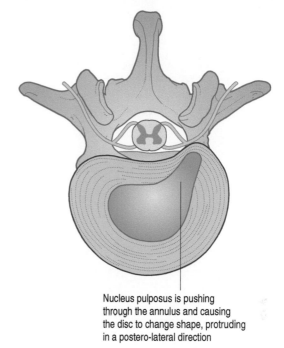

Nucleus pulposus is pushing through the annulus and causing the disc to change shape, protruding in a postero-lateral direction

Figure 9.9 Herniated nucleus pulposus pressing toward a nerve root.

a bulge) the disc has changed shape, but the majority of the annulus fibrosus is still intact. Another type of disc protrusion is called a prolapse. In a prolapse the nucleus has not yet broken through the outer barriers of the annulus, but only the outermost fibers of the annulus are containing the nucleus. In an extrusion, the disc material has pushed through the outer border of the annulus, but is still connected to the nucleus in the center of the disc. The final stage of degeneration is the sequestration. In this stage, the disc material has actually separated from itself, and portions of the disc material can be floating freely in the spinal canal.

One of the apparent clinical challenges is trying to decipher when disc herniation is actually a cause of back pain. LBP can be a co-existing symptom along with disc herniation, but not necessarily caused by the disc herniation itself. A number of recent studies using magnetic resonance imaging (MRI) have examined low back structure in people without back pain. These studies show that herniated discs are often present in asymptomatic

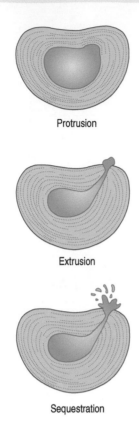

Protrusion

Extrusion

Sequestration

Figure 9.10   Different types of disc herniation.

individuals, which indicates that disc pathology is often not the source of LBP.[44–48]

When a lumbar disc protrudes against a nerve root, it is likely to cause symptoms in the distribution of that nerve root. Therefore, symptoms that are not neurological in nature and confined to the back are less likely to be coming from a disc pressing on a nerve root. However, if the symptoms are in the lower extremity and in characteristic dermatomes or myotomes, there is a greater likelihood of nerve root involvement.

Treatment

Traditional approaches

The HNP is usually treated conservatively with rehabilitative exercises. The exercise program developed by New Zealand physiotherapist Robin McKenzie has been quite effective for relieving symptoms thought to be originating from disc herniation.[38,49,50] In many cases, postural retraining along with rehabilitative exercise is sufficient for resolving the symptoms of disc herniation.[51]

Corticosteroid injections have been used with some success. There does appear to be some short-term pain relief with their use, although whether or not there is a long-lasting benefit is questionable.[35] Inflammation can be present, but is usually not a dominant aspect of this condition. The primary benefit of corticosteroid injections is pain relief more than reduction of inflammation.

Another procedure that has been used with some degree of success is chemonucleolysis.[52,53] In this procedure, a derivative of the papaya enzyme is injected into the area of the protruding disc. The papaya enzyme breaks down the protruding disc material reducing the likelihood of its pressing on nearby nerve roots. This treatment is used less now due to problems with allergic reactions to the papaya derivative.[54,55]

One of the more recent treatment methods is percutaneous laser disc decompression (PLDD).[56–58] This is a procedure in which a reduction in disc pressure is achieved through a laser treatment. A needle is first inserted into the nucleus pulposus under local anesthesia. A small amount of the nucleus pulposus is vaporized with the laser energy. As a result there is a sharp decline in pressure within the disc and the herniation moves away from the nerve root. This procedure is performed on an outpatient basis, and requires no general anesthesia and greatly reduces rehabilitation time.[59]

Surgical approaches for treating disc herniation have been used extensively, although this trend is decreasing. Traditional procedures are laminectomy (removal of a portion of the lamina) or discectomy (removal of a portion of the protruding disc).[60] Because it appears that people can have herniated discs and no back pain, the need for surgery seems less urgent. In fact, some have suggested the need for disc surgery to be about 2% of the individuals with a diagnosis of herniated nucleus pulposus.[61]

There is increasing concern about the use of surgery for low back problems, particularly because there is no clearly defined pathological process in a large number of cases.[62] In the United States the rate of surgery for back pain is at least 40% higher than in any other country.[63] It appears that back surgery increases as the supply of orthopedic and neurosurgeons in the country increases. Whether there is excessive surgery or if those in other countries are suffering from lack of surgery is yet to be determined.[63] What can be said is that in many cases conservative and less invasive treatments are more effective than surgical intervention for symptoms of disc herniation.

Soft-tissue manipulation

General guidelines Soft-tissue treatment is not necessarily contraindicated for HNP, but should be used with caution. It is always a good idea to have the client evaluated by another health professional if a disc herniation is suspected. Determining the level of disc herniation will determine what level of soft-tissue treatment is acceptable.

Massage does not directly reduce disc herniation. However, disc herniation often results from chronic compressive loads over time and hypertonic lumbar muscles can be a major factor in producing these loads. Addressing the muscular components of the compressive loads can help reduce factors that aggravate the disc herniation.

Suggested techniques and methods The focus of massage treatment for disc herniations is to reduce the role that muscle tightness plays in the disc pathology. Attention is focused on low back muscles that contribute to the compressive forces on the spine. Any of the techniques discussed in the previous section on neuromuscular back pain could be used to address the muscular components that aggravate a disc herniation.

Rehabilitation protocol considerations

- The primary focus of treatment is to reduce compression on neurological structures. Massage can be performed concurrently with other traditional conservative treatments such as manipulation or mobilization. Massage is a valuable adjunct for those treatments and is especially valuable if performed prior to those treatments. Reduction in muscle and soft-tissue tension allows these other techniques to be applied with greater ease and less resistance.

- Movement reeducation to reduce postural stress is an important aspect of treatment and can also be performed concurrently with massage treatment.

- If there is an acute disc herniation, significant muscle spasm can result. Protective muscle spasm should be addressed first in order to reduce the perpetuation of dysfunctional muscular activity.

- Massage is also a valuable adjunct treatment in post-surgical rehabilitation. After surgery massage treatment should not be used anywhere near surgical incision sites, but is effective in reducing excess muscle tension and restoring proper neuromuscular activity in the affected muscles.

- If the disc herniation has become a chronic situation, slightly more aggressive massage treatment can be attempted, but treatment should never aggravate the client's symptoms.

Cautions and contraindications Because the symptoms that can occur with herniated discs involve neurological sensations such as paresthesia, numbness, or motor disturbance in the lower extremity, other causes of these problems should be investigated as well. If symptoms are bilateral, a cauda equina syndrome (pressure directly on the spinal cord) could exist and should be immediately referred to a physician for proper evaluation.

Massage should not aggravate symptoms of disc herniation, so if there is an increase in neurological sensations after massage treatment, the treatment should be adjusted accordingly. Use caution when performing techniques close to the spine. The location of disc herniation is not vulnerable to massage treatment because the transverse processes of the spine protect the region. However, any technique that puts anteriorly directed pressure on the spine could move vertebrae in a way that aggravates nerve-root compression.

ZYGAPOPHYSIAL (FACET) JOINT IRRITATION

Description

The zygapophysial, or facet joints, are responsible for guiding the degree and orientation of movement in different regions of the spine. In the lumbar region, the angle of the facet joints is mostly vertical (parallel with the sagittal plane), so there is more movement allowed in flexion and extension. Further up the spine in the thoracic region, the facet joints are more obliquely aligned, which allows for less flexion and extension, but more rotation in the thoracic region. A functional unit of the spine is composed of two vertebrae and the intervertebral disc between them. There is a good indication that facet joint pain may be at least partially occurring from a lack of proper mobility in the functional units of the lumbar spine.[64]

In the spine, the vertebral body is the primary weight-bearing structure. The intervertebral disc sits directly on the body of the vertebra and acts as a cushion. There is some weight-bearing capacity of the posterior arch of the vertebrae. Thus, the contact points between adjacent vertebrae (the facet joints) are a partial weight-bearing joint. During extension, the center of gravity moves in a posterior direction. As a result, the posterior vertebral structures – the lamina, pedicle, pars interarticularis, posterior portion of the intervertebral disc, and facet joints – carry an increased percentage of weight. These structures are not designed for the weight increase and spinal pathology, such as facet joint dysfunction, disc herniation, spondylolysis, or spondylolisthesis, can result.

The amount of weight carried by the facet joints increases when the spine is in extension. When the spine is in extension, the center of gravity is more posterior, and this causes the facet joints to carry a greater load. There is greater weight carried by the facet joints in regions of the spine that have lordotic curvatures because the joints are already in extension. Due to the greater lordotic curvature, the low back region carries the greatest load. As a result, facet joint irritation is more common in this area than in other regions. Exaggerated lumbar lordosis increases the likelihood of facet joint irritation.

No specific tissue has been identified as the primary cause of pain in facet joint dysfunction, but there are several commonly suggested. The joint capsule is richly innervated, and certain postural strains on the facet joints can stretch or pinch capsular fibers causing significant pain. Chondromalacia of the joint surfaces, as well as capsular or synovial inflammation, has also been suggested as a cause of pain.[31]

Facet joint pain can be similar to pain that originates from other lumbar structures. For example, injection of a fluid irritant into the facet joints causes referred pain patterns similar to those of lumbar disc pathology.[65] There are certain signs and symptoms that appear consistent with facet joint irritation. However, there is no gold standard for identifying facet joint pain and, therefore, it remains difficult to accurately identify and treat.[66]

Treatment

Traditional approaches

Oral anti-inflammatory medication is often prescribed for facet joint irritation. However, the purpose of anti-inflammatory medication is unclear, as the presence of inflammation is not always demonstrated in facet dysfunction. This could be the reason for variable effectiveness with anti-inflammatory medication.

Other conservative forms of treatment include instruction in body mechanics, stretching, and strength training. Instruction in body mechanics is helpful if the individual has a tendency toward an exaggerated lumbar lordosis. The client will benefit by reinforcing the postural corrections on a regular basis, otherwise treatment results generally do not last. Because excessive lordosis compresses the facet joints further, improvement of this postural distortion is one of the most important parts of a therapeutic approach.

Cryotherapy is sometimes used to address inflammatory processes in the facet joints. The effectiveness of this approach may be limited, because the presence of inflammation is not a consistent finding in facet joint dysfunction.[67,68] Facet joint injections may be used for diagnostic as well as treatment procedures. However, there is controversy about the effectiveness of this procedure, despite the fact that use of these injections is widespread. Corticosteroid injections into the facet joints have not been found to be of much value in treatment.[69] The lack of agreement in treatments for facet joint problems suggests that more research is needed to identify effective approaches.

Soft-tissue manipulation

General guidelines   A challenge for the soft-tissue practitioner treating facet joint dysfunction is how to restore proper joint biomechanics without increasing further trauma or aggravation in the area. Massage treatment has limited effectiveness in directly affecting joint biomechanics. However, a number of techniques can help to improve proper joint function and, thus, reduce the aggravation of facet joint dysfunction.

Soft-tissue treatment begins with improved body mechanics that decrease irritation on the aggravated joint structures. Soft-tissue manipulation is enhanced if instruction in proper body mechanics is consistently followed during the treatment. As there is no clear-cut cause of a majority of facet joint dysfunction, the ideal treatment protocol remains unclear. However, reducing tension in the intrinsic spinal muscles is an important treatment goal as tightness in these muscles can contribute to facet joint dysfunction.

The muscular components of postural distortion that perpetuate excessive lumbar lordosis and increased facet joint compression must also be addressed. Massage treatment should emphasize the lumbar extensors, iliopsoas, and the rectus femoris, which all contribute to excessive lumbar lordosis. These muscles are effectively treated with techniques such as deep longitudinal stripping and active-assisted stretching procedures.

Stretching is helpful to reduce chronic muscular tension. At home the client should emphasize stretching in forward flexion and lateral flexion of the lumbar region. These are the areas, when hypertonic, that are most likely to aggravate facet joint compression.

Suggested techniques and methods

A. Deep longitudinal stripping to spinal extensors Deep stripping techniques are applied to the erector spinae and spinal extensor muscles. Use a broad contact surface of pressure at the outset, especially if there is a greater degree of tension in these muscles. Once the muscles have begun to relax, more specific muscle treatment can be applied using stripping techniques with a small contact surface such as the finger tips, thumb, or pressure tool (Fig. 9.3).

B. Deep longitudinal stripping on quadratus lumborum The client is in a prone or side-lying position. Use the thumb or fingertips to perform a longitudinal stripping technique on the QL (Fig. 9.4). Use stripping motions from the iliac crest to the transverse processes, iliac crest to twelfth rib, and transverse processes to twelfth rib as the QL has fibers running in all these directions. When treating from lateral to medial on the fibers running from the iliac crest to the transverse processes, apply pressure deep enough to work up under the lateral edge of the erector spinae muscle group. However, use caution not to apply too much pressure directly against the tips of the transverse processes.

C. Deep stripping in lamina groove Use the thumb, finger tip, or pressure tool to apply deep longitudinal stripping techniques to the muscles in the lamina groove. A hand position that uses two thumbs is the most effective way to perform this technique. This technique can be performed moving in a superior or inferior direction. The thumbs are positioned at almost right angles to each other. One thumb applies pressure against the spinous processes, while the other is applying pressure down and forward in the direction that the hands are moving (Fig. 9.6). Pause and repeat short stripping movements on areas where increased muscle tension is palpated or the client reports greater tenderness. Increased tension in the intrinsic spinal muscles is likely to be near the facet joint compression, so spend more time treating these areas. Some practitioners advocate working in an inferior to superior direction (opposite the direction of facet joint compression due to gravity) in order to decrease compression between adjacent vertebrae. However, there is no clear evidence that one is better than the other.

D. MET for iliopsoas The client is in a supine position with one thigh hanging off the side of the table. The client holds the opposite thigh in a fully flexed and bent knee position. The client attempts hip flexion of the hanging thigh, while the practitioner offers resistance. The client holds the contraction for about 5–8 seconds, and then releases the contraction. As the client releases the contraction, the practitioner pushes the thigh into extension to stretch the iliopsoas muscle (Fig. 9.11). If the client experiences discomfort, instruct the client to further flex the opposite hip, which will increase rotation of the pelvis, straighten the spine, and reduce facet joint compression.

Rehabilitation protocol considerations

- In some cases facet joint dysfunction results from other conditions affecting spinal biomechanics, such as intervertebral disc degeneration. In these cases the dysfunctional spinal biomechanics or

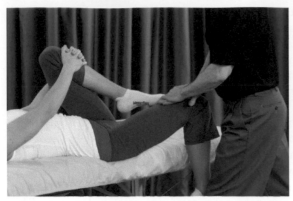

Figure 9.11   MET in Thomas test position.

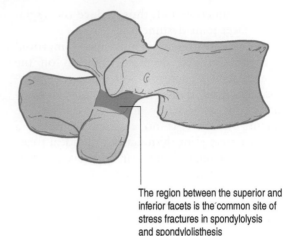

The region between the superior and inferior facets is the common site of stress fractures in spondylolysis and spondylolisthesis

Figure 9.12   Lateral view of a lumbar vertebra showing the pars interarticularis – site of stress fractures.

positions will need to be addressed sufficiently in order to resolve the facet joint dysfunction. Massage can be performed simultaneously with those other approaches.

- Stretching is a valuable adjunct for improving postural strain that leads to facet joint irritation. Stretching procedures are more helpful if soft-tissue treatment, such as massage, is performed prior to the stretching.

- Strength training and conditioning can be helpful in establishing new movement patterns in the lumbar and trunk muscles. These approaches are most effective if there have been a number of massage treatments and reinforced postural changes prior to initiating the strengthening program. Otherwise, the benefits of soft-tissue treatment can be eliminated when the person walks out the door if they immediately adopt dysfunctional postural patterns.

Cautions and contraindications Symptoms of facet syndrome can be the same as many other back disorders, some of which are more serious. If symptoms get worse as a result of treatment, cease that approach and reinvestigate the problem. The client may need to be referred to another health care provider for further evaluation.

SPONDYLOLYSIS AND SPONDYLOLISTHESIS

Description

While these are two separate conditions, they are closely related to one another and are treated the same, so they are described here together. By definition, spondylolysis is a breakdown of the vertebral body. The breakdown is a stress fracture to a region of the vertebra called the pars interarticularis (Fig. 9.12). The stress fracture results from repeated loads placed on the posterior aspect of the lumbar vertebrae. Most problematic are increased loads while the spine is in extension.[70]

The majority of weight is carried through the lumbar spine by the main body of each vertebra. However, during extension, the center of gravity moves in a posterior direction, and the posterior vertebral structures carry an increased percentage of that weight. Increased weight bearing, especially with repetitive or high-intensity loads, can lead to the development of stress fractures. Stress fractures produce pain themselves, but they also create problems as they progress into spondylolisthesis.

Spondylolisthesis is a forward slippage of one vertebra in relation to another and is often the result of bilateral spondylolysis. Once the stress fractures have occurred, on each side, forward slippage of the vertebra is more likely to occur. A common location for spondylolisthesis is at the L5–S1 junction (Fig. 9.13). Clients with spondylolisthesis report lumbar pain that is aggravated by strenuous activities, especially repetitive flexion and extension or hyperextension movements of the spine.

Spondylolisthesis is particularly common in the adolescent athletic population. The higher incidence of the condition in this group can be related

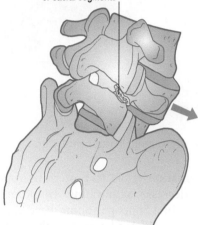

Bilateral stress fractures at the pars interarticularis have expanded allowing the body of the lumbar vertebra to migrate forward in relation to the adjacent vertebral or sacral segments

Figure 9.13 Spondylolisthesis at the L5–S1 junction.

to significant loads on the spine during skeletal immaturity. In adolescence bones are still developing some of their structural integrity and may not be ready to handle the load demand of vigorous athletic activities involving spinal extension.

In both conditions pain is diffuse in the lower lumbar and upper sacral regions. Pain is also common at the sacroiliac joint and there may be symptoms of radiating nerve pain with spondylolisthesis. Neurological sensations result from traction on the lower lumbar nerve roots and the cauda equina as a result of the anteriorly shifted vertebra.[31,71] Forward slippage of a vertebra also causes spinal stenosis (narrowing of the intervertebral foramen) at that vertebral level, which can increase the likelihood of nerve root impingement.[72]

One factor that makes the cause of pain confusing in spondylolysis and spondylolisthesis is that the severity of symptoms does not necessarily correlate with the degree of slippage.[33] An individual can have significant forward slippage with minimal pain where someone else may have only minor slippage, but experiences more pain.

Hamstring tightness is present in many individuals with spondylolisthesis. There is a strong proprioceptive function of the hamstrings as the body attempts to adjust to the forward slippage of the lower lumbar vertebra. The hamstrings tighten in an effort to posteriorly rotate the pelvis. The posterior pelvic rotation decreases the potential for forward slippage of the lower lumbar vertebra and helps stabilize the lumbar region.[73,74]

Treatment

Traditional approaches

Treatment for spondylolysis is controversial. Because a stress fracture is involved, an important factor is reducing cumulative stress on the area so the fracture can heal appropriately. Activity modification is usually sufficient to reduce the cumulative trauma in the area. Some clinicians advocate rigid braces if bone scans reveal a greater severity of injury.[70] However, others question this protocol and propose rest from offending activities and stabilization exercises that emphasize flexion instead of extension (such as Williams flexion exercises) as a more valuable treatment.[75]

Treatment for spondylolisthesis follows the same protocol as that for spondylolysis. In most instances, conservative treatment is effective, and there is no need for surgery. If conservative treatment fails, surgery may be needed. Lumbar fusion is a procedure that is used in more severe cases.[72] Yet, some of the recent clinical evidence suggests that lumbar fusion may not be any more effective than the current methods of conservative treatment.[60] Additional research is needed to establish more definitive treatment guidelines for this problem.

Soft-tissue manipulation

General guidelines Positioning on the treatment table is an important consideration in soft-tissue treatment for spondylolysis and spondylolisthesis. Back treatments are usually performed in a prone position, and include significant pressure applied to the lumbar area. A primary concern in these conditions is anterior translation of the lumbar vertebra. Caution is advised with techniques that put pressure on the lumbar area in an anterior direction as these could aggravate the problem. The client usually reports increased pain with pressure levels that aggravate the condition. Putting the client in a partially flexed position on the treatment table is helpful to reduce lumbar stress. Bolsters, pillows, or a number of commercially

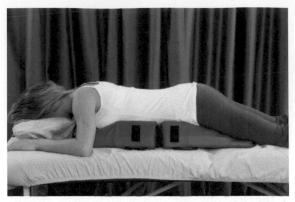

Figure 9.14 Flexion protocol on cushioned support to keep the lumbar region in a partially flexed position.

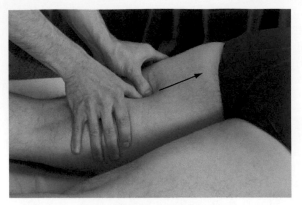

Figure 9.15 Deep stripping to hamstrings.

available support cushions are useful for this positioning (Fig. 9.14).

The primary problem in these conditions involves structural deficiency in the bones, which soft-tissue manipulation can not change. The focus of soft-tissue treatment is to encourage restoration of biomechanical patterns that help reduce anterior vertebral translation.

Suggested techniques and methods

A. Effleurage and sweeping cross fiber Effleurage is performed with long gliding strokes parallel to the muscle fiber direction. The cross fiber techniques sweep diagonally across the primary fiber direction in different regions of the back (Fig. 9.2). Increasing levels of pressure are used to access deeper muscles. Use caution and relax pressure if the strokes increase the client's symptoms.

B. Deep longitudinal stripping to spinal extensors Deep stripping techniques are applied to the erector spinae and spinal extensor muscles. Use a broad contact surface of pressure at the outset, especially if there is a greater degree of tension in these muscles. Once the muscles have begun to relax, apply the stripping techniques with small contact surface pressure such as the finger tips, thumb, or pressure tool to work on specific regions of any particular muscle (Fig. 9.3).

C. Deep longitudinal stripping to hamstrings Reduction of hamstring tension can help aid the overall lumbo-pelvic balance. Start with a broad contact surface of pressure and then eventually perform the stripping techniques with a small contact surface (Fig. 9.15). Hamstring tightness is a result

of a compensation effort to posteriorly rotate the pelvis and decrease aggravating symptoms from anterior vertebral slippage. Some have suggested that massage should not be used on the hamstrings as it could reduce their ability to posteriorly rotate the pelvis and protect against anterior vertebral slippage. It is unlikely that reduction of tension in the hamstrings will decrease their effectiveness in making these biomechanical alterations. Once the individual stands and moves around, the body perceives a need for greater stability. At this time an appropriate protective contraction in the hamstrings is likely, even if they have been previously relaxed with massage treatment.

Rehabilitation protocol considerations

- Massage techniques are most helpful when they are performed in conjunction with exercise and activity modification. Massage can slightly alter soft-tissue proprioception. If massage is performed shortly before exercise, the client should slowly work into the exercise movements, allowing the nervous system time to integrate the new movement patterns.

- If the condition is severe, pressure on low-back muscles can aggravate pain too much and massage is not recommended. The bone and other soft-tissue damage will need time to heal prior to engaging soft-tissue therapy.

Cautions and contraindications Because the symptoms of spondylolysis and spondylolisthesis can mimic other lumbar pathologies, it is important to accurately identify these problems before initiating treatment. Palliative care can be given to the individual as long as the practitioner avoids any activity that aggravates the symptoms. Use great caution in applying pressure techniques to the lumbar area as these could further encourage anterior vertebral translation.

POSTURAL DISTORTIONS

The next section includes a number of structural and postural disorders of the lumbar and thoracic spine. These disorders are not considered injury conditions, as are the prior conditions in this chapter. However, they can produce considerable stress on other tissues or structures and contribute to their dysfunction. Massage is not always used to correct these postural deviations, but it may be a helpful approach to restoring appropriate biomechanical balance in the region.

EXAGGERATED LUMBAR LORDOSIS

Description

There is a natural lordotic curve in the lumbar region that is necessary for shock absorption. The lordotic curve is exaggerated during extension and is reduced during flexion. The primary muscles that produce spinal extension are the erector spinae group, quadratus lumborum, and several small intrinsic spinal muscles including the multifidi, rotatores, interspinales, and intertransversarii. LBP and myofascial trigger points can develop from hypertonicity in these muscles and exaggerate the lordosis.

In a normal lumbar lordosis the vertebral body is the primary weight-bearing structure. With an excessive lumbar lordosis, more of the body's weight is transferred to the posterior portion of the vertebrae. Increased weight is then borne by posterior vertebral arch structures such as the lamina, pedicle, pars interarticularis, posterior portion of the intervertebral disc, and facet joints. These structures are not designed for the weight increase and spinal pathology such as facet joint dysfunction, disc herniation, spondylolysis, or spondylolisthesis can result. Increased lumbar extension also narrows the intervertebral foramen and can lead to spinal nerve root compression.[74]

Dysfunctional patterns of muscular activation and poor posture can perpetuate an excessive lordosis. An example is the lower crossed syndrome, originally described by Vladimir Janda.[76] He categorizes the body's muscles into two groups: postural or phasic muscles, which differ in their fiber type and activation patterns.[77] When overused and fatigued, postural muscles tend to become hypertonic, while phasic muscles tend to become weak and inhibited. The phasic muscles are antagonists to postural muscles. Because postural muscles tend toward hypertonicity, they create a functional weakness in the phasic muscles through the process of reciprocal inhibition.[26]

Postural muscles in the lumbar spine include the erector spinae, quadratus lumborum, and iliopsoas. Phasic muscles in this region include the abdominals, gluteus maximus and medius. An exaggerated lumbar lordosis also produces an anterior pelvic tilt and a postural distortion called the *lower crossed syndrome*. A graphical comparison of the functional and positional relationships of certain lumbopelvic muscles shows how they interact and where the term lower crossed syndrome originates from (Fig. 9.16). See the section in Chapter 8 on anterior pelvic tilts for additional descriptions of the lower crossed syndrome and reciprocal inhibition.

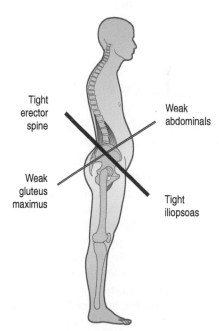

Tight erector spine

Weak abdominals

Weak gluteus maximus

Tight iliopsoas

Figure 9.16   Lower crossed syndrome (from Chaitow L, DeLany J. Clinical Application of Neuromuscular Techniques. Vol 1. Edinburgh: Churchill Livingstone; 2000).

Treatment

Traditional approaches

Traditional treatment approaches for exaggerated lumbar lordosis and the resulting lower crossed syndrome are the same as those described under the section on anterior pelvic tilt in Chapter 8.

Soft–tissue manipulation

Soft-tissue treatment and rehabilitation protocol considerations for an excessive lumbar lordosis are the same as those described for anterior pelvic tilt in Chapter 8.

Cautions and contraindications   Use caution with any iliopsoas treatment technique that uses direct pressure through the abdomen. There is a risk of adverse vascular responses with the external iliac artery if an aortic aneurysm exists. Some clients may report increased back pain or discomfort with MET stretching techniques for the iliopsoas performed from the supine position. To reduce client discomfort, have the client increase the level of flex in the opposite hip, which posteriorly rotates the pelvis, straightens the spine, and reduces facet joint compression.

Box 9.2   Clinical Tip

One of the errors that health professionals make is looking at problems in certain regions as isolated mechanical or structural disorders. An excessive lumbar lordosis, for example, creates numerous patterns in other regions of the body. There is mechanical stress in the low back to be certain. However, the biomechanical ramifications of this postural distortion can produce numerous other pathologies. The excessive lumbar lordosis produces an anterior pelvic tilt. That anterior pelvic tilt causes increased length in the hamstring muscles. The increased hamstring length in an anterior pelvic tilt is associated with a higher incidence of hamstring strains. Therefore, preventive treatment of hamstring strains may need to focus on the low back region.

KYPHOSIS

Description

There is a natural slight kyphotic curvature in the thoracic region located between the lordotic curves of the cervical and lumbar spine. The primary function of this curve is shock absorption. Kyphosis occurs when the curvature is exaggerated and a subsequent postural distortion develops (Fig. 9.17). Kyphosis, also called hunchback, routinely occurs with advanced age and can also develop from chronically poor posture or degenerative changes such as osteoporosis.[78] The condition can adversely affect other physiological processes such as digestive function and breathing.[79]

When the thoracic kyphosis is increased, the head naturally tilts toward the floor. At the same time the body's righting reflex attempts to keep

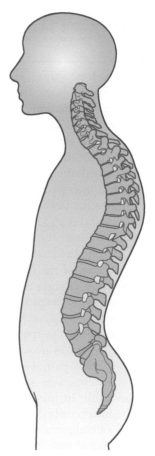

Figure 9.17   Kyphosis in the upper thoracic spine.

the eyes horizontal by contracting the cervical extensor muscles. The attempted postural compensation produces exaggerated compressive loads on the anterior aspect of the thoracic vertebrae and the posterior aspect of the cervical vertebrae. In some cases, the increased loads are enough to create vertebral stress fractures.[80]

An individual with kyphosis is likely to have an exaggerated cervical lordosis and forward head posture. Biomechanical patterns of muscular dysfunction, such as the upper crossed syndrome discussed in Chapter 10, are common in the client with kyphosis. In addition, there is increased tensile load on ligaments and muscle tissues in the posterior thoracic region.

Pathological kyphosis that causes clinical problems usually results from trauma, tumors, infection, tuberculosis, chronic postural stress, developmental disorders, rheumatoid arthritis, or other systemic conditions.[81] Bone weakness pathologies, such as osteoporosis or Scheuermann's disease, are also common causes of kyphosis. Osteoporosis involves a loss of bone density and is most prevalent in the elderly. Scheuermann's disease is a hereditary condition involving vertebral end-plate weakening and predominantly affects juveniles.[82]

Kyphosis can either produce or be caused by hypertonicity in the anterior chest muscles, such as the pectoralis major. Tightness in the anterior chest muscles pulls the arm into medial rotation and a corresponding scapular protraction develops. The altered scapular position limits function in the shoulder girdle, reducing range of motion and contributing to structural problems, such as shoulder impingement syndrome.[83]

Kyphosis does not necessarily produce pain or discomfort, but prolonged postural stress or more severe cases can produce a number of symptoms. Myofascial trigger points are typical in the upper thoracic or posterior cervical muscles and produce characteristic referral patterns. Pain in the upper thoracic region is typical and due to fatigue and overexertion in the upper thoracic spinal muscles.[74]

Treatment

Traditional approaches

Because kyphosis is a disorder of postural distortion, it is commonly treated using exercise and postural re-education. The emphasis is on reducing the forward head posture, lifting the anterior chest region, and straightening the upper back. In more severe cases of structural kyphosis, such as those that result from Scheuermann's disease, surgical implantation of rods to straighten the spine may be used.[84]

Soft-tissue manipulation

General guidelines This discussion of soft-tissue treatment for kyphosis assumes that the condition is primarily one of degenerative posture due to habitual neuromuscular patterns and not the result of problems with bony structure such as Scheuermann's disease or osteoporosis. In conditions of major bone structure deformity, massage can be used as palliative care or support for new neuromuscular patterns in the area, but it will not change the structural deformity.

Massage treatment for kyphosis focuses on the tissues that are short and hypertonic in the upper chest region, as well as those tissues that are fatigued from being held too long in an over-lengthened position in the upper back. On the anterior torso, attention is focused on the anterior deltoid, and pectoralis minor and major. In the upper back there are several layers of muscles that are emphasized in treatment including the rhomboids, middle and lower trapezius, serratus posterior superior, and intrinsic spinal muscles. These muscles are effectively addressed with a variety of techniques including static compression, deep longitudinal stripping, and active engagement methods.

Suggested techniques and methods

A. Sweeping cross fiber to anterior chest muscles Treatments aimed at the anterior chest muscles reduce the medial shoulder rotation, scapular protraction, and thoracic kyphosis. This technique helps reduce tension in superficial fibers of pectoralis major and anterior deltoid. Stand facing the client's feet with the fingers anchored in the client's axilla. Use the thumb to perform sweeping cross fiber movements on the pectoralis major (Fig. 9.18). During the sweeping motion the pectoralis major is sifted between the fingers. Similar sweeping cross fiber techniques are applied to the anterior deltoid while facing in the same position (toward the client's feet).

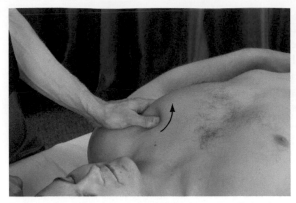

Figure 9.18   Sweeping cross fiber on pectoralis major.

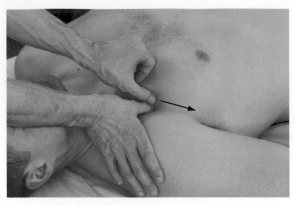

Figure 9.20   Deep stripping on pectoralis major.

B. Static compression for anterior chest muscles Apply static compression to areas of tension found in the pectoralis major when performing general warming and gliding techniques. Trigger points or areas of muscle hypertonicity are treated with both broad and small contact surface static compression methods (Fig. 9.19). Hold pressure on trigger points or areas of muscle tightness for about 5–8 seconds, or until a tissue release is felt.

C. Deep stripping on pectoralis major Use the thumbs, finger tips, or pressure tool to perform deep stripping techniques to the pectoralis major. Treatment can move from medial to lateral or lateral to medial (Fig. 9.20).

D. Deep stripping on pectoralis minor Perform a deep longitudinal stripping technique on the pectoralis minor beginning at the coracoid process of the scapula and moving inferiorly to its attachments on ribs 3, 4, & 5 (Fig. 9.21). Performing this technique requires work directly through the pectoralis major, so use care in the amount of pressure applied as this region can be tender.

E. Effleurage and sweeping cross fiber to upper back muscles Use the palm, thumb, back of the hand, or other broad contact surface to apply effleurage and sweeping cross fiber strokes to the rhomboids and middle trapezius between the spine and the vertebral border of the scapula (Fig. 9.22). There are several layers of muscles being treated in this region, so it is advantageous to apply both the effleurage and sweeping cross fiber movements in multiple directions.

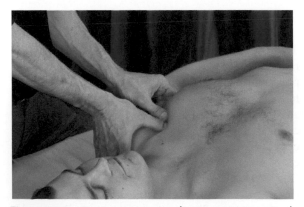

Figure 9.19   Static compression (small contact surface) on anterior chest muscles.

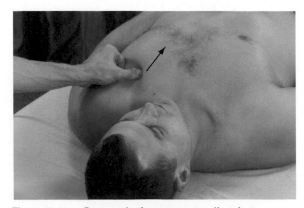

Figure 9.21   Deep stripping on pectoralis minor.

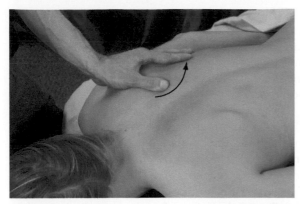

Figure 9.22   Sweeping cross fiber to rhomboids and mid trapezius.

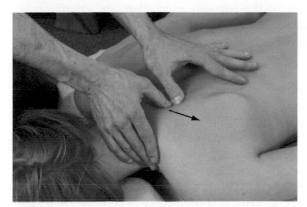

Figure 9.23   Deep stripping to rhomboids, trapezius, serratus, etc.

F. Deep stripping to posterior back muscles
Perform deep longitudinal stripping techniques with a small contact surface to the rhomboids, mid trapezius and serratus posterior superior muscles (Fig. 9.23). There are likely to be myofascial trigger points in these areas and localized areas of tight fibers and increased tenderness. The tightness felt in these tissues is not from shortened muscles, but from taut muscles held for prolonged periods in a lengthened position. Static compression with a small contact surface can be applied to these tight focal regions to neutralize the muscle tissue dysfunction.

Rehabilitation protocol considerations
- In both the upper chest and upper back regions, there are several layers of muscles being treated.

It is important to relax the superficial muscles first prior to using greater pressure on the deeper muscles.

- Some people advocate that the shortened side (anterior chest muscles) should be treated prior to addressing the over-lengthened side (upper back). Generally this is a good guideline to follow. However, some individuals with kyphosis complain of much greater pain in the upper back region. Relieving pain in the back first appears to have beneficial effects on reducing tension in the anterior chest muscles. It is not clear that there is a firm guideline about which order to treat these areas, so experiment with both and communicate with the client.

Cautions and contraindications   Some cases of kyphosis are caused by weakness and degeneration in bony structures as in osteoporosis. Many people develop their kyphotic posture with age as gravity gradually takes a toll on the upright vertical structure. In either case, especially that of osteoporosis, there can be fragility in the skeletal structures. Use caution when working in these areas, especially with techniques that use greater pressure, such as the deep stripping or static compression methods.

SCOLIOSIS

Description

Scoliosis is a lateral/rotary curvature in the spine and is relatively common, especially in children.[81] Most children grow out of scoliosis without need for further intervention. If the condition persists into adulthood, it can become seriously debilitating. The condition is caused by various diseases or muscular distortion.

There are two types of scoliosis: structural and functional. Structural scoliosis is caused by a fixed bony deformity, which can be inherited or acquired. A structural scoliosis is hard to correct and has detrimental long-term effects on spinal mechanics. The deformity could result from structural irregularities in the spine or a number of systemic disorders or neuromuscular

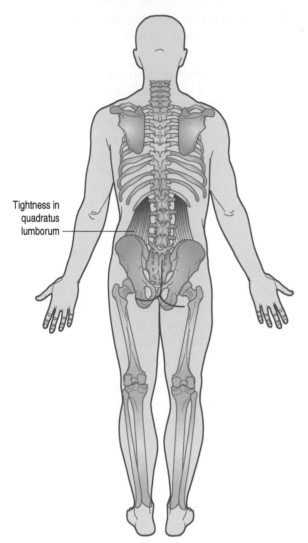

Tightness in
quadratus
lumborum

Figure 9.24 Functional scoliosis develops in the lumbar spine as a result of muscle tightness.

The rib hump is often visible when the client is in a prone position and results from lateral curvature of the spine that also causes rotation of the individual vertebrae. The vertebrae rotate toward the side that is higher when the client is in a prone position.

If there is a single scoliotic curve, it is called a C curve. In other cases two curves are convex in opposite directions; this distortion is called an S curve. The scoliotic curve is named for the convex side of the curve. If, for example, the right quadratus lumborum is in spasm and the pelvis tilts to the left, a functional scoliosis in the lumbar region results that is convex on the left and concave on the right. When the convex side of the curve is to the left, the condition is called a levoscoliosis. If the convex side of the curve is to the right the condition is called a dextroscoliosis.[74]

While many cases of scoliosis begin as mild structural disorders, they can progress to more serious complaints because of the functional adaptation of muscles to the distorted postures. There is a focus on the role of paraspinal muscles and the quadratus lumborum in creating or perpetuating the lateral bending. The small intrinsic spinal muscles should not be overlooked, however, as critical components of scoliosis. Muscles such as the multifidi, rotatores, and transversospinalis govern spinal rotary movement and can play an important role in developing the condition.

pathologies such as an upper or lower motor neuron lesion.[43]

Functional scoliosis develops from excessive muscle tension and not from deformity in the bones of the spine. For example, hypertonicity in the quadratus lumborum and iliocostalis lumborum produce a lateral pelvic tilt to the opposite side, creating a functional scoliosis in the lumbar region (Fig. 9.24).

In severe cases of scoliosis, especially structural forms, there is a characteristic rib hump visible in which one side of the back appears more pronounced in a posterior direction than the other.

Treatment

Traditional approaches

Structural scoliosis can often be prevented by detection early in life and use of corrective braces. If the scoliosis is severe and does not respond to braces or other conservative approaches, surgery might be suggested to straighten the spine. Surgical procedures used include spinal fusion and implantation of corrective devices such as Harrington rods. These are rods placed along each side of the spine and attached to the vertebral bodies to help keep the spine straight. The rods correct the lateral/rotary curvature and prevent the curvature from affecting other structures, such as spinal nerve roots or internal organs.

In certain cases a functional disorder involves skeletal structures, as in a structural leg-length discrepancy. The leg-length discrepancy can be corrected with orthotics and will help the scoliosis as well. Skeletal imbalances must be addressed first and then muscular compensations can be treated with massage.

Soft-tissue manipulation

General guidelines Treatment of a functional scoliosis requires identification of biomechanical factors that led to the distortion. Massage is used to lengthen muscles that are shortened. In massage treatment of scoliosis emphasis is placed on those muscles on the concave side of the curve because they are shortened. For example, if the functional scoliosis results from a lateral pelvic tilt caused by muscular hypertonicity, attention should focus on reducing tightness or myofascial trigger points in the muscles on the concave side of the curve.

Massage treatments for scoliosis have not been adequately researched. Yet, there is reason to believe that treating hypertonic muscles on the concave side of the curvature is beneficial. Massage is also valuable for reducing general hypertonicity and pain associated with this postural disorder.

Suggested techniques and methods For the following techniques it is assumed that they will be applied in the lumbar region on the concave side of the scoliotic curvature. It may be beneficial to also apply the techniques to the convex side of the scoliotic curve, but emphasis in treatment should be on the concave side.

A. Deep longitudinal stripping to spinal extensors Deep stripping techniques are applied to the erector spinae and spinal extensor muscles. Use a broad contact surface of pressure at the outset, especially if there is a greater degree of tension in these muscles. Once the muscles have begun to relax, apply the stripping techniques with small contact surface pressure such as the finger tips, thumb, or pressure tool to work on specific areas of tightness in the muscles (Fig. 9.3).

B. Deep longitudinal stripping on quadratus lumborum The client is in a prone or side-lying position. Use the thumb or finger tips to perform a longitudinal stripping technique on the QL (Fig. 9.4). Use stripping motions from the iliac crest to the transverse processes, iliac crest to twelfth rib, and transverse processes to twelfth rib as the QL has fibers running in all these directions. When working from lateral to medial on the fibers running from the iliac crest to the transverse processes, apply pressure deep enough to treat under the lateral edge of the erector spinae muscle group. However, use caution not to apply too much pressure directly against the tips of the transverse processes.

C. Deep stripping in lamina groove Numerous intrinsic muscles of the spine are difficult to treat unless deep specific work using a small contact surface is applied. Use the thumb, finger tip, or pressure tool to apply deep longitudinal stripping techniques to the muscles in the lamina groove. A hand position that uses two thumbs is the most effective way to perform this technique. The thumbs are positioned at almost right angles to each other. One thumb applies pressure against the spinous processes, while the other applies pressure down and forward in the direction that the hands are moving (Fig. 9.6). Pause and repeat short stripping movements on areas where increased muscle tension is palpated or the client reports greater tenderness. This technique can be performed in a superior or inferior direction.

Rehabilitation protocol considerations

- If the scoliosis is a more advanced structural scoliosis, consult with the client's physician or other health care provider about strategies being employed to address the structural disorder. It is important that massage approaches work in conjunction with these other treatments.

- If the scoliosis is predominantly a functional scoliosis resulting from postural disorders such as a lateral pelvic tilt, be sure to address all components of those disorders as well as treating the lateral curvature in the spine.

Cautions and contraindications Some people with a congenital scoliosis may already have rods or implanted stabilizing devices along the spine. Use caution when performing any specific massage treatments along the spine for anyone with surgically implanted instrumentation.

Box 9.3   Case Study

Background

Dennis is a 49-year-old construction contractor. This season has been a particularly hard winter which has meant a lot more snow shoveling. A week ago there were three straight days of heavy snow, and Dennis had to shovel his driveway each of those 3 days. He also helps the elderly couple next door by shoveling their driveway. He is in good physical condition but hurt his back with all this snow removal work over the last week.

His injury started when he had been working on snow removal for about 45 minutes. He had a moderately heavy pile of snow on his shovel and had turned in a bit of an awkward position to lift it up and away from his car in the driveway. When he turned and lifted his shovel he felt a sudden sharp pain in his back. He immediately fell to his knees and had a hard time getting up. The injury forced him to miss work for several days because he was in such pain. He put ice on it right after the injury and that helped a little with the pain. He has also been taking over the counter anti-inflammatory medication for the last week to deal with the pain and discomfort.

It has been hurting ever since, but decreasing a little in intensity with time.

Questions to consider

- What are several possible conditions that could be causing Dennis' back pain?
- Do you think he should see another health professional for evaluation prior to receiving massage? If so, who do you think he should see?
- What are several factors in his case that indicate a likely biomechanical overload on various structures in his lumbar spine?
- If his condition turns out to be primarily a muscular injury, such as muscle spasm, would massage treatment be helpful? If so, what techniques would be most appropriate?
- Based on the limited information you have about Dennis, what are several muscles that you think might be injured in this condition?
- Do you think his injury might be neurological, such as a herniated disc? If so, is this something you think should be treated with massage?

References

1. Waddell G. The Back Pain Revolution. Edinburgh: Churchill Livingstone; 1998.
2. Frymoyer JW, Cats-Baril WL. An overview of the incidences and costs of low back pain. Orthop Clin North Am. 1991;22(2):263–271.
3. Dagenais S, Caro J, Haldeman S. A systematic review of low back pain cost of illness studies in the United States and internationally. Spine J. 2008;8(1):8–20.
4. Nguyen TH, Randolph DC. Nonspecific low back pain and return to work. Am Fam Physician. 2007;76(10):1497–1502.
5. Pai S, Sundaram LJ. Low back pain: an economic assessment in the United States. Orthop Clin North Am. 2004;35(1):1–5.
6. van der Roer N, Goossens ME, Evers SM, van Tulder MW. What is the most cost-effective treatment for patients with low back pain? A systematic review. Best Pract Res Clin Rheumatol. 2005;19(4):671–684.
7. Maetzel A, Li L. The economic burden of low back pain: a review of studies published between 1996 and 2001. Best Pract Res Clin Rheumatol. 2002;16(1):23–30.
8. Lorusso A, Bruno S, L'Abbate N. A review of low back pain and musculoskeletal disorders among Italian nursing personnel. Ind Health. 2007;45(5):637–644.
9. Lorusso A, Bruno S, L'Abbate N. Musculoskeletal complaints among Italian X-ray technologists. Ind Health. 2007;45(5):705–708.
10. Feng CK, Chen ML, Mao IF. Prevalence of and risk factors for different measures of low back pain among female nursing aides in Taiwanese nursing homes. BMC Musculoskelet Disord. 2007;8:52.
11. Violante FS, Fiori M, Fiorentini C, et al. Associations of psychosocial and individual factors with three different categories of back disorder among nursing staff. J Occup Health. 2004;46(2):100–108.
12. Eriksen W. The prevalence of musculoskeletal pain in Norwegian nurses' aides. Int Arch Occup Environ Health. 2003;76(8):625–630.
13. Cherkin DC, Deyo RA, Wheeler K, Ciol MA. Physician variation in diagnostic testing for low back pain. Who you see is what you get. Arthritis Rheum. 1994;37(1):15–22.

14. Cherkin DC. Primary care research on low back pain. The state of the science. Spine. 1998;23(18):1997–2002.
15. McPhillips-Tangum CA, Cherkin DC, Rhodes LA, Markham C. Reasons for repeated medical visits among patients with chronic back pain. J Gen Intern Med. 1998;13(5):289–295.
16. Mense S, Simons DG. Muscle Pain: Understanding Its Nature, Diagnosis, & Treatment. Baltimore: Lippincott Williams & Wilkins; 2001.
17. Simons D. New aspects of myofascial trigger points: etiological and clinical. Journal of Musculoskeletal Pain. 2004;12(3/4).
18. Ernst E. Massage therapy for low back pain: A systematic review. J Pain Symptom Manage. 1999;17(1):65–69.
19. Cherkin DC, Eisenberg D, Sherman KJ, et al. Randomized trial comparing traditional Chinese medical acupuncture, therapeutic massage, and self-care education for chronic low back pain. Arch Intern Med. 2001;161(8):1081–1088.
20. Furlan AD, Brosseau L, Imamura M, Irvin E. Massage for low-back pain: a systematic review within the framework of the Cochrane Collaboration Back Review Group. Spine. 2002;27(17):1896–1910.
21. Hernandez-Reif M, Field T, Krasnegor J, Theakston H. Lower back pain is reduced and range of motion increased after massage therapy. Int J Neurosci. 2001;106(3–4):131–145.
22. Preyde M. Effectiveness of massage therapy for subacute low-back pain: a randomized controlled trial. CMAJ. 2000;162(13):1815–1820.
23. Tsao JC. Effectiveness of massage therapy for chronic, non-malignant pain: a review. Evid Based Complement Alternat Med. 2007;4(2):165–179.
24. Janda V. Rational therapeutic approach of chronic back pain syndromes. Paper presented at: Chronic back pain, rehabilitation, and self-help, 1985; Turku, Finland.
25. Chaitow L. Modern Neuromuscular Techniques. New York: Churchill Livingstone; 1996.
26. Chaitow L, DeLany J. Clinical Application of Neuromuscular Techniques. Vol 1. Edinburgh: Churchill Livingstone; 2000.
27. Simons D, Travell J, Simons L. Myofascial Pain and Dysfunction: The Trigger Point Manual. Vol 1. 2nd ed. Baltimore: Williams & Wilkins; 1999.
28. Panjabi M, White A. Biomechanics in the Musculoskeletal System. New York: Churchill Livingstone; 2001.
29. Gracovetsky S. Is the lumbodorsal fascia necessary. Paper presented at: Fascia Research Congress, 2007; Harvard Medical School, Boston, MA.
30. Trudeau M. The contribution of the thoracolumbar fascia to the spine's stiffness. Paper presented at: Fascia Research Congress, 2007; Harvard Medical School, Boston, MA.
31. Cailliet R. Low Back Pain Syndrome. Philadelphia: F.A. Davis; 1988.
32. Nordin M, Frankel V. Basic Biomechanics of the Musculoskeletal System. 2nd ed. Malvern: Lea & Febiger; 1989.
33. Liebenson CE. Rehabilitation of the Spine. Baltimore: Williams & Wilkins; 1996.
34. Slipman CW, Lipetz JS, Jackson HB, Vresilovic EJ. Deep venous thrombosis and pulmonary embolism as a complication of bed rest for low back pain. Arch Phys Med Rehabil. 2000;81(1):127–129.
35. Carette S, Leclaire R, Marcoux S, et al. Epidural corticosteroid injections for sciatica due to herniated nucleus pulposus. N Engl J Med. 1997;336(23):1634–1640.
36. Fadale PD, Wiggins ME. Corticosteroid Injections: Their Use and Abuse. J Am Acad Orthop Surg. 1994;2(3):133–140.
37. vanTulder M. Randomized trial comparing interferential therapy with motorized lumbar traction and massage in the management of low back pain in a primary care setting – Point of view. Spine. 1999;24(15):1584.
38. Busanich BM, Verscheure SD. Does McKenzie therapy improve outcomes for back pain? J Athl Train. 2006;41(1):117–119.
39. Preyde M. Effectiveness of massage therapy for subacute low-back pain: a randomized controlled trial. Can Med Assn J. 2000;162(13):1815–1820.
40. Schleip R. Fascial plasticity – a new neurobiological explanation Part 2. Journal of Bodywork and Movement Therapies. 2003;7(2):104–116.
41. Mixter WJ, Barr JS. Rupture of the intervertebral disc with involvement of the spinal canal. N Engl J Med. 1934;211:210–215.
42. Buckwalter JA. Aging and degeneration of the human intervertebral disc. Spine. 1995;20(11):1307–1314.
43. Magee D. Orthopedic Physical Assessment. 3rd ed. Philadelphia: W.B. Saunders; 1997.
44. Haig AJ, Geisser ME, Tong HC, et al. Electromyographic and magnetic resonance imaging to predict lumbar stenosis, low-back pain, and no back symptoms. J Bone Joint Surg Am. 2007;89(2):358–366.
45. Haig AJ, Tong HC, Yamakawa KS, et al. Spinal stenosis, back pain, or no symptoms at all? A masked study comparing radiologic and electrodiagnostic diagnoses to the clinical impression. Arch Phys Med Rehabil. 2006;87(7):897–903.
46. Jarvik JG, Hollingworth W, Heagerty PJ, Haynor DR, Boyko EJ, Deyo RA. Three-year incidence of low back pain in an initially asymptomatic cohort: clinical and imaging risk factors. Spine. 2005;30(13):1541–1548; discussion 1549.
47. Boden SD, Davis DO, Dina TS, Patronas NJ, Wiesel SW. Abnormal magnetic-resonance scans of the lumbar spine in asymptomatic subjects. A prospective investigation. J Bone Joint Surg Am. 1990;72(3):403–408.
48. Jensen MC, Brant-Zawadzki MN, Obuchowski N, Modic MT, Malkasian D, Ross JS. Magnetic resonance imaging of the lumbar spine in people without back pain. N Engl J Med. 1994;331(2):69–73.
49. Clare HA, Adams R, Maher CG. A systematic review of efficacy of McKenzie therapy for spinal pain. Aust J Physiother. 2004;50(4):209–216.
50. McKenzie R. Understanding centralisation. J Orthop Sports Phys Ther. 1999;29(8):487–489.

51. Bush K, Cowan N, Katz DE, Gishen P. The natural history of sciatica associated with disc pathology. A prospective study with clinical and independent radiologic follow-up. Spine. 1992;17(10):1205–1212.

52. Couto JM, Castilho EA, Menezes PR. Chemonucleolysis in lumbar disc herniation: a meta-analysis. Clinics. 2007; 62(2):175–180.

53. Guha AR, Debnath UK, D'Souza S. Chemonucleolysis revisited: a prospective outcome study in symptomatic lumbar disc prolapse. J Spinal Disord Tech. 2006; 19(3):167–170.

54. Chicheportiche V, Parlier-Cuau C, Champsaur P, Laredo JD. Lumbar Chymopapain Chemonucleolysis. Semin Musculoskelet Radiol. 1997;1(2):197–206.

55. Nordby EJ, Javid MJ. Continuing experience with chemonucleolysis. Mt Sinai J Med. 2000;67(4):311–313.

56. Maksymowicz W, Barczewska M, Sobieraj A. Percutaneous laser lumbar disc decompression – mechanism of action, indications and contraindications. Ortop Traumatol Rehabil. 2004;6(3):314–318.

57. McMillan MR, Patterson PA, Parker V. Percutaneous laser disc decompression for the treatment of discogenic lumbar pain and sciatica: a preliminary report with 3-month follow-up in a general pain clinic population. Photomed Laser Surg. 2004;22(5):434–438.

58. Sobieraj A, Maksymowicz W, Barczewska M, Konopielko M, Mazur D. Early results of percutaneous laser disc decompression (PLDD) as a treatment of discopathic lumbar pain. Ortop Traumatol Rehabil. 2004;6(3): 264–269.

59. Choy DS. Percutaneous laser disc decompression (PLDD): twelve years' experience with 752 procedures in 518 patients. J Clin Laser Med Surg. 1998;16(6):325–331.

60. Gibson JN, Grant IC, Waddell G. The Cochrane review of surgery for lumbar disc prolapse and degenerative lumbar spondylosis. Spine. 1999;24(17):1820–1832.

61. Deyo RA, Cherkin DC, Loeser JD, Bigos SJ, Ciol MA. Morbidity and mortality in association with operations on the lumbar spine. The influence of age, diagnosis, and procedure. J Bone Joint Surg Am. 1992;74(4):536–543.

62. Nachemson AL. Newest knowledge of low back pain. A critical look. Clin Orthop. 1992;(279):8–20.

63. Cherkin DC, Deyo RA, Loeser JD, Bush T, Waddell G. An international comparison of back surgery rates. Spine. 1994;19(11):1201–1206.

64. Maitland GD, Banks K, English K, Hengeveld E. Maitland's Vertebral Manipulation. 6th ed. Edinburgh: Elsevier; 2001.

65. Mooney V, Robertson J. The facet syndrome. Clin Orthop. 1976(115):149–156.

66. Dreyer SJ, Dreyfuss PH. Low back pain and the zygapophysial (facet) joints. Arch Phys Med Rehabil. 1996;77(3):290–300.

67. Dreyfuss PH, Dreyer SJ, Herring SA. Lumbar zygapophysial (facet) joint injections. Spine. 1995; 20(18):2040–2047.

68. Schwarzer AC, Aprill CN, Derby R, Fortin J, Kine G, Bogduk N. Clinical features of patients with pain stemming from the lumbar zygapophysial joints. Is the lumbar facet syndrome a clinical entity? Spine. 1994;19(10): 1132–1137.

69. Carette S, Marcoux S, Truchon R, et al. A controlled trial of corticosteroid injections into facet joints for chronic low back pain. N Engl J Med. 1991;325(14):1002–1007.

70. Reeves RK, Laskowski ER, Smith J. Weight training injuries part 2: diagnosing and managing chronic conditions. Physician Sportsmed. 1998;26(3).

71. McCulloch J, Transfeldt E. Macnab's Backache. 3rd ed. Baltimore: Williams & Wilkins; 1997.

72. Bassewitz H, Herkowitz H. Lumbar stenosis with spondylolisthesis: current concepts of surgical treatment. Clin Orthop. 2001(384):54–60.

73. Amundson G, Edwards C, Garfin S. Spondylolisthesis. In: Herkowitz H, Garfin S, Balderston R, Eismont F, Bell A, Wiesel S, eds. Rothman–Simeone: The Spine. Vol 1. 4th ed. Philadelphia: W.B. Saunders; 1999:835–885.

74. Lowe W. Orthopedic Assessment in Massage Therapy. Sisters, OR: Daviau–Scott; 2006.

75. Torg J, Shephard R. Current Therapy In Sports Medicine. 3rd ed. St. Louis: Mosby; 1995.

76. Janda V. Muscles as a pathogenic factor in back pain. Paper presented at: IFOMT, 1980; New Zealand.

77. Janda V. Postural and Phasic Muscles in the Pathogenesis of Low Back Pain. Paper presented at: XIth Congress ISRD, 1968; Dublin.

78. Dorland's Illustrated Medical Dictionary. Philadelphia: Saunders; 2003.

79. Di Bari M, Chiarlone M, Matteuzzi D, et al. Thoracic kyphosis and ventilatory dysfunction in unselected older persons: an epidemiological study in Dicomano, Italy. J Am Geriatr Soc. 2004;52(6):909–915.

80. Neumann DA. Kinesiology of the Musculoskeletal System. St. Louis: Mosby; 2002.

81. White A, Panjabi M. Clinical Biomechanics of the Spine. 2nd ed. Philadelphia: Lippincott Williams & Wilkins; 1990.

82. Nowak J. Scheuermann Disease. September 1, 2004; www.emedicine.com. Accessed May 26, 2005.

83. Bullock MP, Foster NE, Wright CC. Shoulder impingement: the effect of sitting posture on shoulder pain and range of motion. Man Ther. 2005;10(1):28–37.

84. Lonner BS, Newton P, Betz R, et al. Operative management of Scheuermann's kyphosis in 78 patients: radiographic outcomes, complications, and technique. Spine. 2007;32(24):2644–2652.

Chapter **10**

Cervical spine

CHAPTER CONTENTS

The cervical spine is susceptible to numerous soft-tissue disorders. The structural mechanics of this region are designed primarily to provide maximum mobility to the head. It is crucially important for survival that the head, where our primary sensory organs are located, is able to move around easily. Balance receptors that affect the whole body are also located in the head, so the role of various tissues in the neck is to maintain simultaneous stability and mobility.

The head of an adult can weigh close to 10 pounds. From a skeletal standpoint, this weight is balanced on a small contact surface (the surface area of the atlanto-occipital joint). To keep a weight this heavy balanced on such a small contact surface while it moves around in all different directions is challenging to say the least. The soft tissues of the cervical region are responsible for guiding this movement and providing stability.

Muscles, tendons, and ligaments have complex mechanical interactions that help produce the motion of the head and neck and maintain the head in an upright position. Due to biomechanical challenges in this region, muscle conditions involving chronic hypertonicity and myofascial trigger points are common. Nerve compression and tension syndromes are also common because of the brachial plexus and other sensitive neurological tissues, which are vulnerable to compression in the area. Pain and/or neurological sensations from these conditions can be felt in the neck or down the upper extremity.

Poor posture, faulty ergonomics, overuse, and stress can all cause various pathological conditions of the neck, as can injuries such as impact trauma and whiplash. There are also several genetic conditions that can produce problems in this region. Massage is an excellent treatment choice for addressing these disorders because the soft tissues play a role in these pathologies.

INJURY CONDITIONS

NEUROMUSCULAR NECK PAIN

Description

The challenge of maintaining the head in an upright position places postural strain on muscles and other soft tissues of the cervical region. In neuromuscular neck pain there is hypertonicity either throughout the entire muscle or in localized areas, such as with myofascial trigger points. In the neck it takes very little muscular dysfunction to set off a cascading process of neuromuscular dysfunction, known as the *pain–spasm–pain cycle*.[1]

Postural distortions, such as a forward head posture, are a result of neuromuscular dysfunction and the constant effort to fight the pull of gravity on the head. If the head is maintained directly on top of the cervical spine, there is very little muscular effort needed to keep it in that position. Once the head moves forward of the center of gravity, even if it is just a few degrees, there is a significant increase in muscle activity to hold the head upright.[2] This constant muscle tension can lead to muscular hypertonicity and the development of myofascial trigger points.

Once these distortions develop, they cause a perpetuation of biomechanical dysfunction. As with other regions of the spine, primary health care providers often place emphasis on structural considerations, particularly joint pathology, as the source of most disorders. However, many of these problems are not structural but instead muscular in nature.[3]

Myofascial trigger points in muscles such as the posterior cervical muscles can become a constant source of pain if they are not properly neutralized. A sudden and awkward loading movement or trauma, as can happen in a motor vehicle accident, often activates these trigger points. The sudden loading of these muscles stimulates excessive neurological activity in related muscles, and produces symptoms in other areas such as the temporomandibular joint.[4]

Because many cervical muscles maintain constant isometric contractions during the day just to keep the head erect, the patterns of dysfunction are facilitated by the very act of attempting to hold the head upright. These movement patterns and their dysfunctional fixations follow a pattern. Once they are set they tend to recur in the same region any time the individual is exposed to further stress. The stress does not have to be an excessive force to activate the pattern of neuromuscular pain or dysfunction; psychological or chemical stressors are just as likely to start a cascade of neuromuscular distress.

Treatment

Traditional approaches

The main approach to treating neuromuscular dysfunction in the cervical region is rest from offending activities. However, rest does not mean immobilization. In the past, a cervical collar was frequently advocated as a means of treating neuromuscular pain or muscle strain in the cervical region. Research has shown that long periods of immobilization are detrimental to the rehabilitation process unless the condition is severe and joint hypermobility is a serious concern. Rest from offending activities means going about normal daily functions, but being careful to avoid movements that aggravate the pain problem.

Various forms of physical therapy are used to address neuromuscular neck pain. These approaches include stretching, therapeutic exercise, or the various soft-tissue manipulation methods. Anti-inflammatory medication may be advocated for these problems as well. There is not an inflammatory process occurring in many cases, but these medications are effective in pain management and that is their primary benefit.

High-velocity manipulation/mobilization is used to treat neuromuscular dysfunction. However, muscle spindles can respond to the rapid rate of change in muscle length causing further contraction due to the myotatic (stretch) reflex. That is one reason why some manipulative therapy practitioners are moving away from high-velocity manipulation adjustments in favor of various *low-force* techniques.[5]

Soft-tissue manipulation

One of the most effective ways to address neuromuscular neck pain is with soft-tissue manipulation. The massage practitioner's ability to sense hypertonic regions and precisely locate myofascial trigger points or dysfunctional muscle tissue is a hallmark of effective massage. For the massage practitioner, numerous methods are effective in treating neuromuscular neck pain. Gentle effleurage and myofascial approaches are used initially if the condition is acute or involves excessive muscle spasm. Active-assisted stretching methods are also a way to begin treating muscles that are in pain or spasm. With muscle tension that is chronic, a slightly more aggressive treatment approach is appropriate. Effective techniques with chronic neuromuscular pain include static compression, deep stripping, and active engagement methods.

Suggested techniques and methods

A. Myofascial approaches Myofascial techniques encourage fascial and muscular relaxation and enhance their pliability. The primary goal is to place moderately light pressure on the subcutaneous fascia while pulling the fascia in multiple directions. Place the hands lightly on the client's neck where the myofascial stretch is to be applied. Pull the hands apart to take the slack out of the tissue and apply a light degree of tensile (pulling) force between the hands (Fig. 10.1). Once there is a slight degree of pull between the hands, hold this position until a subtle sensation of tissue release is felt. This technique can be applied to muscles of the posterior, anterior, and lateral cervical region. To retain the best contact between the client and the practitioner's hands, generally no creams or lotions are used.

B. Effleurage and sweeping cross fiber These techniques are effective for reducing tension in neck muscles. Effleurage is performed with long gliding strokes parallel to the muscle fiber direction. Cross fiber techniques sweep diagonally across the primary fiber direction of muscles; the direction of the movement changes depending on the muscles being addressed (Fig. 10.2). Use care with effleurage or sweeping cross fiber motions across tissues of the lateral and anterior neck region due to the superficial vascular structures in this area.

C. Deep longitudinal stripping to cervical extensors Deep stripping techniques are applied to the cervical erector spinae and extensor muscles. Due to the practitioner's hand size and the small region of the neck to be treated, it is not as easy to use a broad contact surface in this area. After reducing tension in superficial muscles with effleurage and cross fiber methods use small contact surface stripping techniques such as the finger, thumb, or pressure tool (Fig. 10.3). Stripping techniques can be performed in a caudal or cephalad direction and the client may be supine, prone, or in a side-lying position.

These same stripping techniques can be applied to muscles of the lateral neck region such as the

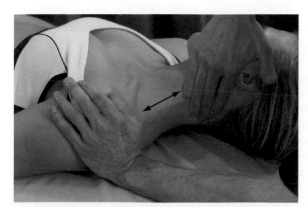

Figure 10.1   Myofascial stretching on the neck.

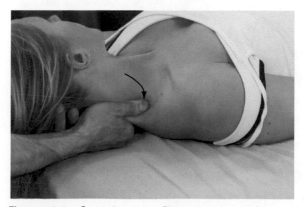

Figure 10.2   Sweeping cross fiber to neck muscles.

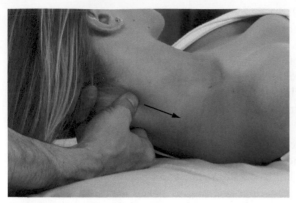

Figure 10.3 Deep stripping on posterior cervical muscles (small contact surface).

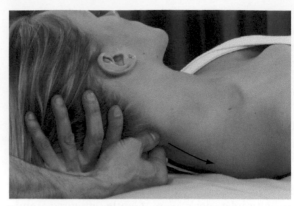

Figure 10.5 Deep stripping in lamina groove on posterior neck region.

upper fibers of the levator scapulae and posterior scalene. Use caution when applying stripping techniques near the anterior neck region due to the proximity of sensitive vascular structures and the brachial plexus.

D. Static compression To reduce muscular hypertonicity in a specific location, use static compression methods. Treat localized areas of tension or specific myofascial trigger points with small contact surface pressure (Fig. 10.4). Pressure maintained for 8–10 seconds is usually sufficient to achieve a reduction of muscle tension.

E. Deep stripping in lamina groove After working through tension in more superficial muscles, treat the deep intrinsic muscles of the cervical spine. Use the thumb or finger tip to apply deep

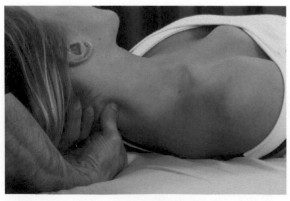

Figure 10.4 Static compression on cervical muscles.

longitudinal stripping techniques to the muscles in the lamina groove. One hand holds the head while the other hand performs the stripping technique in the lamina groove (Fig. 10.5). It is easiest to treat these muscles if the thumb is used. If it feels difficult to keep the thumb's interphalangeal joint straight, brace the thumb with the other fingers as pressure is applied in this stroke. Pause and repeat short stripping movements on any areas where increased muscle tension is palpated or the client reports greater tenderness.

F. Massage with active engagement to cervical extensors An effective way to treat chronic muscle tension in deeper neck muscles is using active engagement lengthening techniques. The client is in a supine position. Use one hand to hold the head and the other hand to perform the stripping technique on the cervical muscles, as in the deep stripping techniques in C and E. Instruct the client to push their head down with a moderate amount of effort into the practitioner's hand that is holding their head. Once a moderate isometric contraction is established, instruct the client to slowly let go of the contraction and gradually lift their head into full flexion. While they are releasing the contraction and the head is moving in flexion, perform a deep stripping technique on the cervical extensor muscles. It is easiest to perform this stroke moving down the neck in an inferior direction (Fig. 10.6).

G. Massage with active engagement to lateral neck flexors The same technique described in F

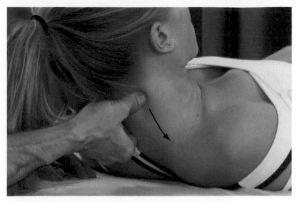

Figure 10.6 Stripping with active engagement on posterior cervical muscles.

above can be performed on the lateral neck flexors instead of the cervical extensors by altering the position slightly. Have the client attempt to laterally flex the neck to the side that is being treated while resistance is offered to that action. Instruct the client to slowly let go of the contraction. As the client slowly releases the contraction, gradually pull (or push) the head to the opposite side. As the client's head is slowly moving to the opposite side, perform a stripping technique on the lateral flexor muscles (Fig. 10.7). Use caution with pressure applied on the lateral side of the neck to avoid applying pressure to cervical vascular structures or the brachial plexus.

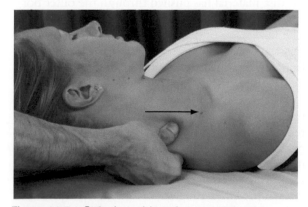

Figure 10.7 Stripping with active engagement on lateral flexor muscles.

Rehabilitation protocol considerations

- There can be a number of serious pathologies in the cervical region so perform a thorough assessment to rule out serious pathologies that need to be referred to another health professional.

- Neuromuscular pain and postural distortions are established by constant reinforcement. It is important to encourage changes in these movement or postural patterns early in the treatment process as muscle tension is addressed.

- Stretching and flexibility enhancement are essential components of treating neuromuscular neck pain. Stretching is most effective when performed after soft-tissue manipulation so the benefits of enhanced tissue pliability can be maximized.

- Certain techniques are more effective or appropriate at particular phases of the rehabilitation process. Techniques such as active engagement methods described in F and G are not suggested in acute or severe neuromuscular pain cases. These techniques can be intense for the client so they are used in the later stages of rehabilitation.

Cautions and contraindications Just as with the back, neuromuscular pain can resolve while the client is on the treatment table, only to return post massage. Decreasing pain-producing tension in the muscular soft tissues alters muscular proprioception. When the individual moves around after treatment there are different muscular recruitment patterns used, which can overtax tissues that have not adapted to the new patterns. The body's reaction to the sudden overload can be muscle spasm. The best way to avoid this situation is to move slowly when getting up from a massage treatment and shortly afterward so the body has time to integrate the new muscular proprioceptive patterns.

Some individuals are particularly sensitive to having their head and neck moved, which can have a profound effect on the treatment results. They may brace with protective muscle guarding as various movements or massage techniques are performed in this region. Be aware of these potential guarding patterns and make sure the quality of touch and the therapeutic environment created by the treatment encourages relaxation.

HERNIATED NUCLEUS PULPOSUS

Description

Intervertebral discs in the cervical region are exposed to compressive forces primarily from weight of the head. Other impacts can produce excess compression on the cervical discs, such as falling on the ground or having a load hit directly on top of the head. A common example where this occurs is someone diving into a shallow pool and hitting their head on the bottom of the pool.

The normal compressive load on the cervical spine is nowhere near that of the lumbar spine. Yet, there can still be enough compressive load to adversely affect the spinal structures. Because the cervical intervertebral discs are significantly smaller than their lumbar counterparts, it takes a smaller load to create damaging levels of compressive stress.

An accumulation of compressive forces on the cervical spine can cause degeneration of the intervertebral disc. Stenosis (narrowing) of the intervertebral foramen often accompanies these degenerative changes. Neurological symptoms can develop as nerve roots are compressed within the narrowing space around them. Muscle weakness and sensory symptoms including paralysis in the upper extremity occur in patients with spinal stenosis.[6]

Herniation technically means pushing through. The primary problem in this condition occurs because degeneration of the annulus fibrosus allows the nucleus to push through it (see Fig. 9.9). As the nucleus continues to exert pressure on the annulus, it causes the annulus to change shape. Eventually, if not halted, the nucleus can push all the way through the annulus. Degeneration of the annulus can be the result of numerous factors, including poor disc nutrition, loss of viable cells, loss of water content, and others.[7–9] Most of these problems originate from excessive compressive loads on the spinal structures over time.

These factors cause the intervertebral disc to lose some of its thickness prior to the process of herniation. When a disc has lost some of its thickness it is common for an individual to be given a diagnosis of degenerative disc disease. Essentially, this means the disc has lost thickness and the vertebrae in the region are closer together. However, this does not necessarily mean that pathological symptoms follow. There are often no symptoms with degenerative disease of the spine and there may be no pathology related to the condition.[10,11]

There are several names given to the different degrees of disc herniation. While these names are not always consistent in the literature, they do offer a greater degree of specificity as to the severity of the disc herniation.[12] Figure 9.10 in the previous chapter illustrates the different degrees of disc herniation. In a disc protrusion (also called a bulge), the disc has changed shape, but the majority of the annulus fibrosis is intact. This disc is considered prolapsed if only the outer-most fibers of the annulus are still containing the nucleus. In an extrusion, the disc material has pushed through the outer border of the annulus, but it is still connected to itself. The final stage of degeneration is sequestration. In this stage the disc material has actually separated from itself, and portions of the disc material may be freely floating in the spinal canal.

Herniation of the nucleus pulposus in the cervical region is similar to that which occurs in the lumbar region. Yet, there are several reasons why cervical discs are not as vulnerable to disc herniations as those in the lumbar region. The ligament (Fig. 10.8) protects protrusions in the cervical region better than it does in the lumbar region, because it is proportionately wider in the cervical region. In the cervical region the posterior longitudinal ligament covers

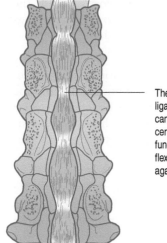

The posterior longitudinal ligament runs inside the spinal canal against the bodies of the cervical vertebrae. Its primary function is to prevent excessive flexion but it also provides restraint against posterior disc protrusions

Figure 10.8   Posterior longitudinal ligament.

the majority of the posterior aspect of the disc. In addition, the nucleus is situated farther anteriorly in the cervical region, making the possibility of a posterior protrusion less likely.[13]

In the cervical region disc herniations are most likely to affect the nerve roots that make up the brachial plexus. Symptoms from compression of these nerve roots are felt down the length of the upper extremity. Pain can also come from the disc pressing on the posterior longitudinal ligament, dura mater, or spinal cord.[13] It is possible, though not common, for cervical pain associated with disc herniations to come from the disc itself without it pressing on nerve roots. Anatomical investigations have shown that the discs have nerve fibers and mechanoreceptors that can produce pain just from excessive pressure.[14–17]

Treatment

Traditional approaches

Conservative treatment is advocated for this condition prior to surgical intervention. Conservative treatment consists of rest, physical therapy modalities such as ice, heat, ultrasound, electrical stimulation, exercise, and traction. Manipulation and mobilization techniques are also used to reduce pressure on the disc. Cervical traction units come in various styles and are often effective for addressing disc pathology. Because a primary part of the problem is excessive compression on the disc,

reversing that compression through traction can provide effective relief. Anti-inflammatory medication may be used in pain management, although it is not always evident that inflammation is present.

If conservative treatment fails, surgery may be used to treat the problem. However, there is increasing controversy about when surgery should be used. Similar to problems in the lumbar spine, many asymptomatic individuals have been found with disc herniations in the cervical region.[10] Assuming the necessity of cervical disc surgery on the presence of disc herniation alone could lead to unnecessary surgery. New treatment approaches encourage a finding of adequate clinical signs showing disc pathology to warrant surgical intervention.

Laminectomy and vertebral fusion are some of the more common surgical approaches for treating cervical disc herniation. However, some of the procedures, such as cervical fusion, may place additional levels of strain on the other vertebral segments.[18] For that reason, newer and less invasive surgical procedures such as percutaneous laser disc decompression (PLDD) may be tried. A reduction in disc pressure is achieved through laser energy in this procedure.[19]

Soft-tissue manipulation

General guidelines   Soft-tissue treatments can be helpful in reducing symptoms in the area, but use caution not to aggravate the symptoms through pressure or movement applied to the area. Cervical disc pathologies may activate myofascial trigger points in the cervical muscles.[20] These activated trigger points can then be perpetuated by other factors. The resultant myofascial pain pattern can then linger long after the disc herniation symptoms have subsided. Massage is effective in addressing these patterns of dysfunctional muscular hypertonicity.

Disc protrusions onto cervical nerve roots can also produce upper-extremity neurological symptoms because of increased neural tension. The increased neural tension can make various regions of the upper extremity more susceptible to neurological pathology. For that reason, thorough soft-tissue treatment of the upper extremity is an important aspect of addressing neural pathology in the cervical region.

Suggested techniques and methods The focus of massage treatment for disc herniations is to reduce the role that muscle tightness plays in the disc pathology. Attention is focused on neck muscles that contribute to the compressive forces or postural distortion of the cervical spine. Any of the techniques in the previous section on neuromuscular neck pain could be used to address the muscular components that are aggravating a disc herniation.

Be careful of any technique that puts excessive pressure in the area or moves the neck in any way that aggravates symptoms. In some muscular pain conditions a degree of pain can be expected and even considered therapeutically helpful. Working deep tension out of muscles can be uncomfortable, but is often described as a sensation of pain that feels pleasant. Massage treatment of neurological conditions, such as a disc herniation, should not increase symptoms because that would indicate further pressure or aggravation of the nerve.

Rehabilitation protocol considerations

- The primary focus of treatment is to reduce compression on neurological structures. Massage can be performed at the same time as other traditional conservative treatments such as manipulation or mobilization. Massage is a valuable adjunct for manipulation or mobilization treatments and is especially valuable if performed prior to these treatments. Reduction in muscle and soft-tissue tension allows these other techniques to be applied with greater ease and less resistance.

- Movement re-education to reduce postural stress is an important aspect of treatment and can be performed along with massage treatment.

- If there is an acute disc herniation, significant muscle spasm is likely to result. Muscle spasm should be addressed first in order to reduce the perpetuation of dysfunctional muscular activity.

- Massage is a valuable adjunct treatment in post-surgical rehabilitation. After surgery, massage is effective in reducing excess muscle tension and restoring proper neuromuscular activity in the affected muscles. Treatment should not be used anywhere near surgical incision sites.

- If the disc herniation has become chronic, slightly more aggressive massage treatment can be attempted, but always work within the client's symptom parameters so that neurological symptoms are not increased.

Cautions and contraindications Watch for any indication of symptom aggravation. If the procedure increases neurological symptoms, discontinue that treatment immediately. It is beneficial to have the client evaluated by another health care provider. Be particularly aware of any symptoms that are bilateral, as this may indicate a central protrusion onto the spinal cord.

Use caution when performing techniques close to spine. The location of disc herniation should not be vulnerable to massage treatment because the transverse processes of the spine protect the region. However, techniques that put anteriorly directed pressure on the spine could move spinal structures in a way that aggravates nerve-root compression by the disc.

Some clients demonstrate protective muscular guarding in their cervical region. Pain from a cervical disc herniation can produce anxiety and fears about treatment, which add to the muscle splinting and hypertonicity. To reduce the client's apprehension thoroughly describe the gentle nature of the soft-tissue treatment and make sure gentle, compassionate touch is conveyed though manual treatment. With these clients, it is best to begin with gentle techniques.

THORACIC OUTLET SYNDROME

Description

Thoracic outlet syndrome (TOS) is not a single pathology, but a term that encompasses several pathologies involving compression of arteries, veins, or nerves near the thoracic outlet (though the compression does not necessarily occur within the thoracic outlet). TOS is a complex condition and is often overlooked or misdiagnosed due to the difficulty in distinguishing between its variations.[21,22]

One area of confusion with this condition is the name thoracic outlet. In some anatomy texts, this region is referred to as the thoracic inlet. However, both names refer to the same general area. The thoracic outlet/inlet is the area where structures either exit (thoracic outlet) or enter (thoracic inlet) the upper border of the thoracic rib cage. Therefore, whether the area is called the thoracic outlet or inlet depends upon the anatomical structure being discussed.

Thoracic outlet syndromes (TOS) were originally described in the medical literature as circulatory problems created by pressure on the arteries and veins in the upper-shoulder region. For that reason, many of the physical examination tests performed to evaluate this problem focus on circulatory responses. The pathology is sometimes defined as arterial (involving compression of the subclavian artery), venous (involving compression of the subclavian ven), or neurogenic (caused by compression of the brachial plexus). It is generally agreed upon today that the vast majority of symptoms from TOS, possibly as much as 90%, arise from neurological impairment.[23,24] For no known reason middle-aged women appear to be more susceptible to TOS than other groups.[25]

Four different pathologies can go by the name TOS. The first is a condition called true neurologic (or neurogenic) TOS. True neurologic TOS is caused by the presence of an unusual anatomical structure called a cervical rib, and is relatively rare (Fig. 10.9). The cervical rib is a pathological

extension of the transverse process of the seventh cervical vertebra. It can be either a fibrous or an osseous structure and often connects the seventh cervical transverse process with the first rib. When the rib is present, the nerves of the brachial plexus must pass over it and, therefore, its presence can lead to neurological compression pathology.

The other three conditions that go by the name TOS are all neurovascular compression pathologies in regions near the thoracic outlet. They include anterior scalene syndrome, costoclavicular syndrome, and pectoralis minor syndrome. In anterior scalene syndrome, the neurovascular structures are compressed between the anterior and middle scalene muscles (Fig. 10.10). In costoclavicular syndrome they are compressed between the clavicle and first rib (Fig. 10.11). In pectoralis minor syndrome the neurovascular structures are compressed between the pectoralis minor muscle and the upper rib cage (Fig. 10.12).

The medial, lateral, and posterior cords of the brachial plexus are its three primary divisions in the thoracic outlet region. Of those three, the medial cord is the most inferior, which makes it most susceptible to compression against the bones that are underneath it. As a result, symptoms are common in the nerves derived from fibers in the medial cord. Most of these fibers make up the ulnar nerve; therefore, it is usual for symptoms from the various forms of TOS to be felt first and foremost in the cutaneous distribution of the ulnar nerve. The cutaneous distribution of the ulnar nerve is pictured in Figure 10.13.

Several factors can lead to the development of TOS. Its onset can be acute or chronic. However, acute onset TOS is rare, and is usually the result of serious trauma, such as a direct blow to the clavicular region. A clavicular dislocation may change the structural arrangement enough to cause compression of the neurovascular structures in the area. An adequate history should provide insight into the onset of the condition.

More common causes of TOS are chronic postural distortions with resultant muscular dysfunction. Tightness or myofascial trigger points in the anterior and middle scalene muscles can be enough to make them press against the brachial plexus. Tightness in the coracobrachialis and

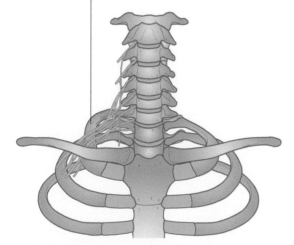

The bony extension of the transverse process of the 7th cervical vertebra will usually have a fibrous attachment to the first rib. The brachial plexus must travel over it before going underneath the clavicle

Figure 10.9   The cervical rib.

Figure 10.10 Anterior scalene syndrome. Compression of neurovascular structures between the anterior and middle scalene muscles.

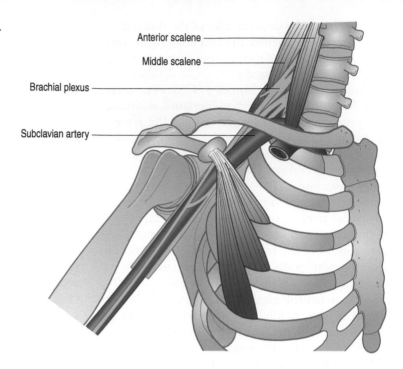

biceps brachii can pull the coracoid process in an anterior/inferior direction. If this occurs, the pectoralis minor is in a shortened position. It may become hypertonic in this shortened position and compress the brachial plexus against the upper rib cage (pectoralis minor syndrome).

Either of these postural distortions can lead to costoclavicular syndrome. Postural or movement patterns that put affected muscles under prolonged contraction also play a part in these pathologies. Examples include maintaining long periods of abduction in the shoulders, such as

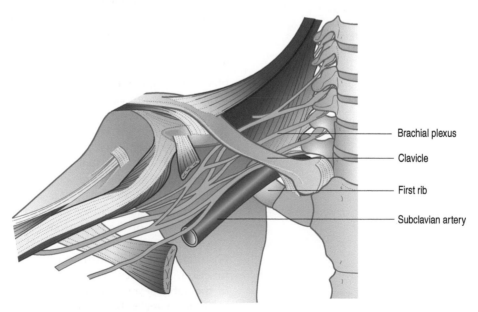

Figure 10.11   Costoclavicular syndrome. Neurovascular structures are compressed between the clavicle and first rib.

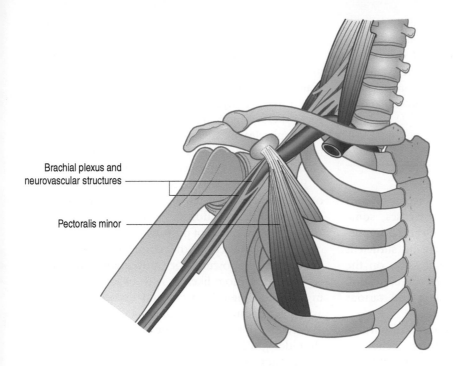

Figure 10.12 Pectoralis minor syndrome. Neurovascular compression under the pectoralis minor muscle.

Brachial plexus and neurovascular structures

Pectoralis minor

in hair styling, or the position a violinist must keep while playing their instrument. Wearing a heavy backpack or carrying heavy objects in the affected upper limb could aggravate symptoms as well.

Symptoms that clients experience include pain or paresthesia down the arm into the hand, feelings of heaviness in the upper limb, coldness or discoloration of the upper limb, or muscular atrophy of the thenar muscles of the hand. The pain, aching, or paresthesia that is felt in the arm and hand is usually in the distribution of the ulnar

nerve or the medial antebrachial cutaneous nerve along the ulnar side of the forearm.

Problems in the thoracic outlet region are commonly involved in double crush injuries (see Chapter 2 for additional information on the double crush phenomenon). There are several locations in the upper extremity where compression

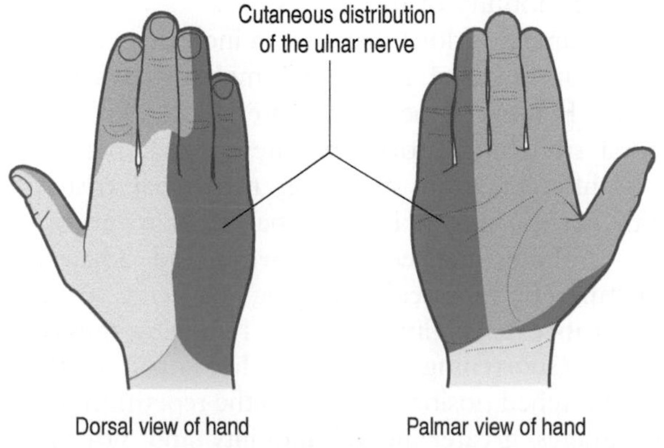

Cutaneous distribution of the ulnar nerve

Dorsal view of hand   Palmar view of hand

Figure 10.13 Cutaneous distribution of ulnar nerve.

Box 10.2   Clinical Tip

The ulnar nerve is the one most commonly involved in the different variations of thoracic outlet syndrome. However, it is important not to overlook the other major nerves of the upper extremity, which can also be involved. A more comprehensive physical examination with functional testing will be required to determine which nerves are primarily responsible for the adverse symptoms. Regardless of which nerve(s) appear to be at fault, it is advantageous to treat the entire neck and upper extremity as if the thoracic outlet nerve entrapment were affecting any or all nerves in the area. The enhanced mobility of all nerves in the upper extremity is valuable in reducing the potential for double crush injuries.

pathologies routinely occur so the likelihood of involvement of at least one, if not more, of these areas is increased. Common postural distortions can adversely affect more than one nerve compression site near the thoracic outlet, so double crush symptoms are common from thoracic outlet pathologies.[26]

Treatment

Traditional approaches

Conservative treatment is usually successful with TOS variations. In the majority of cases, some form of postural re-education is of crucial importance because postural change may be sufficient to remove the dysfunctional compression on the neurovascular structures. Postural re-education can be enhanced through stretching and various strength training methods as well.

If conservative treatment is unsuccessful, surgery may be the next option. Surgical approaches are most effective when dealing with compression caused by a cervical rib. Excision (removal) of the cervical rib often brings immediate relief of symptoms. However, there are those that question the necessity of surgery for this problem, even if a cervical rib exists.[27] If an individual with a cervical rib has made it through their life without symptoms, it is questionable whether the surgery is absolutely necessary. More research is needed to determine which conservative treatments are most effective in treating a neurogenic TOS caused by a cervical rib.

Surgery can be used to treat some of the other soft-tissue variations of TOS. The anterior scalene syndrome is sometimes treated surgically by removing some of the scalene muscles or a portion of the first rib.[28] However, removal of the muscles or the first rib is likely to have other detrimental effects on muscular function in the region.[29]

Soft-tissue manipulation

General guidelines   Particular attention is paid to treating the soft tissues involved in the specific region of compression. It is helpful to treat all of these areas regardless of where the primary site of compression is occurring, because more than one site may be involved. It is beneficial to treat these other areas, even if they are not directly involved in the compression pathology.

If neurological or vascular symptoms are increased during treatment, move to another region, as it is likely that nerve compression is being increased. Several muscles, including the pectoralis major, latissimus dorsi, teres major, and subscapularis, can have myofascial trigger points that mimic some TOS symptoms. It is advantageous to treat these muscles in the process as well. If they are holding dysfunctional trigger points, their treatment helps restore proper muscular balance.

Because these neurovascular compression disorders are often caused by postural distortion, it is important to address postural dysfunctions. A critical component of postural correction for these disorders is to repeat the corrections frequently. The more a postural or movement pattern is repeated, the more likely it is to become ingrained in the neurological system and become a natural aspect of posture or movement.

Stretching muscles of the cervical region and shoulder girdle is an important part of treating all the variations of TOS. When stretching muscles take the muscle to the point of mild pain or discomfort and hold it there until the pain or discomfort subsides. In doing this, the connective tissue component of the muscle is elongated, and the neuromuscular component changes the rate of stimulation in the muscle to reduce tightness. In the process of stretching, the client may report an exacerbation of neurological symptoms in certain positions. This is ordinarily due to stretching of nerve tissue in these positions. If there is adverse neural tension throughout any of the nerves in the upper extremity due to one of these problems, some degree of neural stretching may be helpful to improve mobility of the nerves.

The same positions that give an increase in symptoms can be used for neural mobility enhancement. However, be very careful in the way neural stretching procedures are applied, because it is different from stretching myofascial tissues. With nerve tissue it is more beneficial to encourage mobility between the nerve and adjacent structures by repeatedly bringing the nerve to the end of its extensibility, and then removing tension from it (shortening it) without holding it in the fully stretched position.[30,31] It is the repetition that encourages greater neural mobility and not the tensile load on the nerve.

Holding the nerve in its fully stretched position is likely to increase the symptoms, and does not achieve a significant increase in mobility. The primary function of neural stretching procedures is not to increase the length of nerve tissue as it is with an elastic tissue like muscle. The primary goal is to increase the mobility between the nerve and adjacent structures. Neural mobility procedures are more effective when the soft tissues along the entire path of the nerve are as relaxed and pliable as possible.

Suggested techniques and methods   The following techniques may be effective for addressing one variation of TOS, but not for another variation. They are categorized in different groups for ease of presentation. It is still valuable to treat all the potentially involved tissues regardless of the variation that exists.

True neurogenic thoracic outlet syndrome   No soft-tissue treatment technique can remove the obstruction of the cervical rib. Massage treatment for a true neurogenic TOS focuses on reducing the likelihood of additional neurovascular compression in the area and enhancing neural mobility. The techniques described below in the other categories are valuable for this approach.

Anterior scalene syndrome and costoclavicular syndrome

A. Myofascial approaches   Myofascial techniques encourage fascial and muscular relaxation. Gentle pressure is placed on the fascia in multiple directions. Relaxing the fascia has benefits in reducing muscular tension and decreasing restrictions on neural mobility. The primary goal is to place a moderately light pressure on the subcutaneous fascia. Pulling the fascia in multiple directions appears to enhance its pliability the most. Place the hands lightly on the client's neck where the myofascial stretch is to be applied. Pull the hands apart to take the slack out of the tissue and apply a light degree of pulling force between the hands (Fig. 10.1). Once there is a slight degree of pull between the hands, hold this position until a subtle sensation of tissue release is felt. These approaches are effective when applied to muscles of the posterior, anterior, and lateral cervical region.

B. Effleurage and sweeping cross fiber   These techniques are effective for reducing tension in neck muscles that may be contributing to neurovascular

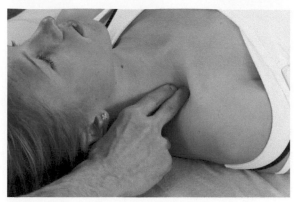

Figure 10.14   Static compression on anterior scalenes.

compression. Effleurage is performed with long gliding strokes parallel to the muscle fiber direction. Cross fiber techniques sweep diagonally across the primary fiber direction of muscles in different regions of the neck (Fig. 10.2). Use care with effleurage or sweeping cross fiber motions across tissues of the lateral and anterior neck region due to the superficial vascular structures in this area.

C. Static compression   Use small contact surface static compression to reduce muscular hypertonicity or treat myofascial trigger points in specific muscles, such as the scalenes, that can be compressing neurovascular structures (Fig. 10.14). Pressure maintained for 8–10 seconds is usually sufficient to achieve a reduction of muscle tension.

D. Deep stripping on scalenes   Due to the location of the scalene muscles deep to the sternocleidomastoid and other neck muscles, they are not easy to access along their whole length. Do not exert a great deal of pressure in the anterior neck region as the brachial plexus and vascular structures are superficial in this area. The client is in a supine position with the head turned slightly away from the side being treated. Use the finger tips or thumb to perform a longitudinal stripping technique on the anterior and middle scalene muscles, just lateral to the lateral edge of the clavicular head of the sternocleidomastoid (SCM) (Fig. 10.15). The entire length of the muscle is not accessible with this stripping technique so just treat the accessible fibers. If the client reports an increase in neurological or vascular symptoms, immediately cease the technique as there may be additional pressure on the primary region of pathology.

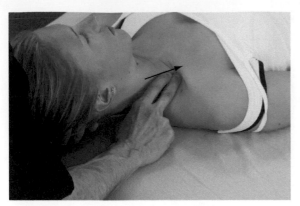

Figure 10.15   Deep stripping on scalenes.

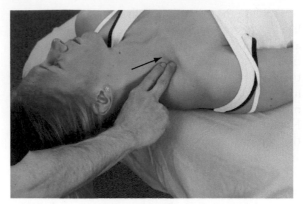

Figure 10.16   Stripping with active engagement (lengthening) on scalenes.

E. Stripping with active engagement It can be difficult to apply adequate and effective pressure on the scalene muscles with stripping techniques because of the sensitivity of this region and the delicate structures nearby. Adding active engagement increases the effectiveness of the stripping technique. The client is in a supine position with the head partially rotated to the opposite side and off the end of the table. If the client does not feel comfortable with the head off the end of the table, use a bolster or pillow under the upper back so there is room to move the head in hyperextension.

Hold the client's head with one hand while the other hand is prepared to apply the stripping technique. Ask the client to lift the head slightly and hold it there for a few seconds (the practitioner's hand keeps light contact with the client's head, but the client is now holding their own head up). After holding that contraction for 5–8 seconds, instruct the client to slowly let go of the contraction. As the contraction is slowly released, gently guide their head into hyperextension with one hand while the other hand performs a stripping technique on the anterior and middle scalenes as in D above (Fig. 10.16). Repeat this technique several times for maximum effectiveness. Do not perform this technique if there is a concern about vertebrobasilar insufficiency (see the cautions and contraindications below).

F. Muscle energy technique for anterior/lateral neck muscles and fascia In some cases additional pressure in the region of the brachial plexus is uncomfortable for the client because it aggravates neurological or vascular symptoms. In those cases

this MET procedure is an effective way to enhance lengthening in the scalene muscles without putting direct pressure on them. This technique is best performed without lubricant on the client's skin. The client is in a supine position and in a position like E above where the head can be relaxed off the end of the table or over a bolster. One hand holds the client's head and the other hand is positioned over the scalene muscles or their distal fascial connections. Ask the client to lift their head out of the hand and hold it there for a few seconds (the practitioner's hand keeps contact with the client's head, but the client is now holding the weight of their own head). After holding that contraction for 5–8 seconds, instruct the client to slowly let go of the contraction. As they slowly let go of the contraction let their head drop back into extension while applying an inferiorly directed traction force to the scalenes and the fascial tissues connected with them (Fig. 10.17). The force of the fingertips pulls on the skin and superficial fascia more than pressing down into the scalenes. Repeat this technique several times and apply at different points along the length of the scalene muscles or their distal fascia. Do not perform this technique if there is a concern about vertebrobasilar insufficiency (see the cautions and contraindications below).

Pectoralis minor syndrome

A. Deep stripping on pectoralis minor The client is in a supine position. Perform sufficient warming techniques, such as effleurage and sweeping cross fiber, to reduce tension in the pectoralis

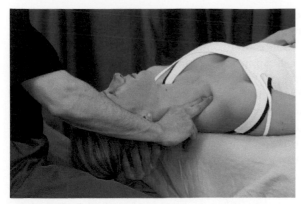

Figure 10.17   MET for scalenes and their fascial connections.

major muscle so the pectoralis minor is more easily accessible. Perform a deep longitudinal stripping technique on the pectoralis minor beginning at the coracoid process of the scapula and moving inferiorly to its attachments on ribs 3, 4, and 5 (Fig. 10.18). Pressure is applied directly through the pectoralis major muscle and this region can be somewhat tender, so use care in the amount of pressure that is applied. Immediately move off the area if the technique reproduces or exacerbates neurological symptoms.

B. Pin and stretch for pectoralis minor The client is in a supine position. The practitioner is at the level of the client's head facing their feet. Place a thumb or finger tip in contact with the pectoralis minor muscle but not on any area that exaggerates or reproduces neurological symptoms when pressure is applied. Instruct the client to

reach as far toward their toes as possible. This motion depresses the scapula and puts the pectoralis minor in a shortened position. With the muscle in this position apply moderate to significant pressure (within the client's comfort tolerance) to the pectoralis minor muscle. Then instruct the client to hike the shoulder up as if bringing it as close to the ear as possible. While they are elevating the shoulder girdle, apply static compression or a short stripping technique to the pectoralis minor muscle (Fig. 10.19). Repeat this technique several times to encourage lengthening of the pectoralis minor.

C. Neural mobilization technique Neural mobilization is helpful to reduce binding or restriction on nerves of the upper extremity that could be affected by regions of entrapment near the thoracic outlet. Most thoracic outlet variations affect the ulnar nerve so this neural mobility technique emphasizes the ulnar nerve. The client is in a supine position with the arm at the side. Hyperextend the client's wrist and fingers and bring the forearm into position of elbow flexion. From that position abduct the shoulder so it appears the client's hand is coming close to covering the ear (Fig. 10.20). At the far end of this movement instruct the client to laterally flex the head to the opposite side as the hand is brought up near the side of the head. Do not hold the final stretch position. Bring the shoulder and elbow back to neutral positions. Immediately repeat this series of movements several times. The idea is to repeatedly pull on the nerves of the brachial plexus and reduce binding or restriction between the nerves and adjacent tissues.

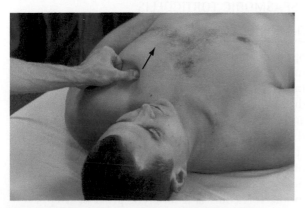

Figure 10.18   Deep stripping on pectoralis minor.

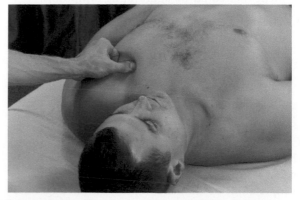

Figure 10.19   Pin and stretch on pectoralis minor.

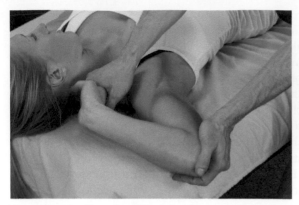

Figure 10.20   Neural mobilization for ulnar nerve.

Rehabilitation protocol considerations

- Strength training for shoulder or neck muscles is sometimes advocated to address postural distortions that contribute to neurovascular compression. Postural retraining should be initiated and routinely reinforced prior to significant strength training activities so dysfunctional patterns are not strengthened or reinforced.

- In more severe cases, some of the suggested treatment techniques are not recommended because the neurological symptoms are severe and any additional pressure on the region aggravates the symptoms. In those cases, simply reduce the pressure applied in the techniques and focus on treatment methods such as the MET technique described above that doesn't put additional pressure on the neurovascular structures.

- Be sure to treat the entire upper extremity as part of the TOS treatment strategy because there can be multiple regions of nerve entrapment that could be aggravating symptoms.

- The neural mobility technique described in C under Pectoralis minor syndrome treatment above should be performed after the entire upper extremity has been treated. Neural mobility procedures are more effective when the soft tissues along the entire path of the nerve are as relaxed and pliable as possible.

Cautions and contraindications   The practitioner should be cautious about applying pressure in any of the affected regions. Because TOS involves nerve compression, additional compression can aggravate the problem. The practitioner should stay in close communication with the client about symptoms so treatment can be immediately modified.

Some of the neural stretching procedures can create an immediate increase of symptoms. Exacerbation of symptoms can be kept to a minimal level if treatment is ceased when symptoms increase. Do not overstretch neural structures when performing neural mobility techniques. If symptoms recur prior to the ending position of the described movements, do not pursue additional movements past the point where symptoms recur.

The position with the client supine and head moving into hyperextension described in E and F under anterior scalene syndrome and costoclavicular syndrome above can produce an adverse effect in some people. This position with the head turned to the side while it is being hyperextended can compress the vertebral artery and decrease blood flow to the brain causing dizziness, vertigo, blurred vision, or fainting. This is a condition called *vertebrobasilar insufficiency.* Prior to performing this technique it is helpful to perform the vertebral artery test to see if the client is potentially susceptible to this compression. With the client in a seated position ask them to look up and over their shoulder so the head is in hyperextension and rotation. Hold that position for about 30 seconds. If the client begins to feel sensations of dizziness, vertigo, nausea, vision problems, or other neurological symptoms, this is a positive result and indicates they are susceptible to vertebral artery compression. If that is the case, those treatment techniques should be avoided.

SPASMODIC TORTICOLLIS

Description

Spasmodic torticollis is a condition of continual muscle spasm that affects the extensor and rotator muscles of the neck. It usually makes the individual's head turn to the side in lateral flexion and/or rotation with some hyperextension as if they were attempting to look over their shoulder. It is most common on one side only. Another form of torticollis, congenital torticollis, arises from difficulty in traveling through the birth canal. Spasmodic torticollis is a different process; it appears to be a central nervous system dysfunction.

This condition is also called wry neck or cervical dystonia. Dystonia is a neurological movement disorder characterized by involuntary muscle contractions that force the body into abnormal and sometimes painful movements or postures. The cause for spasmodic torticollis is unknown, although there does seem to be some central nervous system dysfunction. In spasmodic torticollis, muscles develop a degree of fibrotic change and contracture within the tissue. Pain in this condition may not be limited to the muscles alone, but may involve dysfunctional central nervous system responses.[32]

Some individuals may develop spasm in cervical muscles. These spasms can happen as the result of sleeping in an awkward position for long periods or even from having a cool draft on the cervical region during the night.[20] Spasmodic torticollis is different as the degree of spasm in the muscles is much greater with torticollis, and torticollis is often harder to resolve than a muscle spasm that results from long periods of awkward positioning.

Treatment

Traditional approaches

Stretching and various physical therapy modalities are commonly used for treatment of spasmodic torticollis. A primary focus is on the level of muscle dysfunction, as well as attempting to normalize any contributing factors from the central nervous system. Medications are sometimes used to address the muscle spasms. Biofeedback and hypnosis have also been used with some clinical success.

When conservative measures are not effective, another treatment that is used is injection therapy. In this procedure, a small amount of botulinum toxin A (known by its commercial name, BOTOX®) is injected into the affected muscles. BOTOX® is a neurotoxic substance that essentially prevents the release of acetylcholine, which interrupts muscle function.[33] The interruption of muscle function is an effective means of reducing the spastic contractions in the neck muscles. The amount of botulinum toxin used in this procedure is well below the level that is poisonous to a human.

In addition to botulinum toxin injections, surgical procedures may also be used. Surgery will focus on denervating the involved muscles so they do not perpetuate their dysfunctional spasm. Surgery alone is generally not as effective as surgery combined with the injection therapy.[34]

Soft-tissue manipulation

General guidelines The primary focus of massage treatment for torticollis is to reduce the chronic muscle spasms that occur in this condition. It is not clear if massage can help with the aspects of this condition that are mediated by the central nervous system. However, due to the systemic effects of massage in lowering stress levels and overall neuromuscular tension, massage might be beneficial for the central nervous system components of the disorder as well.

Always strive to work gently within the client's comfort zone. Any increased tonus level that is stimulated through excessive pressure may cause an increased central nervous system response. This will be detrimental to the primary goal of treatment. The foremost aim of treatment is to reduce muscle spasms and excess central nervous system activity that is contributing to the disorder. A treatment environment that is conducive to overall relaxation is desirable for achieving those outcomes. The cumulative effect of environmental factors on reducing central nervous system stress should not be ignored; for example, a long treatment session (more than 45 minutes), a dimly lit room, and relaxing music. The factors that contribute to nervous system relaxation should be maximized as much as possible.

Suggested techniques and methods

A. Myofascial approaches Myofascial techniques encourage fascial and muscular relaxation. Gentle pressure is placed on the fascia in multiple directions. Relaxing the fascia has benefits in reducing muscular tension and decreasing any restrictions on neural mobility. The primary goal is to place a moderately light pressure on the subcutaneous fascia. Pulling the fascia in multiple directions appears to enhance its pliability the most. Place the hands lightly on the client's neck where the myofascial stretch is to be applied. Pull the hands apart to take the slack out of the tissue and apply a light degree of pulling force between the hands (Fig. 10.1). Once there is a slight degree of pull between the hands, hold this position until there is a subtle sensation of tissue release. Apply these fascial techniques specifically to the muscles in the neck that are engaged in spasm due to torticollis.

B. Effleurage and sweeping cross fiber These techniques are effective methods for reducing tension in superficial neck muscles. Effleurage is performed with long gliding strokes parallel to the muscle fiber direction. The cross fiber techniques sweep diagonally across the primary fiber direction of muscles in different regions of the neck (Fig. 10.2). Use care with the pressure level in effleurage or sweeping cross fiber motions as there are sensitive vascular structures that are superficial in the anterior neck region. Emphasize long gliding strokes with the muscles that are in spasm as these long strokes help reduce excess neurological activity.

C. Pin and stretch on sternocleidomastoid The SCM is one of the primary muscles that maintain the dysfunctional torticollis position when in spasm. The SCM can be difficult to treat. Due to the layers of soft tissues and sensitive structures underneath the SCM, significant pressure should not be used. Depending on the severity of the torticollis, the head may not be able to move much. Perform what is within the client's comfort tolerance and gradually work towards improvement. The description below assumes a greater range of motion is possible.

This pin and stretch technique allows direct pressure and stretching on the SCM without pushing down into anterior neck structures. This technique can be performed actively with the client moving their own head or passively with the practitioner moving the client's head. Place one hand underneath the client's head in a position where their head can adequately be moved in a number of different directions. Move their head into a position of flexion and contralateral rotation (e.g. turning left if treating the right SCM). This position puts the SCM in a fully shortened position. Grasp the SCM muscle between the thumb and fingers. Either actively or passively rotate the client's head into extension and ipsilateral rotation, as if they are looking up over their shoulder (Fig. 10.21). Do not perform this technique if there is a concern about vertebrobasilar insufficiency (see the cautions and contraindications below).

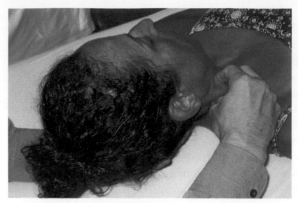

Figure 10.21   Pin and stretch on sternocleidomastoid (SCM).

D. MET using reciprocal inhibition for neck rotators In many cases muscle spasm does not respond well to direct manipulation, but active-assisted stretching using reciprocal inhibition can achieve beneficial results by using appropriate neurological principles. This technique assumes attention is focused on the SCM, a contralateral neck rotator muscle. The technique can be modified to address the contributions of other muscles, such as the flexors or lateral flexors of the neck that may be contributing to the disorder. The description assumes the right side is being treated. Reverse the instructions to address the left side SCM. The client is in a supine position. Place one hand gently on the right side of the client's forehead. Instruct the client to attempt to rotate the head to the right while offering resistance for about 5–8 seconds. This resisted action engages the left SCM (and the right side ipsilateral rotators). When they contract there is decreased neurological activity in our target muscle, the right SCM. Instruct the client to release the contraction. As they let go of the contraction gently attempt to turn the head in same direction that they were attempting (to the right). This will stretch the SCM on the right side (Fig. 10.22).

Rehabilitation protocol considerations

- Depending on the severity of the spasm in torticollis, different massage techniques are used. In a severe case, there may be very little that direct soft-tissue manipulation can do due to client pain. In these cases, begin with less invasive

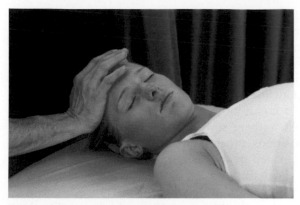

Figure 10.22 MET with reciprocal inhibition for cervical contralateral rotators.

techniques such as the MET with reciprocal inhibition described in D above.

- Myofascial techniques have clear effects on reducing neuromuscular activity through mild tensile loads applied to the tissues. Due to their gentle intervention, these techniques are advantageous in more severe cases when there is a significant amount of muscle spasm.

Cautions and contraindications There may be significant pain and discomfort associated with spasmodic torticollis. Be aware of the client's reported level of discomfort and adjust treatments accordingly. It is more beneficial to work slowly on improving central nervous system effects over a number of treatments, rather than trying to reduce all the symptoms in one or two sessions.

Special precautions should be taken with massage treatment for a client who is currently receiving botulinum injection therapy. No studies have been published on the effects of massage in conjunction with botulinum toxin injections. Because of the potential that massage treatments have to enhance circulation, there may be some adverse interference with the local administration of the medication. It is best to get clearance from a physician about massage treatment in this area for a client who is currently receiving injection therapy.

The position with the client supine and head moving into hyperextension described in C can produce an adverse effect in some people. This position with the head turned to the side while it is being hyperextended can compress the vertebral artery and decrease blood flow to the brain causing dizziness, vertigo, blurred vision, or fainting. Prior to performing this technique, perform the vertebral artery test to see if the client is potentially susceptible to this compression. With the client in a seated position ask them to look up and over their shoulder so the head is in hyperextension and rotation. The client holds the position for about 30 seconds. If the client begins to feel sensations of dizziness, vertigo, nausea, vision problems, or other neurological symptoms, they are susceptible to vertebral artery compression and those treatment techniques should be avoided. Depending on the severity of the torticollis the client may not be able to make these movements in a position that would be enough to compress the vertebral artery. However, as greater motion is achieved it could be an issue.

WHIPLASH

Description

Whiplash is a frequently misunderstood condition, as it is not a single condition. Whiplash is an injury that occurs as the result of a sudden acceleration or deceleration of the head and neck in relation to the torso. Numerous problems can result from whiplash. Consequently, it is not appropriate to speak of whiplash as an isolated condition. It is more appropriate to describe it as a broad spectrum of possible disorders. It is now commonly referred to as whiplash associated disorder (WAD), indicating that whiplash is the mechanism of injury, but numerous tissues could be injured as a result.

One of the most important classifications of WAD published to date came from the Quebec Task Force on Whiplash-Associated Disorders.[35] They have classified WAD into four categories of severity:

Category 1: Neck complaint without musculoskeletal signs such as loss of mobility.
Category 2: Neck complaint with musculoskeletal signs such as loss of mobility.
Category 3: Neck complaint with neurological signs.
Category 4: Neck complaint with cervical fracture or dislocation.

It is apparent from looking at this classification that various pathologies fall under the description of whiplash – from simple musculoskeletal irritation, all the way to cervical fracture and severe neurological impairment. Assessment of the injury level is crucial for any practitioner attempting to treat whiplash disorders.

The approach to classifying whiplash and designing appropriate treatment protocols has been challenging because of the different symptoms that occur some time after the initial incident. Although the Task Force has set up a helpful system for classifying whiplash problems, their conclusions are not without controversy. There is still a call for a better understanding of WAD.[36,37]

Whiplash injuries can cause damage to muscles, neural structures, ligaments, tendons, fascia, facet joints, bones, intervertebral discs, or vascular structures. Pain may be local in the neck, or it may radiate into the head, shoulder, or upper extremity. Some people suffering from whiplash experience impairment of memory, concentration, or sleep, as well as fatigue, depression, and various forms of psychological distress.[38,39] The practitioner should be on the lookout for any of these symptoms if their client has suffered a whiplash trauma.

A challenging aspect of WAD is matching the onset of symptoms to the actual structures that are damaged. It is common for whiplash symptoms to emerge days, weeks, or even months after the initial trauma. Explanations for this delay of symptoms include delayed inflammatory effects or altered mechanics that take a while to produce symptoms. There is also evidence of increased central nervous system sensitivity that could be playing a role in delayed onset of tissue sensitivity.[40,41]

If not severe, whiplash conditions are generally limited to soft-tissue injury. Cervical muscles can be strained or under protective spasm. Ligaments of the cervical region can be sprained from excess joint motion. In many instances, myofascial trigger points develop in the cervical muscles following the injury. Trigger points lead to patterns of facilitated muscular dysfunction that often linger for months or years after the initial trauma.[20]

Treatment

Traditional approaches

As with other conditions, rest from offending activity is essential, especially in the early phases after the injury. It is common practice to begin rehabilitation of whiplash injury as soon as the inflammatory phase has subsided. This may be difficult to identify in many cases, however, because visible inflammation is mostly absent. A general guideline of 48–72 hours after the initial incident is a common period for the inflammatory stage. When there is relief of symptoms from various positions other than static rest, some degree of managed treatment can begin.[5]

For years, the cervical collar was a mainstay of treatment for whiplash, and the practice persists. However, health care practitioners now realize that unless there is a severe level of damage, early, protected mobilization is more beneficial than immobilization in a collar.[42–45] When cervical collars are used, whether soft or hard collars, they can cause further complications from the initial trauma. It is common for temporomandibular dysfunction, joint adhesions, muscle atrophy, and myofascial trigger points to develop from long periods of immobilization in a cervical collar.[46]

Various drugs, such as anti-inflammatory medications or muscle relaxants, may be used to treat whiplash symptoms. Cervical traction units may also provide relief for symptoms. This will be especially true in instances where there is compression of the vertebral bodies or facet joints.[47] Remember that numerous tissues can be the source of whiplash pain so evaluation of these potential problems should be thorough.

Soft-tissue manipulation

General guidelines   If a specific tissue injury can be identified as the source of pain, such as a strain to the splenius capitis, massage treatment focuses directly on that tissue injury. Use comprehensive orthopedic assessment to clarify the nature of the tissue injury as accurately as possible. Without identification of a specific tissue that is damaged, soft-tissue treatments are more general in nature. For example, it is difficult to treat some ligaments of the cervical spine that are sprained because they are deep along the cervical spine or near the atlanto-occipital joint and too deep to access. However, the resultant muscular dysfunction that occurs from excessive neurological activity and movement restriction can become a serious part of the whiplash-associated disorder, and this muscular dysfunction is treatable with massage.

The appropriate form of massage depends greatly upon what tissues are injured. Techniques such as effleurage, sweeping cross fiber, active engagement, as well as active-assisted massage are useful at various stages of whiplash rehabilitation. Gentle stretching in the cervical region is also an integral part of the treatment process.

Suggested techniques and methods Depending on the exact nature of the injury, which is determined by proper assessment, any of the techniques A–G described in the section Neuromuscular neck pain can be valuable in treating WAD. In some cases the muscles or other soft tissues of the cervical region are too sensitive for direct soft-tissue manipulation. The additional techniques included below can be used in the early stages of rehabilitation when it is too early for other soft-tissue work.

Because there are a number of tissues that can be injured in a whiplash injury, it may be difficult to identify the severity or nature of the injury. In cases that appear to be more than a mild muscular whiplash disorder referral to a physician is strongly recommended to screen for more serious pathologies.

A. MET with reciprocal inhibition for cervical extensors This technique emphasizes muscular dysfunction in the cervical extensors following the whiplash injury. The client is in a supine position to begin. Gently cradle one hand behind the client's head and place the other hand on the client's forehead. Instruct the client to slowly lift the head off the treatment table against resistance. Hold the contraction for about 5–8 seconds. Depending on the severity of the whiplash injury, engaging the cervical muscles in a contraction may be uncomfortable or cause further pain. Only engage this muscle contraction within the client's pain or comfort tolerance. Instruct the client to release the contraction. As they release the contraction gently push the head farther into flexion to stretch the posterior cervical muscles (Fig. 10.23).

B. MET with reciprocal inhibition for lateral flexors The client is in a supine position. Instructions for this technique assume that the lateral rotators on the right side of the neck are being

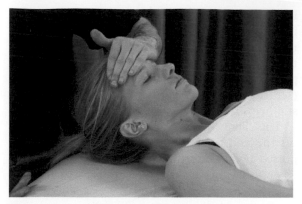

Figure 10.23 MET with reciprocal inhibition for cervical extensors.

treated. Place one hand against the left side of the client's head and the other against the client's right shoulder. It might be more helpful to cross the arms and have the right hand underneath the client's head with fingers on the side of their head and the left hand on the client's shoulder. Instruct the client to hold this position as the practitioner attempts to laterally flex the client's head to the right (the client engages the left lateral flexors to resist this motion). The client holds that contraction for about 5–8 seconds. Instruct the client to release the contraction and as the contraction is released, move the head into left lateral flexion to stretch the lateral flexor muscles on the right side (Fig. 10.24).

C. MET with reciprocal inhibition for anterior neck flexors Deep flexors of the neck, such as the

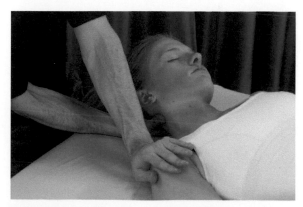

Figure 10.24 MET with reciprocal inhibition for lateral neck flexors.

longus colli and longus capitis, are commonly injured in rear-impact whiplash incidents. These muscles are deep in the neck and lie very close to the cervical spine. This MET procedure avoids pressure on the baroreceptors in the carotid sinus (see this important contraindication below), but still helps treat the deep neck flexor muscles.

The client is in a supine position with the head off the end of the table or the upper back supported by a bolster so the head can move back in extension. Both of the practitioner's hands are holding the head. Holding the head with both hands is important to give the client maximum confidence that no sudden or forceful neck movement will result. Starting in a neutral position instruct the client to gently push their head into the hands for about 5–8 seconds as resistance is offered. After holding that contraction, instruct the client to let go of the contraction and gently let the head drop back into further extension stretching the deep neck flexors on the anterior side of the neck (Fig. 10.25). Only perform this stretch within the client's comfort tolerance. Do not perform this technique if there is a concern about vertebrobasilar insufficiency (see the cautions and contraindications below).

Rehabilitation protocol considerations

- WAD runs the gamut from mild muscular irritation to severe and life-threatening cervical injury. Accurate assessment of the injury is crucial to determine the severity of tissue damage and what types of massage treatment are appropriate or potentially contraindicated.

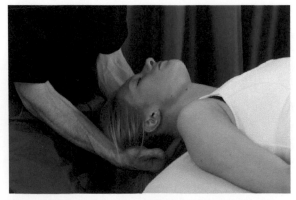

Figure 10.25 MET with reciprocal inhibition for deep anterior neck flexors.

- In the early stages of the injury use gentle techniques that emphasize neurological responses without putting excess pressure on muscle and other soft tissues. Myofascial approaches and active-assisted stretching procedures, such as the MET with and without reciprocal inhibition, are particularly well suited to the early stages of a whiplash injury

- Positional release is also a good treatment choice in the early stages of whiplash injury because it does not require invasive pressure and uses gentle neurological responses to achieve treatment objectives.

- Due to excessive neuromuscular tension following WAD injuries, thermal modalities are useful adjuncts to soft-tissue treatment. Ice and cold applications are preferable in the immediate aftermath of the injury to reduce inflammatory effects. However, ice is also valuable in the later stages with muscular spasm because of its ability to slow nerve conduction velocity and interrupt muscle spasm. If the WAD has moved into the sub-acute or chronic phase, individuals respond well to heat applications because they reduce neuromuscular tension and settle down excessive sympathetic nervous system activity.

- Early mobilization and gentle exercise is a mainstay of WAD treatment. More vigorous movement retraining, strengthening, and conditioning are also a part of WAD treatment to restore proper strength and resilience to the tissues in this area. However, due to the heightened neurological stress in the area following this type of injury and the increased central nervous system sensitivity, it is best to wait later in the rehabilitation process for significant strength-training activities. Strength training or conditioning that is begun too soon can cause reactive muscular spasms as the body is readjusting to proprioceptive feedback from the injured muscles.

Cautions and contraindications   One of the concerns in working with clients with a WAD injury is identifying what the problem really is. Because symptoms can be delayed, do not perform any treatment technique that is going to make the condition worse. It is not unusual for clients to go through therapy, massage and other types, for whiplash treatment and come out feeling worse. In these cases, the practitioner may have been too aggressive with the treatment, or simply used an approach that was improper for the nature or stage of the injury.

Acquire thorough and complete information from the client related to the symptoms they have experienced and those they are currently experiencing in order to make responsible clinical decisions. Watch for symptoms that indicate the need for intervention of another health professional for further and more complete evaluation. If there is uncertainty of the severity or nature of the whiplash injury, it is best to refer that person out for a more comprehensive evaluation prior to treatment. Underlying dysfunctions such as severe joint instability may not be immediately apparent due to protective muscle spasm. Overly enthusiastic stretching or movement techniques could then cause joint subluxation or dislocation.

Some treatment techniques for the deep neck flexors, such as the longus colli and longus capitis, advocate direct treatment of the muscles. This direct deep treatment usually involves displacing the trachea to the side so muscles in the anterior neck can be directly accessed. Unfortunately these muscles are also very close to sensitive tissues such as the thyroid gland and vascular structures such as the carotid artery and carotid sinus. The carotid sinus contains sensitive neurological receptors called baroreceptors that are important in regulating blood pressure. Attempts at putting pressure on the deep neck flexors could inadvertently put pressure on the baroreceptors and cause an unintentional alteration of blood pressure with adverse effects. Indirect treatment techniques such as active-assisted stretching (see the MET procedures described in C above) avoid direct deep pressure in the anterior neck region, but still provide effective treatment of these important muscles.

The position with the client supine and head moving into hyperextension described in MET with reciprocal inhibition for anterior neck flexors can produce an adverse effect in some people. This position can compress the vertebral artery and decrease blood flow to the brain causing dizziness, vertigo, blurred vision, or fainting (a condition called vertebrobasilar insufficiency). Prior to performing this technique it is helpful to perform the vertebral artery test. With the client in a seated position ask them to look up and over their shoulder so the head is in hyperextension and rotation. The client holds the position for about 30 seconds. If the client begins to feel sensations of dizziness, vertigo, nausea, vision problems, or other neurological symptoms, this is a positive result and indicates they are susceptible to vertebral artery compression. If that is the case, this treatment technique should be avoided.

POSTURAL DISORDERS

This section includes a discussion of forward head posture, the most common postural distortion in the cervical region. It is not considered an injury condition, as are the prior conditions in this chapter. However, it can produce considerable stress on other tissues or structures and contribute to their dysfunction. Massage is a valuable tool in addressing this postural condition, due to the combination of muscle dysfunctions that create it.

FORWARD HEAD POSTURE

Because humans stand upright in a vertical gravity plane and the head is a heavy weight, we are susceptible to the distortion of a forward head posture. Chronic dysfunctional posture is the likely cause. This condition usually involves muscular distortion in the thoracic and cervical regions. In forward head posture, there is extension in the upper cervical vertebrae and flexion in the lower cervical vertebrae. When the head is positioned forward of the line of gravity, a tensile load is placed on the posterior cervical extensor muscles. These muscles keep the eyes looking straight ahead and prevent the head from falling forward. Even a slight degree of forward head posture increases stress on the posterior neck muscles.

In addition there is an increased compressive load on the posterior vertebral arch structures. For every inch the head moves forward from its normal posture, the compressive load on the lower neck is approximately equal to that number times the weight of the head (e.g. 2 inches forward head posture equals two times the weight of the head).[5]

In a forward head posture the posterior cervical muscles must work harder to keep the head upright. As a result fatigue, tension, and myofascial trigger points develop. Muscle tension and myofascial trigger point referrals can produce pain in the head, neck, upper back, and temporomandibular joint. Muscular irritation from forward head posture is at the root of numerous head and neck pain conditions. For example, myofascial trigger points that develop in the sub-occipital muscles from forward head posture frequently produce headache pain. The increased compressive loads can eventually lead to vertebral stress fractures or cervical facet (zygapophysial) joint irritation.

The previous chapter discussed the lower crossed syndrome, a condition that involves the relationship between postural and phasic muscles in the lumbar region. A similar relationship exists in the cervical region and is referred to as the upper crossed syndrome.[46] The upper crossed syndrome often exists in conjunction with the lower crossed syndrome. Postural and phasic muscles differ in their fiber type and activation patterns. When overused and fatigued, postural muscles tend to become hypertonic, while phasic muscles tend to become weak and inhibited. The phasic muscles are antagonists to postural muscles. Because postural muscles tend toward hypertonicity, they create a functional weakness in the phasic muscles through the process of reciprocal inhibition. A graphical comparison of their position and functional relationships with each other shows how they interact in the upper crossed syndrome (Fig. 10.26).

The postural muscles in the neck prone to hypertonicity include the upper trapezius, levator scapulae, and cervical extensors on the posterior aspect, as well as the pectoralis major and minor in the front.[5] The postural muscles are known to house active myofascial trigger points and refer characteristic sensations when palpated. Phasic muscles that are prone to weakness include the deep neck flexors, such as the longus colli and longus capitis, as well as the lower trapezius and serratus anterior.[5]

Forward head posture results from poor postural habits, such as leaning forward toward a computer screen for long periods. This condition also occurs alongside upper thoracic kyphosis or

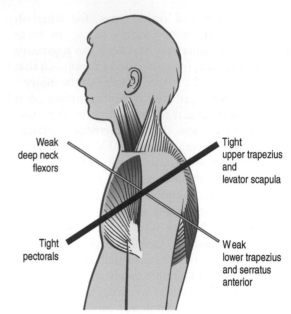

Figure 10.26 Forward head posture and upper crossed syndrome (from Chaitow L, DeLany J. Clinical Application of Neuromuscular Techniques. Vol 1. Edinburgh: Churchill Livingstone; 2000).

excessive lordosis and can be a result of osteoporosis. Due to the postural compensations that naturally occur with age, forward head posture is more prevalent in older adults.

Treatment

Traditional approaches

Traditional treatment focuses on strength training and postural re-education. Ergonomic changes at work play an important role and any method of postural retraining that reinforces correct cervical alignment is beneficial. Certain postural retraining techniques, such as the Alexander technique, are frequently successful in the correction and retraining of forward head posture. Faulty joint alignment of the forward head posture is often treated with manipulation or mobilization.

Soft-tissue manipulation

General guidelines The primary focus of massage treatment in a forward head posture is to reduce tension in the shortened muscles so proper alignment can be regained. Superficial posterior cervical muscles, such as the trapezius, splenius capitis, and semispinalis capitis, are shortened in the condition and should be a focus of treatment. In addition, it is important to treat the four small sub-occipital muscles on each side of the spine. These muscles develop myofascial trigger points from their chronic shortened position and are a frequent cause of muscle tension headaches.

Forward head posture originates not only in the cervical muscles, but also in the corresponding pattern of kyphosis that develops in the upper thoracic region. Treatment emphasizes the shortened muscles of the upper anterior torso and posterior cervical region. These hypertonic muscles often develop myofascial trigger points so they can be treated with static compression, deep longitudinal stripping, and eventually with active engagement methods as well. Certain muscles, such as the rhomboids and mid-trapezius that are held in a lengthened position due to this posture, also become painful from fatigue. Similar techniques can be applied to these muscles.

Suggested techniques and methods Soft tissue treatment and rehabilitation protocol considerations for a forward head posture are the same as those described for kyphosis in Chapter 9. In addition, the techniques listed under neuromuscular neck pain at the beginning of this chapter are valuable for treating forward head posture. Two other techniques that are helpful in treating the suboccipital muscles are also included.

A. Static compression on suboccipital muscles The client is in a supine position. To deactivate myofascial trigger points in the posterior cervical and suboccipital muscles, apply static compression with the fingertips or thumb to the posterior cervical and suboccipital region one side at a time (Fig. 10.27). Hold the static compression on these regions until the client reports a decrease in the irritability of the muscle tension (about 5–8 seconds).

B. Static compression with head rotation This technique is a variation of the one described above. It allows for an alternating amount of pressure to the suboccipital muscles. The practitioner is to the side of the client's head. Gently rotate the client's head to the opposite side with one hand. With the other hand place the thumb on the

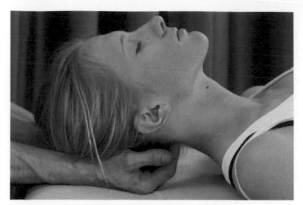

Figure 10.27   Static compression on suboccipital muscles.

suboccipital muscles so that it is pressing up into the muscle tissue just below the occiput. With the hand that is holding the head, gently rotate the head onto the thumb of the other hand, which gradually applies more pressure to the suboccipital muscles (Fig. 10.28). Hold the static compression until there is some sensation of tissue release in the suboccipital muscles or the client reports a reduction in pain sensations.

Cautions and contraindications Forward head posture and kyphosis are related. Some cases of kyphosis are caused by weakness and degeneration in bony structures as in osteoporosis. People often develop their kyphotic posture with age as gravity gradually takes a toll on the upright vertical structure. In either case, especially that of osteoporosis, there can be fragility in the skeletal structures. Use caution when working in these

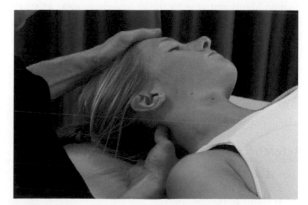

Figure 10.28   Static compression on suboccipital muscles with head turned into thumb.

areas, especially with techniques that use greater pressure, such as the deep stripping or static compression methods.

When treating the suboccipital muscles be cautious of treatment techniques that apply pressure into the suboccipital region bilaterally at the same time. These techniques can potentially produce compression of the vertebral arteries and reduce cranial blood flow (vertebrobasilar insufficiency). A way to avoid the potential of arterial insufficiency is to only treat the suboccipital region on one side of the head at a time. That way there is still an opportunity for normal blood flow on one side.

If there is concern that the client might have adverse arterial compression with treatment, evaluate their susceptibility with the vertebral artery test. With the client in a seated position ask them to look up and over their shoulder so the head is in hyperextension and rotation. Hold that position for about 30 seconds. If the client begins to feel any sensations of dizziness, vertigo, nausea, vision problems, or any other neurological symptoms, they are susceptible to vertebral artery compression, and extra care should be exercised when treating the suboccipital region.

Box 10.3 Case Study

Background

Miriam is a 52-year-old who is in good physical condition. She spends a good deal of her day at the computer doing freelance writing projects for the local magazines and newspaper. Three weeks ago she was in an automobile accident where someone ran a traffic light and hit her on the passenger side of her car. She was not hurt badly in the accident and was able to walk away. However, she did go see a doctor the next day because she was having neck and arm pain. The doctor said there were no fractures or serious joint trauma and most likely her pain was related to soft-tissue injury.

The neck and arm pain has persisted since her injury. She has also been experiencing regular headaches that come on about halfway through her day. She is not able to spend anywhere near as much time at her computer now because the headaches as well as neck and arm discomfort prevent long periods of her writing. She reports that ice applications have been helpful initially with managing the pain.

Questions to consider

- Due to the mechanics of the injury in the automobile accident, what are several different tissues that could have been injured?
- She reported that ice has been helpful in pain management. What are the primary physiological effects of ice applications that are likely to be helping reduce her pain?
- She was hit broadside from the passenger side of her car. Which side of her neck received the initial tensile stress from the immediate force of the collision?
- What are several factors that may help you decide if it is appropriate to treat Miriam with massage?
- What are several questions you would want to ask Miriam in your initial evaluation with her?
- If it turns out that she has a sudden tensile stress injury to the brachial plexus from the collision, is this something that can be treated with massage?

References

1. Mense S, Simons DG. Muscle Pain: Understanding Its Nature, Diagnosis, & Treatment. Baltimore: Lippincott Williams & Wilkins; 2001.
2. Neumann DA. Kinesiology of the Musculoskeletal System. St. Louis: Mosby; 2002.
3. Janda V. Rational therapeutic approach of chronic back pain syndromes. Paper presented at: Chronic back pain, rehabilitation, and self-help, 1985; Turku, Finland.
4. Friedman MH, Weisberg J. The craniocervical connection: a retrospective analysis of 300 whiplash patients with

cervical and temporomandibular disorders. Cranio. 2000;18(3):163–167.

5. Liebenson Ce. Rehabilitation of the Spine. Baltimore: Williams & Wilkins; 1996.

6. Pavlov H, Torg JS, Robie B, Jahre C. Cervical spinal stenosis: determination with vertebral body ratio method. Radiology. 1987;164(3):771–775.

7. Buckwalter JA. Aging and degeneration of the human intervertebral disc. Spine. 1995;20(11):1307–1314.

8. Le Maitre CL, Freemont AJ, Hoyland JA. Accelerated cellular senescence in degenerate intervertebral discs: a possible role in the pathogenesis of intervertebral disc degeneration. Arthritis Res Ther. 2007;9(3):R45.

9. Podichetty VK. The aging spine: the role of inflammatory mediators in intervertebral disc degeneration. Cell Mol Biol (Noisy-le-grand). 2007;53(5):4–18.

10. Boden SD, McCowin PR, Davis DO, Dina TS, Mark AS, Wiesel S. Abnormal magnetic-resonance scans of the cervical spine in asymptomatic subjects. A prospective investigation. J Bone Joint Surg Am. 1990;72(8): 1178–1184.

11. Matsumoto M, Fujimura Y, Suzuki N, et al. MRI of cervical intervertebral discs in asymptomatic subjects. J Bone Joint Surg Br. 1998;80(1):19–24.

12. Magee D. Orthopedic Physical Assessment. 3rd ed. Philadelphia: W.B. Saunders; 1997.

13. Cailliet R. Neck and Arm Pain. Philadelphia: F.A. Davis; 1991.

14. Mendel T, Wink CS, Zimny ML. Neural elements in human cervical intervertebral discs. Spine. 1992; 17(2):132–135.

15. Roberts S, Eisenstein SM, Menage J, Evans EH, Ashton IK. Mechanoreceptors in intervertebral discs. Morphology, distribution, and neuropeptides. Spine. 1995; 20(24):2645–2651.

16. Bogduk N, Windsor M, Inglis A. The innervation of the cervical intervertebral discs. Spine. 1988;13(1):2–8.

17. Bogduk N, Tynan W, Wilson AS. The nerve supply to the human lumbar intervertebral discs. J Anat. 1981; 132(Pt 1):39–56.

18. Matsunaga S, Kabayama S, Yamamoto T, Yone K, Sakou T, Nakanishi K. Strain on intervertebral discs after anterior cervical decompression and fusion. Spine. 1999; 24(7):670–675.

19. Choy DS. Percutaneous laser disc decompression (PLDD): twelve years' experience with 752 procedures in 518 patients. J Clin Laser Med Surg. 1998;16(6):325–331.

20. Simons D, Travell J, Simons L. Myofascial Pain and Dysfunction: The Trigger Point Manual. Vol 1. 2nd ed. Baltimore: Williams & Wilkins; 1999.

21. Sheth RN, Belzberg AJ. Diagnosis and treatment of thoracic outlet syndrome. Neurosurg Clin N Am. 2001; 12(2):295–309.

22. Huang JH, Zager EL. Thoracic outlet syndrome. Neurosurgery. 2004;55(4):897–902; discussion 902–893.

23. Sanders RJ, Hammond SL, Rao NM. Diagnosis of thoracic outlet syndrome. J Vasc Surg. 2007;46(3):601–604.

24. Dawson D, Hallett M, Wilbourn A. Entrapment Neuropathies. 3rd ed. Philadelphia: Lippincott-Raven; 1999.

25. Sucher BM. Thoracic outlet syndrome – a myofascial variant: Part 1. Pathology and diagnosis. J Am Osteopath Assoc. 1990;90(8):686–696, 703–684.

26. Smith TM, Sawyer SF, Sizer PS, Brismee JM. The double crush syndrome: a common occurrence in cyclists with ulnar nerve neuropathy – a case-control study. Clin J Sport Med. 2008;18(1):55–61.

27. Sucher BM. Thoracic outlet syndrome – a myofascial variant: Part 2. Treatment. J Am Osteopath Assoc. 1990;90(9):810–812, 817–823.

28. Baltopoulos P, Tsintzos C, Prionas G, Tsironi M. Exercise-induced scalenus syndrome. Am J Sports Med. 2008; 36(2):369–374.

29. Altobelli GG, Kudo T, Haas BT, Chandra FA, Moy JL, Ahn SS. Thoracic outlet syndrome: pattern of clinical success after operative decompression. J Vasc Surg. 2005;42(1):122–128.

30. Butler D. Mobilisation of the Nervous System. London: Churchill Livingstone; 1991.

31. Shacklock M. Clinical Neurodynamics. Edinburgh:Elsevier; 2005.

32. Kutvonen O, Dastidar P, Nurmikko T. Pain in spasmodic torticollis. Pain. 1997;69(3):279–286.

33. Comella CL, Jankovic J, Brin MF. Use of botulinum toxin type A in the treatment of cervical dystonia. Neurology. 2000;55(12 Suppl 5):S15–21.

34. Smith DL, DeMario MC. Spasmodic torticollis: a case report and review of therapies. J Am Board Fam Pract. 1996;9(6):435–441.

35. Spitzer WO, Skovron ML, Salmi LR, et al. Scientific monograph of the Quebec Task Force on Whiplash-Associated Disorders: redefining "whiplash" and its management. Spine. 1995;20(8 Suppl):1S–73S.

36. Alexander D. Quebec task force on whiplash associated disorders challenged. Journal of Soft Tissue Manipulation. 1998;6(2):2–3.

37. Freeman MD, Croft AC, Rossignol AM. "Whiplash associated disorders: redefining whiplash and its management" by the Quebec Task Force. A critical evaluation. Spine. 1998;23(9):1043–1049.

38. Wallis BJ, Lord SM, Barnsley L, Bogduk N. The psychological profiles of patients with whiplash-associated headache. Cephalalgia. 1998;18(2):101–105; discussion 172–103.

39. Young WF. The enigma of whiplash injury; current management strategies and controversies. Postgrad Med. 2001;109(3):179–186.

40. Petersen-Felix S, Arendt-Nielsen L, Curatolo M. Chronic pain after whiplash injury – evidence for altered central sensory processing. Journal of Whiplash & Related Disorders. 2003;2(1):5–16.

41. Curatolo M, Arendt-Nielsen L, Petersen-Felix S. Evidence, mechanisms, and clinical implications of central hypersensitivity in chronic pain after whiplash injury. Clin J Pain. 2004;20(6):469–476.

42. Mealy K, Brennan H, Fenelon GC. Early mobilization of acute whiplash injuries. Br Med J (Clin Res Ed). 1986; 292(6521):656–657.

43. Gross AR, Goldsmith C, Hoving JL, et al. Conservative management of mechanical neck disorders: a systematic review. J Rheumatol. 2007;34(5):1083–1102.

44. Conlin A, Bhogal S, Sequeira K, Teasell R. Treatment of whiplash-associated disorders – part I: Non-invasive interventions. Pain Res Manag. 2005;10(1):21–32.

45. Schnabel M, Ferrari R, Vassiliou T, Kaluza G. Randomised, controlled outcome study of active mobilisation compared with collar therapy for whiplash injury. Emerg Med J. 2004;21(3):306–310.

46. Chaitow L, DeLany J. Clinical Application of Neuromuscular Techniques. Vol 1. Edinburgh: Churchill Livingstone; 2000.

47. Lord SM, Barnsley L, Wallis BJ, Bogduk N. Chronic cervical zygapophysial joint pain after whiplash. A placebo-controlled prevalence study. Spine. 1996;21(15): 1737–1744; discussion 1744–1735.

Chapter 11

Shoulder

The shoulder has the greatest range of motion of any joint in the body. The shoulder's movement abilities are possible only at the expense of bony stability, requiring the soft tissues to play a more critical role in maintaining joint integrity. This increased responsibility for stabilization places the shoulder at risk for numerous soft-tissue injuries. There are four articulations in the shoulder girdle: the scapulothoracic, sternoclavicular, acromioclavicular, and glenohumeral joints. Disorders involving the glenohumeral articulation are most common. Its range of motion is significant, but it could not function properly without the combined motions at the other three skeletal articulations of the shoulder girdle. The anatomical structure of this area combined with its unique biomechanical demands place a heavy demand on the soft tissues.

Shoulder pain is the third most common musculoskeletal disorder, following low back and cervical spine pain.[1] Acute injuries result from incidents such as blows to the shoulder, falling on an outstretched arm, or forceful movements that dislocate or sublux the joint. Chronic injuries develop from the movement requirements in repetitive upper-extremity activities. Also problematic are activities requiring that the shoulder be held in a position that impinges soft tissues. Shoulder problems and injuries are common in sports, recreation, and assorted occupations.

INJURY CONDITIONS

FROZEN SHOULDER (ADHESIVE CAPSULITIS)

Description

The term frozen shoulder is used to refer to a set of symptoms in the shoulder involving pain and limited motion at the glenohumeral joint and is often used interchangeably with the diagnostic term, adhesive capsulitis. However, adhesive capsulitis refers to a discrete clinical pathology, whereas frozen shoulder refers to a variety of pathologies.[1] The pathologies that may be involved in frozen shoulder include not only adhesive capsulitis, but subacromial bursitis, calcific tendinitis, rotator cuff pathology, and other conditions limiting shoulder motion.[2] More than anything, frozen shoulder describes a functional limitation in range of motion associated with pain and stiffness. In frozen shoulder this limited motion appears directly related to dysfunction of inert tissues such as the glenohumeral joint capsule or coracohumeral ligament.

Adhesive capsulitis involves loss of active and passive motion due to adhesions within the glenohumeral joint capsule.[3] There is a distinction between a stiff and painful shoulder without any capsular involvement (frozen shoulder) and that involving adhesion within the joint capsule (adhesive capsulitis).[4] While the anatomical tissues involved differ between frozen shoulder and adhesive capsulitis, the symptoms, etiology, and clinical characteristics of the pathologies are virtually the same. In this discussion the term frozen shoulder is used unless there is a specific reference to adhesion within the glenohumeral joint capsule, in which the term adhesive capsulitis will be used.

Frozen shoulder is divided into two categories – primary and secondary. In primary frozen shoulder, the problem comes on with no apparent cause. There is some indication that it may be an autoimmune disorder but why the motion limitations develop is still unclear.[1] In a number of cases there seems to be an association between the onset of the condition and serious emotional or psychological trauma, but this connection is controversial.[5] There is a lack of agreement on how to treat the primary frozen shoulder due to the inability to locate its cause.

Secondary frozen shoulder results from another pathology, such as rotator cuff tears, arthritis, bicipital tendinosis or tenosynovitis, surgery, shoulder separation, diabetes, or glenohumeral subluxation.[2,6] The inciting trauma causes problems in the same tissues as primary frozen shoulder, although there is more evidence of capsular adhesion in the secondary variation. In secondary frozen shoulder, scar tissue from the prior trauma causes the axillary folds of the joint capsule to adhere to each other. Some period of shoulder immobilization generally precedes the onset of symptoms.

There are three stages that characterize the progression of frozen shoulder pathology:[6]

- Freezing: the onset may be anywhere from 10 to 36 weeks. There is likely to be pain and a gradual decrease in range of motion.
- Frozen: occurs between 4 and 12 months after the initial onset. Pain is likely to gradually decrease during this time, although motion is likely to remain quite limited.
- Thawing: this is the period characterized by a gradual return of range of motion and decrease in pain. It may be as short as several months, but it is not uncommon for it to last years.

A frequently overlooked cause of secondary adhesive capsulitis is the presence of myofascial trigger points. It appears that trigger point activity in the subscapularis muscle is especially likely to set off the cascade of adhesion in the capsule.[7] The subscapularis muscle appears prone to developing enthesopathy (inflammatory irritation at the attachment site) on the humerus near the joint capsule. The local inflammatory process at the attachment site will often cause fibrous adhesion to develop in the capsule, because the capsule is so close to the tendinous attachment.

One of the primary challenges with adhesive capsulitis is the self-perpetuating nature of the problem. The joint capsule is richly innervated so pain is out of proportion to the amount of tissue damage. As a result, the more it hurts to move the shoulder, the more the person avoids any kind of glenohumeral motion. This pain avoidance causes further problems with increasing limitations to motion. It is well documented that immobility and lack of movement is a primary cause of continued fibrosis.[3] Therefore, even though it hurts, some degree of movement is essential for the individual to improve.

Treatment

Traditional approaches

Traditional treatment for frozen shoulder begins with a conservative approach focusing on increasing range of motion. Gentle protective exercise, such as Codman's pendulum exercises, and regular stretching to improve range of motion are the main components of this approach.[8] Encouraging an increase in range of motion is important but results should not be expected too quickly. If an individual pushes the shoulder too far or too fast, it may tear some of the fibrous adhesion in the capsule and cause further pain avoidance, increase additional fibrous adhesion, and restrict range of motion even further.

Strengthening programs are often used to address frozen shoulder. The theory is that if the surrounding muscles have greater endurance and stamina they can reduce the demand placed on shoulder tissue during various movements. If there is a reduced demand on the shoulder, earlier healing may result. However, overly aggressive strength training methods are likely to make the problem worse by overtaxing the capsule and related structures.[9] Anti-inflammatory oral medications or with intra-articular corticosteroid injections might be used to reduce further inflammation and adhesion in the capsule. However, there is some question as to the long-term effectiveness of these strategies.[10]

When conservative treatment is not successful a more aggressive approach can be tried. Freeing capsular adhesions surgically is one option, but more commonly forced manipulation of the shoulder under anesthesia is tried first. In this procedure the client's shoulder is anesthetized with an injection.

The arm is then forcibly moved into a position that stretches the glenohumeral capsule and breaks the capsular adhesions. The procedure can be effective for immediately increasing the available range of motion. However, it is best reserved for those with a high pain tolerance and strong motivation to exercise and stretch after the treatment. When the anesthesia wears off, the shoulder can be very painful. If not regularly moved, the fibrous adhesion is likely to return.

Soft-tissue manipulation

General guidelines Stretching is a very important part of the treatment process in frozen shoulder. Stretching procedures are aimed at increasing length and pliability in the joint capsule to address the fibrous adhesion in the connective tissues of the joint capsule. Connective tissues, such as the ligamentous tissue that makes up the joint capsule, stretch more effectively when there is a slower rate of stretch tension applied.[11–13] When stretched more rapidly the capsular tissue is more resistant to elongation. Consequently, when stretching capsular tissues in a client with frozen shoulder the practitioner should hold the stretch position for a longer period (20 seconds or more) as opposed to a short duration stretch.

In frozen shoulder fascial connective tissue around the shoulder joint can contribute to the range-of-motion loss and make it more difficult to mobilize and stretch the joint capsule. Myofascial approaches and massage techniques that reduce tension in the surrounding shoulder muscles are particularly helpful. Effleurage, sweeping cross fiber, and even active engagement techniques can be used.

Perform stretching of the deeper capsular structures after improving pliability in the superficial connective tissues with the massage techniques mentioned above. Heating these tissues prior to stretching is helpful as it increases tissue extensibility. Topical heating modalities, such as moist heat Hydrocollator packs are valuable to warm the superficial shoulder tissues. However, these topical applications are not able to increase temperature in the joint capsule due to the joint's depth. A deep heating method, such as ultrasound, is sometimes used to increase heat for improved extensibility in the capsular tissues.

One of the most important factors in the treatment of adhesive capsulitis is the positive support given to the client during treatment. This condition can persist for months and seriously affect an individual's ability to perform many upper-extremity movements. It is easy for the client to become depressed as a result of the prolonged pain and limited motion. Encouraging the client about even the smallest increments of progress in regaining range of motion is beneficial. A goniometer is a helpful way of quantifying small range-of-motion improvements and that information can be shared with the client. Quantifiable evidence of improvement helps the client keep a positive attitude and stay motivated for treatment.

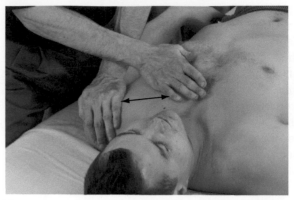

Figure 11.1 Myofascial stretching to anterior shoulder girdle muscles.

Suggested techniques and methods Some of the techniques described for treatment of frozen shoulder involve movement of the affected glenohumeral joint. Any glenohumeral joint movement should be performed carefully and well within the client's pain tolerance. The pain from capsular adhesion in frozen shoulder is significant and reactive muscle splinting or capsular irritation can further impair efforts to gain extensibility in the capsule.

A. Myofascial release of shoulder region Limited motion in the shoulder region from capsular restriction can cause prolonged shortening of fascial tissues. This shortening contributes to further mobility restrictions. Fascial techniques are applied in multiple planes to provide the greatest mobility enhancement. The primary goal is to place a moderately light tangential (tensile) force on the subcutaneous fascia. Pulling the fascia in multiple directions enhances its pliability the most. Place the hands lightly on the client's shoulder region where the myofascial stretch is to be applied. Pull the hands apart to take the slack out of the tissue and apply a light degree of tensile (pulling) force between the hands (Fig. 11.1). Once there is a slight degree of pull between the hands, hold this position until a subtle sensation of tissue release is felt. Apply these myofascial techniques in the anterior as well as posterior shoulder girdle regions.

B. Sweeping cross fiber to anterior chest muscles Treatments aimed at the anterior chest muscles reduce limited motion in the shoulder so joint capsule stretching has the best opportunity to succeed. This technique reduces tension in superficial fibers of the pectoralis major and anterior deltoid. Stand facing the client's feet with the fingers anchored in the client's axilla. Use the thumb to perform sweeping cross fiber movements on the pectoralis major (Fig. 11.2). During the sweeping motion, the pectoralis major is sifted between the fingers. Similar sweeping cross fiber techniques can be applied to the anterior deltoid while facing in the same position (toward the client's feet).

C. Static compression for anterior chest muscles Apply static compression to areas of tension in the pectoralis major found during effleurage and sweeping cross fiber techniques. Trigger points or areas of muscle hypertonicity are treated with both broad and small contact surface static compression

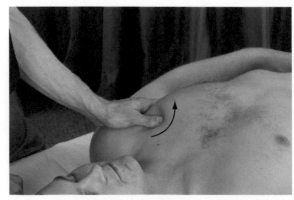

Figure 11.2 Sweeping cross fiber to anterior shoulder muscles.

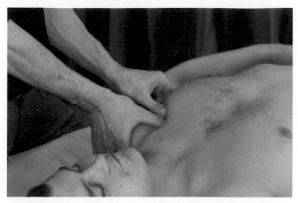

Figure 11.3 Static compression to anterior shoulder muscles.

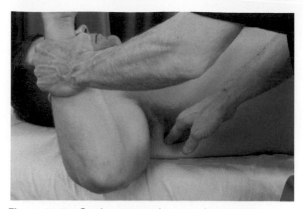

Figure 11.5 Static compression to subscapularis.

methods (Fig. 11.3). Hold pressure on trigger points or areas of muscle tightness for about 5–8 seconds, or until you feel the tissue release.

D. Deep stripping on pectoralis major Use the thumbs, finger tips, or pressure tool to perform deep stripping techniques to the pectoralis major. Treatment can move from medial to lateral or lateral to medial (Fig. 11.4). Variations on this technique, such as pin and stretch, can also be used especially in the later stages of frozen shoulder when mobility has been improved.

E. Static compression on subscapularis The subscapularis is a very important muscle in frozen shoulder treatment because its attachment site is close to the joint capsule and irritation of the attachment site (enthesitis) can contribute to capsular adhesion. Address hypertonicity and myofascial trigger points in subscapularis with static

compression methods. The client is in a supine position. Hold the client's arm slightly away from their body. Use the finger tips of the other hand to apply static compression to the subscapularis muscle (Fig. 11.5). A variation on this technique is to have the client then perform small active medial and lateral rotation movements while pressure is maintained on the muscle.

F. Capsular stretching Stretching of all the shoulder tissues is valuable, but stretching of the joint capsule is particular important. In the capsular pattern of the shoulder, the greatest motion limitation is in lateral rotation first, abduction second, and medial rotation third. Capsular stretching should focus on all of these motions, starting with lateral rotation, then moving to abduction, finally medial rotation. When performing capsular stretching slowly bring the client's shoulder into a position that is just short of the stretch position that causes pain (Fig. 11.6). Hold that stretch position for 20–30 seconds and then gradually come back out of the stretch. This process should be repeated several times. Holding the stretch position longer is valuable because the viscoelastic properties of capsular connective tissue are such that a slower and longer duration stretch does a better job of enhancing pliability in the capsule.

Rehabilitation protocol considerations

- It is crucial to identify the stage of the client's frozen shoulder condition (freezing, frozen, thawing, etc.). If treatment is attempted during

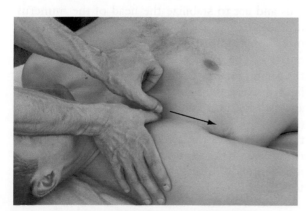

Figure 11.4 Deep stripping to pectoralis major.

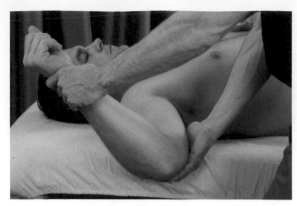

Figure 11.6 Capsular stretching.

the freezing stage, it may not seem to be immediately effective, but it may reduce further joint restriction and capsular adhesion.

- In the later stages of the condition (the thawing stage) more active treatment techniques, such as active engagement and pin and stretch, can be used. Mobility gains may appear more rapid at this time as well.

- Strongly encourage the client with any measurable progress in regaining shoulder motion and note that motion improvement is likely to be slow.

- Consider use of heat modalities prior to or in conjunction with massage treatment methods.

- The client's ability to relax and improve through soft-tissue treatment is directly related to the trust they place in the practitioner. A sense of confidence, compassion, and understanding for the nature of this sometimes intense chronic pain condition will help the client.

Cautions and contraindications Range-of-motion techniques and stretching, while helpful, can also perpetuate the condition or make it worse. Be conservative in the way stretching and range-of-motion techniques are applied. Even though progress may not be as fast, there is less chance of tearing the capsular tissues and causing the condition to worsen. Particular attention should be paid to the client's pain levels with various motions.

ROTATOR CUFF STRAIN

Description

The term rotator cuff tear is common, but it can be an incomplete description of the client's pathology. There are four rotator cuff muscles; any of these four muscles can be involved in the injury. It is rare for all four to sustain a tear at the same time. More than likely it is one or two of these muscles that are involved in a particular shoulder injury. Accurate assessment is essential to determine which of the muscles is involved.

The rotator cuff is composed of the supraspinatus, infraspinatus, teres minor, and subscapularis muscles and their associated tendons. The four tendons form a cuff around the head of the humerus and act to stabilize the head of the humerus in the glenoid fossa. The supraspinatus is the most commonly strained of the four rotator cuff muscles. There are several reasons why injury to the supraspinatus is more common. Due to the limited space, the supraspinatus can be compressed against the underside of the acromion process (Fig. 11.7).[14,15] The repeated compression against the underside of the acromion process contributes to tissue degeneration in the supraspinatus muscle/tendon unit, and eventually leads to fiber tearing.

Another factor that leads to supraspinatus dysfunction is that there is an area of decreased

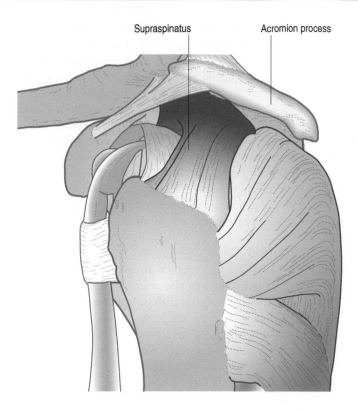

Supraspinatus   Acromion process

Figure 11.7 Lateral view of the left shoulder showing the small space under the acromion process.

vascularity near the insertion site of the supraspinatus tendon.[16] The decrease in vascularity means there is slower healing time for any tissue trauma in the area. In addition to strains, decreased vascularity of this tendon region also contributes to tendinosis, which may precede muscle tearing. Progressive degradation of fibers of the supraspinatus muscle and tendon may lead to calcific tendinitis in the area as well.[17,18] Calcific tendinitis is a deposition of calcium into the tendon tissue most commonly experienced at the supraspinatus tendon.

Rotator cuff tears typically occur as a result of progressive muscle and tendon degeneration over time. Many of these tears are only partial thickness tears where the tendon is not torn all the way through. A more serious injury is a full-thickness tear of the tendon, which is more likely to happen when the load on the tendon is much greater. Acute injuries that involve high force loads to the rotator cuff muscles produce more serious damage like a full-thickness tear.

The infraspinatus and teres minor muscles can also contribute to rotator cuff tendinosis or strain.

However, the mechanism of injury to these muscles is somewhat different. These muscles both play a fundamental role in concentric lateral rotation movements and eccentric medial rotation movements in the shoulder. Injuries to the posterior rotator cuff muscles are common in throwing motions. During the follow-through phase of a throwing motion, the posterior rotator cuff muscles (infraspinatus and teres minor) are the muscles primarily responsible for slowing or decelerating the motion of the arm. Very strong forces are required to slow the arm's momentum in a throwing motion. If these muscles are not equipped for the force demands placed on them, tendinosis and then eventually fiber tearing can result. Fatigue of these muscles accelerates this degenerative process, so strength training and conditioning is a great preventive strategy.

The subscapularis is rarely strained. It is protected from strains because there are several larger muscles that perform the same actions and give mechanical support to the subscapularis. These muscles, such as the pectoralis major, latissimus dorsi, and teres major, are significantly stronger than the subscapularis and assist it significantly. However, subscapularis tears do occur, and often they accompany a more serious injury, such as a glenohumeral dislocation. There appears to be a greater incidence of subscapularis tearing with dislocations in patients who are over 40.[19,20]

Other shoulder pathologies frequently accompany rotator cuff dysfunction. The pain from rotator cuff disorders can create reflex muscular inhibition, which interferes with biomechanical balance around the joint, and can lead to limitations in range of motion. Sometimes it can be difficult to determine if the pain and limitation in range of motion is specifically from a tear or from the reflexive muscular inhibition that results.

Treatment

Traditional approaches

Physical therapy is a common approach for rotator cuff strains, and includes stretching, preventive strength training, and use of modalities such as ultrasound to facilitate healing of the damaged tissues. As with similar conditions, strength training can be a valuable part of the rehabilitation process, but it should not be undertaken too soon as repeated use of damaged muscles may exacerbate the problem.

If conservative treatment is not successful, injection therapy or surgery may be the next course of treatment. Injection of corticosteroids into the subacromial region may be performed to reduce inflammatory activity. There have been numerous reports of tendon weakness and rupture as a result of corticosteroid injection directly into tendons.[21–24] Complications of corticosteroid injection may be prevented if the injection is not given directly into the tendon. Complications are also reduced if the therapy is given at least 3 months apart with no more than two injections and resisted exercise is avoided for at least 1 week after the injection.[25]

Surgical procedures are used if conservative treatment or injection therapy has not had beneficial results. Most rotator cuff surgeries are for treating supraspinatus tears. A common surgery is a subacromial decompression, in which the surgeon increases space between the acromion process and humeral head by shaving off the underside of the acromion. Creating greater subacromial space decreases the likelihood of further supraspinatus fiber degeneration from compression in the area. This surgery is performed as either an open procedure with a larger incision, or as an arthroscopic surgery, which usually has a faster recovery period and less damage to surrounding soft tissues. If there is a full-thickness tear in the muscle–tendon unit, surgical repair is a bit more complicated. A procedure to stitch the tear site is necessary. Appropriate rehabilitation following the surgery is essential in order to gain the best results from any of these procedures.

Soft-tissue manipulation

General guidelines Once proper assessment has determined which of the rotator cuff muscles are at fault, soft-tissue treatment can focus on those particular tissues. As with any muscle strain, treatments are most effective when combined with a cessation or rest from offending activities. Because of the extensive upper-extremity movement in daily activities, it can be challenging for the client to halt or decrease certain offending activities. When treating a rotator cuff tear or tendinosis, it is valuable to treat all the muscles of the shoulder region to help achieve proper biomechanical balance.

If the supraspinatus is the primary problem, treatment with massage is more difficult. Tears are often located near the musculotendinous junction, which is largely inaccessible to palpation because it is underneath the acromion process. There are, however, other ways to treat strains in the supraspinatus. In a supraspinatus tear, there is likely compensating tightness or dysfunction in other soft tissues of the shoulder that should be addressed.

Massage is effective in treating tears or tendinosis in the posterior rotator cuff muscles because these muscles are superficial and easily accessible. Treat the entire shoulder complex to address compensating biomechanical imbalances. Stretching the rotator cuff group and surrounding muscles is also an essential part of the rehabilitative process.

Subscapularis tears are rare, but when present are difficult to treat because the large majority of the subscapularis muscle is inaccessible with palpation. However, the distal musculotendinous junction, where tears typically occur, is accessible to massage treatment. The subscapularis is treated effectively with friction and static compression techniques to the muscle belly.

Suggested techniques and methods
Treatments aimed at supraspinatus and subacromial region

A. Deep stripping to proximal fibers of the supraspinatus Reducing muscle tension on the tear site is crucial for proper tissue healing. Stripping techniques on the supraspinatus reduce pull on the region of torn fibers. The client is in a prone position. Place the thumb or fingertip anterior to the trapezius and on the proximal fibers of the supraspinatus near the vertebral border of the supraspinous fossa. Perform a slow deep stripping technique on the supraspinatus muscle to encourage tissue lengthening and reduction of muscle tightness (Fig. 11.8). This technique can be performed with the client in other positions if those are more comfortable.

B. Deep stripping to the deltoid muscle Hypertonicity in the deltoid can pull the humeral head in a more superior direction and decrease subacromial space. Perform deep stripping techniques on the anterior, middle, and posterior deltoid to help decrease muscle tightness that might contribute to lifting the humerus superiorly in the glenoid fossa and further compressing the supraspinatus tendon (Fig. 11.9).

C. Deep friction to the supraspinatus tendon insertion In some cases, the supraspinatus tear site is closer to the musculotendinous junction. In those cases, the site of injury can be treated with

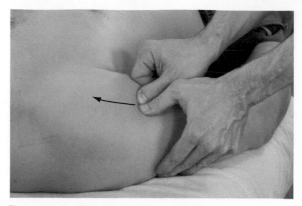

Figure 11.9   Deep stripping on deltoid.

deep friction just lateral and inferior to the acromion process near the supraspinatus insertion on the humerus. Deep friction can stimulate fibroblast activity in the damaged tendon fibers and thereby contribute to a faster recovery rate. Locate the lateral edge of the acromion process of the scapula. With the thumb or finger tip, apply deep friction treatments to the distal supraspinatus tendon (Fig. 11.10). Stretching and joint range-of-motion techniques should be used after the friction treatment.

Treatments aimed at posterior rotator cuff muscles

D. Static compression on infraspinatus and teres minor This technique is used to reduce tension on damaged muscle or tendon fibers. Apply static compression with a finger tip, thumb, or pressure tool to areas of increased tension in the muscles (Fig. 11.11). When applying pressure to the infraspinatus, keep in mind there is a flat bone

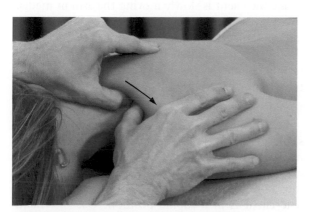

Figure 11.8   Deep stripping on supraspinatus.

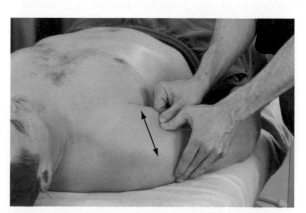

Figure 11.10   Deep friction to distal supraspinatus tendon.

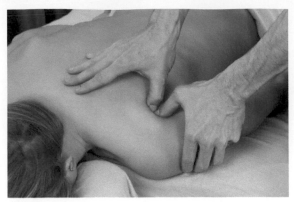

Figure 11.11   Static compression on infraspinatus and teres minor.

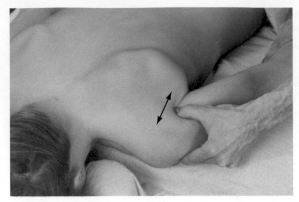

Figure 11.13   Deep friction to posterior rotator cuff tendons.

underneath the muscle so pressure does not have to be strong to generate discomfort from muscle tension. When treating the teres minor, the muscle is not being pressed against a flat underlying bone, so the client can usually tolerate a slightly greater pressure level.

E. Deep stripping on infraspinatus and teres minor With the thumb or fingertips, apply a deep longitudinal stripping technique from the proximal to distal fibers of the infraspinatus and teres minor (Fig. 11.12). Continue the stripping technique several times until all the fibers of the infraspinatus and teres minor have been treated. This technique can also be performed in a distal to proximal direction if the practitioner finds that hand position more comfortable.

F. Deep friction to posterior rotator cuff region Apply deep friction to the region of primary tenderness in the posterior rotator cuff tendons

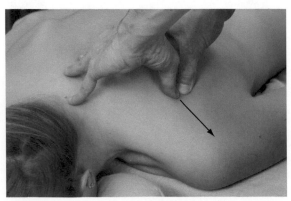

Figure 11.12   Deep stripping on infraspinatus and teres minor.

(Fig. 11.13). This region of tenderness is likely the site of tissue tearing or dysfunction. Friction can be either longitudinal or transverse. It is helpful to include stretching and other techniques such as the active engagement methods mentioned below along with the friction treatment to encourage tissue pliability.

G. Active engagement lengthening to posterior rotator cuff muscles This technique is particularly helpful for encouraging tissue lengthening on the posterior rotator cuff tendons. It is best used in the later stages of rehabilitation or when a posterior rotator cuff injury is not severe. The client is in a prone position with the shoulder abducted to about 90° and laterally rotated as far as possible. Holding the arm in the laterally rotated position engages the lateral rotator muscles isometrically. Instruct the client to slowly drop the forearm and hand toward the floor, which causes an eccentric medial rotation. While the client is slowly moving the arm in medial rotation, perform a deep stripping technique on the infraspinatus and teres minor muscles (like that described in E above) (Fig 11.14). Perform this technique several times until the infraspinatus and teres minor have been adequately treated.

Treatments aimed at subscapularis

H. Static compression on subscapularis The subscapularis is not strained very often and the muscle is difficult to access with palpation. Static compression is used to reduce tension in the muscle to aid in healing fiber tearing or disruption. The client is in a supine position. Use one hand to hold the client's arm slightly away from their body. Use the finger tips of the other hand to

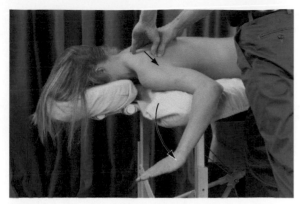

Figure 11.14   Active engagement lengthening with stripping to posterior rotator cuff tendons.

apply static compression to the subscapularis muscle (Fig. 11.5). A variation on this technique is to have the client then perform small active medial and lateral rotation movements while pressure is maintained on the muscle.

I. Deep friction on distal subscapularis Deep friction techniques can be applied to the distal fibers of the subscapularis and its musculotendinous junction, which is a likely site of a tissue tear. The client is in a supine position. Use one hand to hold the client's arm slightly away from their body. Use the finger tips of the other hand to apply deep friction to the distal subscapularis. This technique can also be performed with the thumb instead of the finger tips (Fig. 11.15).

Rehabilitation Protocol Considerations

- Determine the severity of any rotator cuff tendinosis or tear and the primary site of tissue damage prior to engaging in treatment. Do not be vigorous with deep friction techniques if a strain is recent or severe.

- Techniques involving active engagement during treatment should be reserved for the later stages of the rehabilitation process when the client is making progress; start with less intense techniques first.

- Stretching, joint range-of-motion techniques, and activity modifications should be a crucial component of a treatment plan. Stress on the damaged tissues must be reduced in order for soft-tissue treatment strategies to work.

- Inflammation might be present in some rotator cuff strain injuries, especially if they are acute. Topical thermal applications are not particularly helpful for supraspinatus or subscapularis injuries due to the depth of tissues, but effective for posterior rotator cuff disorders.

Cautions and contraindications   Rotator cuff tears can easily masquerade as other shoulder injuries, so accurate assessment of the condition is essential. The practitioner should have a thorough knowledge of the actions of the four rotator cuff muscles. They should be able to discern when the muscles are contracting or stretching during various shoulder movements and assess which is involved in the client's present condition. It is also crucial to determine the severity of the injury as certain massage techniques would not be appropriate at particular stages of the rehabilitation process depending on the severity of tissue injury.

If the client is being treated with other methods such as physical therapy or corticosteroid injections, communicate with the other practitioners about the treatment methods you are using to ensure they work well together. If surgery has been performed for a rotator cuff tear, it is important to wait an appropriate level of time prior to administering any deep soft-tissue therapy in the area. The surgeon should be able to give advice about the appropriate length of time to wait prior to soft-tissue treatment.

SHOULDER IMPINGEMENT

Description

Shoulder impingement involves compression of several different soft-tissue structures underneath

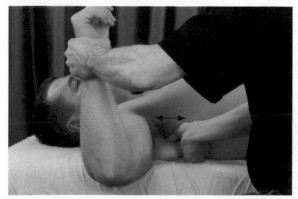

Figure 11.15   Deep friction to subscapularis (performed with thumb while other hand holds up the client's arm).

Figure 11.16   Anterior–lateral view of the shoulder showing the coracoacromial arch.

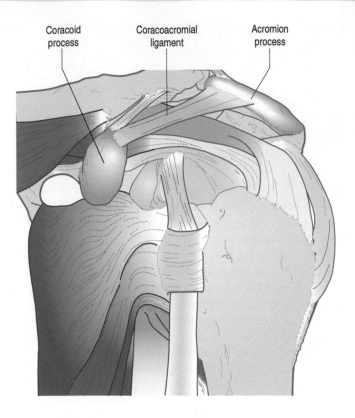

Coracoid process

Coracoacromial ligament

Acromion process

the coracoacromial arch. The acromion process, the coracoacromial ligament, and the coracoid process of the scapula create the coracoacromial arch (Fig. 11.16). Tissues susceptible to compression underneath the arch include the supraspinatus muscle or tendon, subacromial bursa, upper region of the glenohumeral joint capsule, coracohumeral ligament, and the tendon from the long head of the biceps brachii.

There are two types of shoulder impingement: primary impingement and secondary impingement. Primary impingement is characterized by a decrease in subacromial space that is the result of anatomical variations that the individual is borne with. For example, the underside of the acromion process may be flat instead of curved. This does not leave much space underneath the arch and may lead to impingement.[26] If the acromion process were tilted down at an angle instead of being more horizontal, that would also decrease the subacromial space and be a cause of primary impingement. Osteophytes or bone spurs on the underside

of the acromion may also be considered a cause of primary impingement.[27]

Secondary impingement is also called acquired impingement. This type of shoulder impingement is most commonly the result of specific activities that cause compression of the subacromial tissues. For example, repeated overhead motions associated with certain swimming strokes are a frequent cause of secondary impingement. Other biomechanical or physiological factors may also lead to secondary impingement. Decreased vascularity near the supraspinatus tendon insertion may cause additional damage to these tissues when they are compressed against the acromion process.[3] Instability in the shoulder, often the result of a glenohumeral dislocation, can make the head of the humerus hit the underside of the acromion process more easily.[25] As the humerus head hits the underside of the acromion process, soft tissues are likely to be compressed causing a secondary impingent.

Shoulder impingement can occur in several stages. Neer describes three stages of impingement:[28]

1. Inflammation edema and hemorrhage – reversible with conservative treatment;
2. Fibrosis and cuff tendinitis – may be treated with conservative treatment;
3. Bony changes (spurs) – usually requires surgical intervention for tears in the rotator cuff muscles (specifically the supraspinatus).

There is often a vicious cycle of degeneration that occurs with secondary impingement. As the shoulder muscles are further impacted by the compression under the coracoacromial arch, they are much less effective at centering the humeral head in the glenoid fossa. Their inability to keep the humeral head in the glenoid fossa is a further cause of impingement during various motions.[29]

Treatment

Traditional approaches

Strengthening the associated muscles around the rotator cuff is a primary focus of early conservative treatment. This is especially true for problems of secondary impingement as opposed to primary impingement. Improper mechanical function and fatigue of certain muscles contributes to impingement. Therefore, strengthening of those affected muscles is valuable for treatment. However, care should be taken when starting a strengthening program to make sure that the exercises do not further aggravate the condition.

Oral anti-inflammatory medication or subacromial corticosteroid injections are also commonly used to address the inflammatory components of the problem. However, anti-inflammatory medication alone will not address the biomechanical dysfunction that is causing the impingement to begin with. It is most helpful if anti-inflammatory medication is used in conjunction with some other methods that address the mechanical components of the impingement. There are concerns about injecting corticosteroids into the connective tissues in this region because of long-term detrimental effects.

When conservative treatments are not effective with impingement problems, surgery is an option. As with the rotator cuff disorders discussed above, increasing space underneath the acromion process is the prime function of surgical approaches,

acromioplasty is a common procedure. In this procedure, the surgeon will shave off the underside of the acromion process to either reshape it or to remove bone spurs that may be compressing soft-tissue structures.

Soft-tissue manipulation

General guidelines   The effectiveness of massage interventions is directly related to how early intervention occurs in the impingement process and how severe the tissue degeneration is. Due to the anatomy and mechanics of subacromial impingement, treating this condition poses similar problems for the soft-tissue therapist as treating supraspinatus rotator cuff disorders.

Attention is focused on those tissues that may be contributing to the impingement. For example, tightness in the deltoid muscle can contribute to pulling the humeral head higher in the glenoid fossa, especially if the individual has some degree of capsular laxity. As a result, impingement problems with overhead motions of the shoulder are more likely to occur. Decreasing tightness in the deltoid muscle can reduce the impingement. It is also important to address problems with other muscles that are essential for glenohumeral mechanics as their dysfunction can play a role in the impingement problems. For example, weakness or dysfunction in the serratus anterior can decrease the amount of upward scapular rotation during shoulder abduction, leading to an increased risk of subacromial impingement.[14]

Although contributions of the subscapularis to shoulder impingement are rarely mentioned in the orthopedic literature there is evidence that the subscapularis may play a role in certain impingement problems. Myofascial treatment of the subscapularis muscle was found to be an effective aspect of treating shoulder impingement problems.[30] Static compression and other similar techniques described in the rotator cuff disorders section above are a valuable part of the treatment approach for impingement problems. If the tendon from the long head of the biceps brachii is the primary tissue being compressed under the coracoacromial arch, it should be treated to reduce the possibility of tendinosis or tenosynovitis that may develop because of the compression.

Suggested techniques and methods   Treatment approaches and rehabilitation protocol considerations for shoulder impingement are the same as those described in the section above on rotator cuff disorders (especially the section on supraspinatus tears). If the biceps brachii is the primary tissue involved in the impingement, treatment techniques and rehabilitation protocol considerations are the same as those described in the section on biceps tendinosis later in this chapter.

Cautions and contraindications   Use caution with pressure applied in various treatment techniques around the subacromial region with shoulder impingement. Generally, the damaged tissues are under the acromion process and not directly palpable. However, some tissues are more palpable than others. The tendon of the long head of the biceps brachii is easily accessible on the anterior region of the shoulder when it is in a neutral position. Impingement of this tendon does not occur until near the end of forward flexion. The subacromial bursa might be inflamed from impingement and it covers a large section of the humeral head. If the subacromial bursa is inflamed, direct compression techniques over the bursa are discouraged.

Box 11.2   Clinical Tip

In many cases of shoulder impingement or rotator cuff tendinosis/tears, the specific tissue that is at fault is not identified. Not knowing exactly which tissue is involved makes accurate treatment more challenging. In most cases treating these disorders with a broad spectrum of approaches is advised to be sure the primary tissue has been addressed. Additional treatment techniques are often not contraindicated. In fact, the additional treatment methods help achieve biomechanical balance. However, in some cases there are precautions to consider before embarking on a broad encompassing approach. For example in a distal supraspinatus tear or tendinosis, an ideal treatment technique would be deep friction to the affected tendon. If the subacromial bursa is involved in the same condition and inflamed, the friction treatment to the supraspinatus could be detrimental and aggravate the inflamed bursa.

SUBACROMIAL BURSITIS

Description

Bursitis in the shoulder is a common orthopedic diagnosis. Some consider it a 'wastebasket diagnosis', meaning it is used more out of convenience than for accurately labeling a condition of true inflammation in the bursa. Yet, this is a problem that can occur with frequency from excess compression underneath the acromion process, so it should be accurately evaluated.

The primary function of any bursa is to reduce friction between adjacent anatomical structures. The subacromial bursa sits on top of the supraspinatus tendon and is designed to reduce friction between the supraspinatus tendon and the overlying acromion process of the scapula (Fig. 11.17). While the bursa is very thin, it does cover a substantial portion of the humeral head underneath the deltoid muscle. The region of the bursa that extends beyond the acromion process is sometimes called the subdeltoid bursa. In some individuals, there is a division between the subacromial and subdeltoid portions of this bursa.

Subacromial bursitis results from the same mechanical factors that cause shoulder impingement problems – repetitive compression of the tissue underneath the coracoacromial arch. The pain of subacromial bursitis can be identical to that of impingement, but other factors in the assessment process help distinguish bursitis from compression of other tissues. The bursa can also be involved with other conditions involving the supraspinatus, because the inferior layer of the bursa is contiguous with the superior layer of the fascia of the supraspinatus.[31]

Bursitis is most commonly caused by repetitive compression, but there may be other causes as well. Autoimmune diseases, crystal deposition, infection, or hemorrhage may also cause an inflammatory reaction in the bursa.[32] The symptoms of these different causes can be identical, so consider these other causes of shoulder pain, especially in the absence of any clear repetitive compression pathology.

Treatment

Traditional approaches

Anti-inflammatory treatment is a mainstay for treatment of subacromial bursitis. It is important

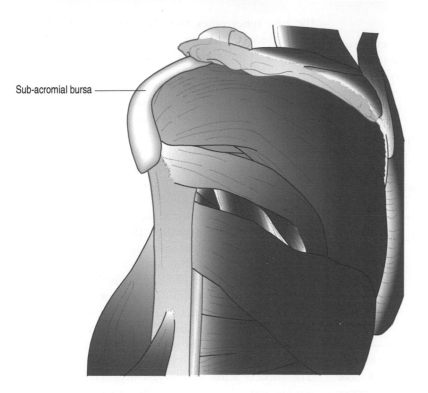

Sub-acromial bursa

Figure 11.17   Posterior–lateral view of the shoulder showing the subacromial bursa.

to identify the factor(s) responsible for the bursa inflammation and address them as well whether that is mechanical compression or systemic dysfunction. Cryotherapy is used to address inflammatory problems. However, ice applications may have limited effectiveness because of the poor penetration depth of thermal modalities in this region. Penetration depth of thermal modalities is limited because the acromion process is between the cold application and the subacromial bursa.

Other anti-inflammatory measures are used more often because of limited effectiveness with cryotherapy. Oral NSAIDs are commonly used to treat this problem. There may be detrimental long-term effects of their use, however.[33] NSAIDs also have a range of adverse side effects. For example, gastrointestinal disturbances are reported from long-term use of NSAIDs.[34–37]

Corticosteroid injections are sometimes used an alternative to oral anti-inflammatory medications. These injections are helpful for reducing inflammation in the bursa. However, there are significant concerns about the long-term use of corticosteroid injections because of their detrimental effect on soft tissues. NSAIDs or corticosteroid injections are not used to heal these injuries but instead are used to reduce symptoms so that clients can engage in rehabilitation activities more fully. Recommendations are no more than three corticosteroid injections in a 12-month period, and these are best spaced at least 30 days apart.[32]

Rotator cuff strengthening programs are used to normalize biomechanical balance in the shoulder girdle. Strengthening exercises should not be performed to the point that there is any aggravation of the pain. Continual exertion that makes the pain worse can exacerbate the problem.

Heat treatment is not an approach that would usually be indicated for an inflammatory condition like bursitis. However, heat application may reduce associated tension in the surrounding shoulder muscles. A local heat application does not appear to aggravate the inflamed bursa in some cases because the heat cannot penetrate the acromion process in order to have an effect on the subacromial bursa.

Soft-tissue manipulation

The bursa becomes aggravated from excessive friction or pressure, so massage treatment on the bursa is contraindicated. The primary goal of the soft-tissue practitioner is reducing any causative factors that might have led to compression of the bursa. For example, muscle tension in surrounding shoulder muscles could be one causative factor in the condition, so treatment of these muscles is beneficial. Any of the massage treatment techniques for the shoulder can be used to address muscle imbalance that may be contributing to the subacromial bursitis. No treatments should be used that aggravate the symptoms from the inflamed bursa.

BICIPITAL TENDINOSIS

Description

Bicipital tendinosis is a condition affecting the tendon from the long head of the biceps brachii. The tendon from the long head travels along the anterior aspect of the arm and between the greater and lesser tuberosities of the humerus (Fig. 11.18). A synovial sheath surrounds the tendon as it passes between the two tuberosities and the tendon is stabilized in the bicipital groove by the transverse humeral ligament. The tendon eventually courses through the glenohumeral joint capsule before attaching to the glenoid labrum and the superior aspect of the glenoid fossa on the supraglenoid tubercle.

As mentioned previously, the common overuse tendon pathologies are now more appropriately called tendinosis rather than tendinitis because they are rarely inflammatory conditions, though tendinitis is still frequently used.[38] A typical symptom with bicipital tendinosis is anterior shoulder pain that is worse during forward flexion of the shoulder. In this position, the tendon can be squeezed under the coracoacromial arch. The pain will usually decrease with rest.

The primary cause of irritation is friction of the tendon in the bicipital groove or underneath the coracoacromial arch. This usually occurs from repeated movements involving shoulder flexion or forearm supination. In some cases friction may be increased because the groove is particularly narrow.[39] The friction leads to collagen degeneration in the tendon and subsequent pain. Because of the synovial sheath surrounding the tendon, tenosynovitis could also be the cause of pain from bicipital tendon overuse.

Figure 11.18 Anterior–lateral view of the shoulder showing the tendon from the long head of the biceps brachii.

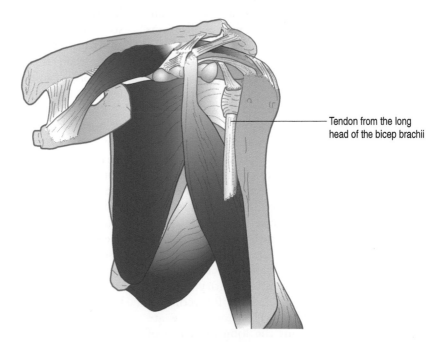

Tendon from the long head of the bicep brachii

If the transverse humeral ligament is not sufficient to keep the tendon in its groove, the tendon may sublux out of the groove in certain shoulder motions. The tendon could also sublux or dislocate because the tuberosities are smaller than normal and cannot hold the tendon as easily within the groove.[40,41] Repeated friction across the tuberosities as the tendon moves in and out of the groove can cause tendinosis.[42]

Treatment

Traditional approaches

Anti-inflammatory medications remain a mainstay of treatment for bicipital tendinosis. However, the effectiveness of this approach is questionable because in many cases this is not an inflammatory condition. Restoring proper flexibility and biomechanical balance around the region will be of prime importance. Stretching exercises are recommended to increase flexibility. It is also essential that any offending activities be reduced or eliminated.

The biceps brachii has three primary actions: shoulder flexion, elbow flexion, and forearm supination. Therefore, repetitive motions in any of these directions could cause an excess amount of tendon irritation. Any strength training activities undertaken during the early rehabilitative phase should avoid excessive use of those motions for that reason.

Use of thermal treatments is advocated by various sources, but they appear only moderately effective. Cold applications are used to reduce inflammatory reaction in the tissues. However, the lack of inflammation in most cases of bicipital tendinosis decreases the need for cold therapy. The greater benefit of cold applications is their use for pain reduction.

Heat applications that would normally be contraindicated for an inflammatory condition can be used effectively for this condition. Heat reduces overall muscular hypertonicity and decreases pain as well. Keep in mind that a true inflammatory tendinitis can exist. If it does, heat applications are not advised. Khan et al provides a comparison of tendinosis and tendinitis which is useful for determining if a true inflammatory condition exists.[43]

Soft-tissue manipulation

General guidelines Massage treatment for bicipital tendinosis focuses on the primary tissue pathology (tendon degeneration), as well as the various contributing musculoskeletal factors such as overuse of the shoulder muscles. There are several goals of treatment. Tendinosis results from excess tension on the tendon; an important goal is to reduce tension on the biceps brachii, which is pulling on the tendon. A variety of massage techniques such as sweeping cross fiber, deep longitudinal friction, and active engagement methods are used to treat the biceps brachii tension. It is also crucial to address the collagen degeneration in the bicipital tendon. Deep friction is used to encourage fibroblast proliferation and encourage collagen synthesis to heal the damaged tendon structure.[44,45]

Treatment of bicipital tendinosis with friction massage is usually applied in a medial–lateral direction. However, if the client has a bicipital groove that is narrow, deep friction administered in a medial–lateral direction could catch the edge of the tendon and cause subluxation of the tendon out of the bicipital groove. This is a situation where a longitudinal friction technique is most beneficial.

Suggested techniques and methods

A. Sweeping cross fiber to biceps brachii Tension reduction in the biceps brachii reduces tension on the bicipital tendon. Apply sweeping cross fiber techniques to the biceps brachii (Fig. 11.19). This technique can be performed with the client's elbow flexed, which keeps the biceps in a shortened position and more pliable.

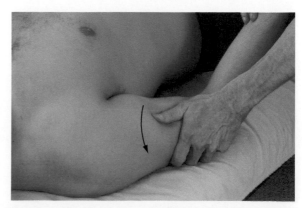

Figure 11.19   Sweeping cross fiber to the biceps brachii.

However, greater muscle tension reduction and fiber spreading is accomplished by applying the sweeping cross fiber technique with the elbow extended so the muscle is in a lengthened position.

B. Deep longitudinal stripping to biceps brachii This technique is an effective means to increase pliability and reduce tension in the biceps brachii. It is most effective when performed after initial therapy begins to increase tissue pliability. With the client's elbow extended, apply deep longitudinal stripping techniques to the biceps brachii working from its distal attachment toward the proximal end. A broad application of pressure can be used initially for more general work. Use a small contact surface of pressure application, such as the thumb or finger tip, to specifically treat the biceps (Fig. 11.20). The muscle belly is not that large on the majority of people so a great deal of pressure is not necessary. Because the proximal tendon is the most common site of tendinosis, the longitudinal stripping technique can trace the path of the muscle fibers and on to the tendon, following the tendon all the way to the shoulder joint. Perform repeated longitudinal strokes on the biceps brachii until the entire muscle has been treated. Keep in mind that the median nerve is running along the biceps brachii, so be cautious about pressing nerve tissue against the underlying bone (the client will likely report sharp neurological sensations).

C. Active engagement shortening Working on the biceps brachii while it is under active contraction magnifies the effect of the pressure applied. The client is in a supine position and is instructed to perform

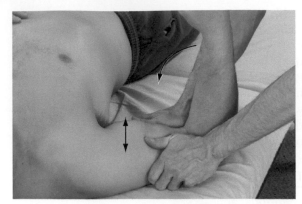

Figure 11.21   Active engagement shortening to biceps brachii.

a repeated elbow flexion and extension movement at a moderate pace. During the shortening phase of elbow flexion, a compression broadening technique is applied to the biceps with the thumbs or thenar eminence of the hand (Fig. 11.21). The broadening technique during elbow flexion is performed repeatedly until the entire muscle is covered.

D. Pin and stretch for biceps brachii Tissue elasticity and pliability is enhanced with pin and stretch techniques to the biceps brachii. The client is in a supine position with the elbow flexed. Grasp the client's distal forearm with one hand while your other hand applies pressure to the biceps with a fingertip or thumb. Pull the client's forearm into full elbow extension while maintaining pressure on the biceps (Fig. 11.22). This technique can be repeated in several places along

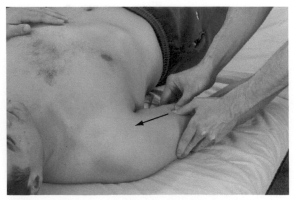

Figure 11.20   Deep stripping on biceps brachii.

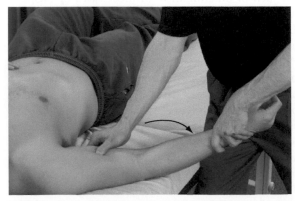

Figure 11.22   Pin and stretch for biceps brachii.

the belly of the biceps. The technique is designed to enhance elongation of the sarcomeres in the muscle fiber, so it is not as effective if applied to the tendon itself.

E. **Active engagement lengthening with additional resistance** The greatest effects of muscle tissue lengthening result from active engagement lengthening techniques. The client is in a supine position. One hand grasps the client's distal forearm, just as in D above. With the client's elbow flexed instruct the client to hold that position while you attempt to pull the forearm into extension. This establishes an initial isometric contraction in the biceps. Once the initial contraction level is established, instruct the client to slowly release the contraction while the client's forearm is pulled into extension, while simultaneously performing a deep longitudinal stripping technique on the biceps (Fig. 11.23). Repeat this whole process until the entire muscle has been adequately covered.

F. **Deep friction to the biceps tendon** Perform deep friction treatments to the tendon of the biceps brachii. The tendon is likely to be tender, so adjust pressure levels to the client's comfort tolerance. Transverse friction applied to the biceps long head tendon could possibly cause subluxation of the tendon (out of the groove), especially if the greater or lesser tuberosities are not very large. Avoid this adverse outcome by performing deep friction techniques longitudinally on the tendon instead of transversely (Fig. 11.24).

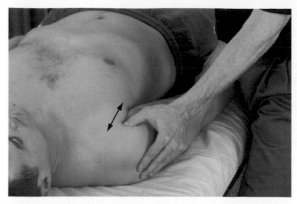

Figure 11.24 Deep friction to biceps tendon long head.

Rehabilitation protocol considerations

- Tendinosis treatment is built on a multi-pronged approach to treatment including reduction of muscle tension, rest from offending activities, and stimulation of fibroblast activity to heal damaged tendon fibers. Stretching approaches are helpful throughout all phases of treatment.

- Thermal applications, such as ice or moist heat, are effective when used in conjunction with the massage approaches mentioned above. Moist heat is helpful in reducing tension in the muscle tissue and enhancing soft-tissue pliability. Cold applications are helpful to reduce any discomfort associated with the deep friction techniques that are applied directly to the affected tendon fibers.

- Techniques such as the active engagement broadening or lengthening may be too intense for a person with a more aggravated tendinosis condition. These techniques can be reserved for a later stage in the rehabilitation process. If the condition is not severe initially, these techniques can be started immediately and adjusted to the client's comfort level and outcome goals.

- Rebuilding the collagen matrix of damaged tendons is a slow process. Encourage the client that persistence in treatment pays off and in the mean time reduction of offending activities is crucial for healing.

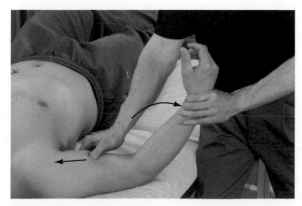

Figure 11.23 Active engagement lengthening with stripping to biceps brachii.

Cautions and contraindications Anti-inflammatory medication is effective at reducing the client's pain in tendinosis conditions. Deep friction massage is frequently given with a pressure level that is close to the pain threshold. If the client is currently taking pain medication, consider reducing the pressure level in friction massage treatments because the client might have an altered pain threshold. As mentioned above, use care when performing friction techniques to the bicipital tendon near the bicipital groove. Transverse friction that is performed vigorously could cause subluxation of the bicipital tendon. Performing deep friction techniques longitudinally on the tendon avoids this potential problem.

Box 11.3   Clinical Tip

There are three main tendons for the biceps brachii. The two proximal tendons include the long head attaching at the supraglenoid tubercle and the short head attaching at the coracoid process. The distal tendon from the muscle belly attaches on the radius. Tendinosis rarely affects the distal tendon or the tendon from the short head. The long head tendon travels over the top of the humeral head and through the bicipital groove. These bony mechanical obstructions in the tendon's path are what primarily contribute to the tendinosis. The tendon is also encased in a synovial sheath as it travels through the bicipital groove and is, therefore, susceptible to tenosynovitis.

Deep friction is a primary treatment method for both tendinosis and tenosynovitis, but for different reasons. In tendinosis, friction is valuable because it helps stimulate fibroblast activity for collagen repair in the damaged tendon. In tenosynovitis, the friction treatment helps break fibrous adhesions between the tendon and its surrounding synovial sheath.

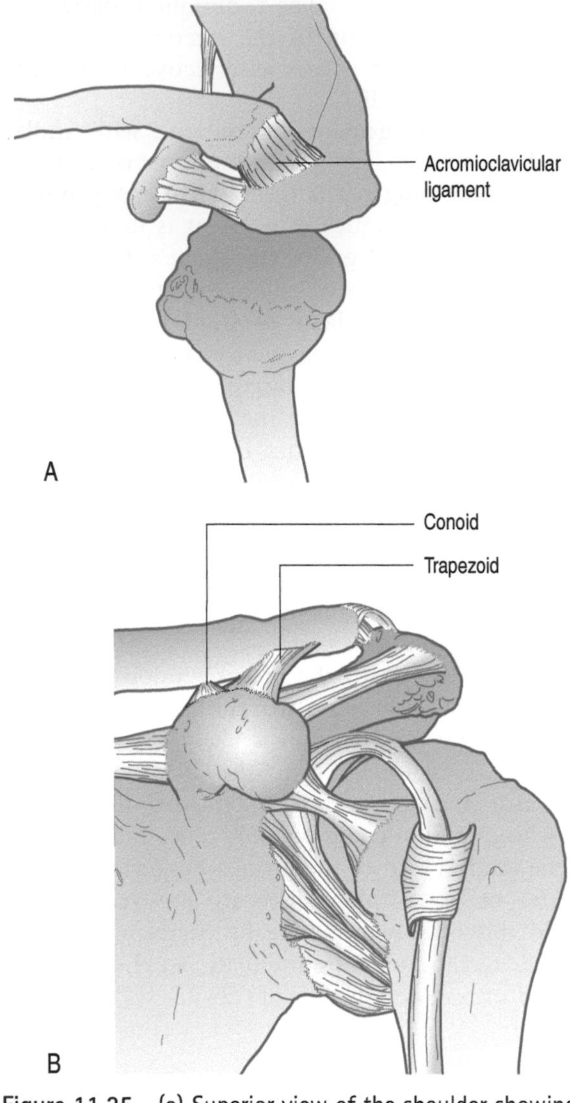

SHOULDER SEPARATION

Description

A shoulder separation is a sprain injury to the ligaments of the acromioclavicular joint. This occurs most often from a direct blow on the shoulder, for example when a person falls on the ground

A

B

Figure 11.25   (a) Superior view of the shoulder showing the acromioclavicular ligament, (b) anterior view showing the two parts of the coracoclavicular ligament.

and lands directly on the anterior/lateral shoulder region or if something falls directly on the lateral shoulder region. There are three primary ligaments that can be injured in a shoulder separation: the acromioclavicular ligament, and the two parts of the coracoclavicular ligament called the conoid and trapezoid (Fig. 11.25). It is not difficult for these ligaments to sustain injury as they are thin and not very strong.

The acromioclavicular ligament is designed to provide anterior/posterior and mediolateral stability. The coracoclavicular ligaments are designed to provide stability against vertical forces. Surrounding muscles and fascia provide additional support for the joint as well. Fibers of the upper trapezius and deltoid muscles insert near this region and lend some additional structural support.[3]

Shoulder separations are divided into three categories, depending upon the particular tissues that are damaged:

- Type 1: there is no fiber disruption to any of the three ligaments, but some degree of ligament stretching.
- Type 2: there is a disruption to the acromioclavicular ligament but the coracoclavicular ligaments are intact.
- Type 3: there is disruption to both the acromioclavicular and coracoclavicular ligaments.

A direct impact blow to the anterior lateral shoulder region usually causes this injury, but any traumatic injury to the shoulder can cause enough mechanical stress on the acromioclavicular articulation to sprain the ligaments. Impact to the clavicle could also cause a compression injury to the neurovascular structures that pass between the clavicle and the first rib. See the discussion of thoracic outlet syndrome for more information about this condition. Other common causes of sprain to the acromioclavicular joint involve falling on an outstretched arm or severe distraction of an abducted arm.[26]

Treatment

Traditional approaches

The primary goal in treating a ligament sprain is to protect the joint against excess motion and to help the damaged ligament tissue heal. Ice and NSAIDs are used as anti-inflammatory treatments for mild sprains. An arm sling is routinely used to keep the area relatively immobile so the ligament can heal properly. However, overuse of the sling can cause problems with excessive fibrosis and development of adhesive capsulitis. To prevent this from occurring early protected motion is a primary treatment goal if the sprain is not severe. Range of motion exercises are gradually incorporated after the sling is no longer being used.

Shoulder separations are generally treated non-surgically even if there is a Type 3 sprain. The Type 3 sprain is likely to leave a cosmetic deformity (protruding clavicle), but there is no strong evidence that surgery for this problem is necessary in many cases.[26] However, each situation is unique, and there are situations where a Type 3 shoulder separation may need surgical intervention. Therefore, it is important to have the condition properly evaluated by a physician to determine if surgery is necessary.

One of the rehabilitation challenges following ligament injury is how to regain stability in the joint when ligaments have been stretched and do not return to their original length. Prolotherapy is a treatment option that is sometimes used in this situation. This treatment involves injection of a dextrose solution into the damaged ligament fibers to stimulate healing of the ligament. In many cases, the injection is able to cause the ligament fibers to heal and tighten to some degree.

Soft-tissue manipulation

General guidelines   Damage to the ligaments of the acromioclavicular joint requires time and protection from additional stress to allow adequate ligament tissue healing. Friction massage is used to stimulate healing properties in tendon and ligament tissue, although adequate studies still need to be performed with human subjects.[46] After the acute stage of the injury has passed (usually after about 72 hours), friction massage of the damaged ligaments can begin. The amount of pressure and length of time the friction massage is applied depends on the severity of the injury and the client's pain tolerance. In general, the rule is – the more recent the injury, the shorter the duration of treatment.

One of the more important roles for the massage practitioner in helping to manage a shoulder separation is preventing excess fibrotic activity in adjacent tissues. This is especially important if the individual is wearing a sling, as prolonged immobilization can lead to tissue fibrosis, especially in the glenohumeral joint capsule. A variety of techniques including sweeping cross fiber and deep longitudinal stripping techniques are valuable to maintain shoulder motion and decrease muscle tension that limits mobility.

Secondary adhesive capsulitis can develop after a shoulder separation, especially if the region is held immobile for long periods. Therefore, it is helpful to encourage range of motion gains, especially in external rotation and abduction, as long as treatment is within the client's pain and comfort tolerance. Some of these motions can cause pain or discomfort at the acromioclavicular joint due to the sprain, so move slowly and cautiously through range-of-motion activities.

General massage to the shoulder girdle is also important. Acute injuries, such as a shoulder separation can produce hypertonicity in numerous muscles around the shoulder. Hypertonicity in these muscles can cause myofascial trigger points or biomechanical imbalance and lead to other soft-tissue dysfunctions. Massage is one of the most effective means of decreasing the compensatory patterns of muscular dysfunction.

Suggested techniques and methods

A. Myofascial release of shoulder region The subtle myofascial techniques can help reduce overall muscle tension around the shoulder and encourage proper healing of the sprain at the acromioclavicular joint. Fascial techniques are applied in multiple planes to provide the greatest mobility enhancement. The primary goal is to place a moderately light tangential (tensile) force on the subcutaneous fascia. Pulling the fascia in multiple directions enhances its pliability the most. Place the hands lightly on the client's shoulder region where the myofascial stretch is to be applied. The practitioner pulls their hands apart to take the slack out of the tissue and to apply a light degree of tensile (pulling) force between the hands (Fig. 11.1). Once there is a slight degree of pull between the hands, the position is held until a subtle sensation of tissue release is felt between the hands. This technique can be applied in various regions of the shoulder, but emphasize the tissues of the anterior shoulder region.

B. Sweeping cross fiber to anterior chest muscles Treatments aimed at the anterior chest muscles help reduce limited motion in the shoulder and reduce tension in shoulder girdle muscles near the acromioclavicular joint. Stand at the head of the table facing the client's feet with the fingers anchored in the client's axilla. Use the thumb to perform sweeping cross fiber movements on the pectoralis major (Fig. 11.2). During the sweeping motion the pectoralis major is sifted between the fingers. Similar sweeping cross fiber techniques can be applied to the anterior deltoid while facing in the same position (toward the client's feet).

C. Deep stripping on pectoralis major Use the thumbs, finger tips, or pressure tool to perform deep stripping techniques to the pectoralis major. Treatment can move from medial to lateral or lateral to medial (Fig. 11.4). Variations on this technique, such as pin and stretch can also be used, especially in the later stages of treatment when the joint is more stable and significant ligament healing has occurred.

D. Deep stripping to proximal fibers of the supraspinatus Muscles near the acromioclavicular joint, such as the supraspinatus, can become tight following a shoulder separation. Stripping techniques on the supraspinatus reduce tension in this muscle. The client is in a prone position. Place the thumb or finger tip anterior to the trapezius and on the proximal fibers of the supraspinatus near the vertebral border of the supraspinous fossa. Perform a slow deep stripping technique on the supraspinatus muscle to encourage tissue lengthening and reduction of muscle tightness (Fig. 11.8). This technique could also be performed in other positions if those are more comfortable for the client.

E. Deep stripping on the upper trapezius The trapezius attaches to the distal clavicle and tension in the trapezius after the sprain can put adverse tension on the joint. Deep stripping can help normalize trapezius tension and decrease any biomechanical dysfunction resulting from the injury. The client is in a prone or side-lying position. After sufficient warming techniques such as effleurage and sweeping cross fiber, perform a longitudinal stripping technique on the upper trapezius. Begin with the fibers in the cervical region and follow the lateral edge of the trapezius out to its attachment on the distal clavicle near the acromioclavicular joint (Fig. 11.26). Perform these stripping techniques repeatedly until the entire upper trapezius has been addressed.

F. Deep friction to the ligaments of the acromioclavicular joint Ligament healing is enhanced with deep friction techniques applied to the damaged fibers. Friction can be applied in multiple directions to create the greatest pliability of the

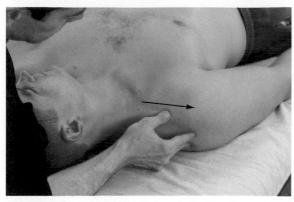

Figure 11.26 Deep stripping on lateral border of upper trapezius.

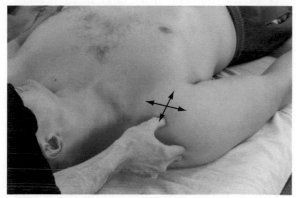

Figure 11.27 Deep friction to the acromioclavicular ligaments injured in shoulder separation.

healing ligament tissue. Apply the deep friction with the finger tips or thumb (Fig. 11.27). Gentle range-of-motion movements can be incorporated with the friction to aid in mobilization of the healing tissue. Motions that should be stressed in these movements include scapular elevation and depression along with horizontal adduction and horizontal abduction. These are the movements that mobilize the acromioclavicular joint the most.

Rehabilitation protocol considerations

- Accurate orthopedic assessment is important to determine the severity of the A–C joint sprain. Some treatment techniques will be modified depending on the severity of the sprain. Deep friction should not be performed directly on the damaged ligaments in a severe sprain or one where there is excessive joint mobility. If there is a Type 3 shoulder separation it is more appropriate to wait a little farther into the healing process before beginning direct friction techniques. Use the client's pain and comfort tolerance as a guide and do not perform friction massage on any injury that is highly painful. A moderate degree of discomfort is common with treatment of any ligament sprain, but avoid treatments that cause a significant pain increase.

- Strength training is sometimes used as an adjunct treatment in rehabilitation of ligament sprains. If exercise is started too early, it can put additional stress on the joint and further aggravate the injury. Strength training should not begin until the later stages of the rehabilitation.

- In the early stages of the injury focus should be on the surrounding muscles and treating the site of ligament injury with short durations of friction. As the injury rehabilitation progresses, increase the time spent working directly on the ligament tear site with vigorous friction.

Cautions and contraindications   Use caution with any techniques or movements that put pressure on or cause movement to the acromioclavicular joint. Pain is an appropriate guide to determine if too much pressure or movement is aggravating the injury. Try not to put too much pressure on the distal end of the clavicle when applying friction techniques to the acromioclavicular joint. This will minimize movement of the clavicle while the ligaments spanning the joint are attempting to heal. If the sprain is severe enough to cause displacement of one end of the clavicle, there may be compression of neurovascular structures in the area so watch for any signs or symptoms that would indicate compression of these tissues.

GLENOHUMERAL DISLOCATION/ SUBLUXATION

Description

The shoulder has the greatest range of motion of any joint in the body. To have this great range, there is very little bony limitation to movement in any direction. As a result, movement restraint at the glenohumeral joint primarily comes from soft tissues. Muscles, along with the ligaments and joint capsule, provide the greatest limitation to excess motion. Because the glenoid fossa is so shallow, the head of the humerus is susceptible to dislocation at this joint.

A rim of cartilage called the glenoid labrum surrounds the glenoid fossa. This cartilage rim helps make the fossa slightly deeper to protect against dislocations. When dislocations do occur they are usually anterior dislocations.[47] In anterior dislocations the head of the humerus is thrust in an anterior direction relative to the glenoid fossa. Anterior dislocations usually occur from the combined motions of shoulder abduction and external rotation.

The joint capsule is contiguous with numerous ligaments that span the glenohumeral joint. However, anatomists have chosen to name some of these ligament structures separately. One of the most important ligament structures for resisting glenohumeral dislocation is the inferior glenohumeral ligament, which is the primary restraint to anterior glenohumeral dislocation (Fig. 11.28).[48] This ligament is pulled or stretched beyond its capacity in anterior dislocations.

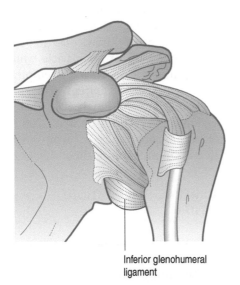

Inferior glenohumeral ligament

Figure 11.28   The inferior glenohumeral ligament.

The inferior glenohumeral ligament attaches to the lower border of the glenoid labrum. With excessive tensile stress it may pull the labrum away from the rim of the glenoid fossa, producing an injury called a Bankart lesion. The Bankart lesion accompanies anterior glenohumeral dislocations, and is a problem that must be addressed once the actual dislocation has been resolved.

Another soft-tissue structure that plays an important role in preventing anterior dislocations is the tendon from the long head of the biceps brachii. This tendon attaches to the supraglenoid tubercle and has fibers that insert into the upper region of the glenoid labrum. The angle of the tendon is such that it comes across the anterior aspect of the humeral head, and helps prevent anterior dislocations of the humerus.[49]

In a situation where an anterior dislocation has occurred, the biceps tendon may put enough tensile (pulling) stress on its attachment site at the supraglenoid tubercle to pull the labrum away from the glenoid fossa. This injury is called a SLAP lesion (superior labrum anterior posterior). It indicates a tear to the superior aspect of the labrum oriented in an anterior to posterior direction. If a SLAP lesion has occurred the biceps brachii is usually less effective in holding the humeral head in its proper position.[50,51] With a decrease of glenohumeral stability from the biceps, there is increased instability in the joint, and future dislocations are even more likely.

Instability is one of the prime factors that both causes and results from dislocations. For example, when a dislocation or subluxation has occurred, the ligaments and joint capsule are further stretched. Once these structures are stretched, the head of the humerus more easily moves around in the glenoid fossa creating joint instability. The more instability in the joint, the greater is the chance of future dislocations.

There are several other problems that result from shoulder instability or glenohumeral dislocation. Continued instability in the shoulder can cause osteoarthritis as the client gets older.[52] Shoulder impingement syndrome or rotator cuff disorders are likely to occur as well. When the humeral head is moving around more in the glenoid fossa, there is a greater chance for it to press the soft tissues that are above it against the underside of the acromion process or the coracoacromial ligament. Subsequently, damage to the supraspinatus, joint capsule, biceps tendon long head, or subacromial bursa may result.

Treatment

Traditional approaches

Restoring a dislocated joint to its proper position is called reducing the dislocation. If a dislocation is serious and has to be reduced, it should only be done by someone who is qualified and trained to reduce dislocations. Serious injury can result by attempting to correct a dislocation if it is performed improperly. The brachial plexus and axillary artery are very close to the lip of the glenoid labrum. If, in attempting to move the humeral head back into the glenoid fossa, the practitioner pinches the brachial plexus or axillary artery between the humeral head and the rim of the glenoid labrum, these neurovascular structures can be severed. In some cases reduction of the dislocation is performed under anesthesia so there is very little muscular resistance to the movement.

Once the dislocated joint has been properly restored to its correct position, attention shifts to the problem of instability and capsular ligament stretching that can cause further complications. If the instability is mild, strengthening of the muscles surrounding the shoulder is initiated so they can aid in glenohumeral stability. Strengthening procedures focus on the rotator cuff, trapezius, and serratus anterior muscles. Any strengthening motions that go near the position of instability are avoided. In addition, strengthening does not emphasize muscles that increase the pull of the humeral head in the unwanted direction. For example, strength training for the pectoralis major is discouraged in an anterior dislocation because it may pull the humeral head in an anterior direction.

If the dislocation is severe, or conservative approaches have been unsuccessful, surgery is an option. A common surgical procedure for dislocations is the capsular shift. In this procedure, an incision is made in the ligamentous capsular tissues and they are pulled up and stitched over one another making a tighter capsule.[27]

A newer procedure that has been gaining interest is thermal capsulorrhaphy. In this procedure, the physician uses a small heat probe with either laser energy or radio frequency generated heat to shrink the capsule and improve stability. Many surgeons have been using this procedure and obtaining good results, although the long-term effectiveness has not yet been determined.[53–56]

Soft-tissue manipulation

General guidelines Massage treatment by itself is not going to restore a dislocated or subluxed joint. However, massage can make a beneficial contribution to treating these disorders. Once the dislocation has been reduced (corrected), massage can aid in the return of proper biomechanical balance and reduction of muscular splinting in the region.

Massage can also be used to target hypertonicity in any muscles that could pull the humeral head in an unwanted direction. For example, various massage techniques to the pectoralis major may help reduce its contribution to further anterior translation of the humeral head.

Reducing other secondary problems such as shoulder impingement resulting from instability is also a goal of massage treatment in this condition. Dislocations could produce excess tension on the tendon from the long head of the biceps brachii, and further aggravate labral damage. Tendon dysfunction, such as bicipital tendinosis or tenosynovitis could also result and massage can be used to address those issues.

Suggested techniques and methods Massage treatments for this condition are not aimed at correcting the dislocation or subluxation. However, hypertonicity or biomechanical dysfunction in muscles of the shoulder can further exacerbate problems resulting from the shoulder instability. The following techniques are helpful in addressing these secondary issues.

A. Sweeping cross fiber to anterior chest muscles Treatments aimed at the anterior chest muscles help restore proper biomechanical balance that can be altered from the dislocation or subluxation. This technique helps reduce tension in superficial fibers of pectoralis major and anterior deltoid. Stand facing the client's feet with the fingers anchored in the client's axilla. Use the thumb to perform sweeping cross fiber movements on the pectoralis major (Fig. 11.2). During the sweeping motion, the pectoralis major is sifted between the fingers. Similar sweeping cross fiber techniques can be applied to the anterior deltoid while facing in the same position (toward the client's feet).

B. Deep stripping on pectoralis major Use the thumbs, finger tips, or pressure tool to perform deep stripping techniques to the pectoralis major. Treatment can move from medial to lateral or lateral to medial (Fig. 11.4). Variations on this technique, such as pin and stretch, can also be used to make pressure penetration more effective. However, use caution with the position of the shoulder during any movement or massage techniques to make sure they do not move close to positions of shoulder instability.

C. Deep stripping on infraspinatus and teres minor Posterior rotator cuff muscles may also be under increased tension as a result of the dislocation. Deep stripping helps normalize tissue tightness in this muscle group. With the thumb or fingertips, apply a deep longitudinal stripping technique from the proximal to distal fibers of the infraspinatus and teres minor (Fig. 11.12). Continue the stripping technique until all the fibers of the infraspinatus and teres minor have been treated. This technique can also be performed in a distal to proximal direction, if a more comfortable hand position is desired.

D. Sweeping cross fiber to biceps brachii Tension reduction in the biceps brachii reduces tension on the bicipital tendon and can help restore proper mechanics of the glenohumeral joint following a dislocation. Apply sweeping cross fiber techniques to the biceps brachii (Fig. 11.19). This technique can be performed with the client's elbow flexed, which keeps the biceps in a shortened position and more pliable. However, greater muscle tension reduction and fiber spreading is accomplished by applying the sweeping cross fiber technique with the elbow extended so the muscle is in a lengthened position.

Numerous other techniques applied to the shoulder region described in this chapter can be helpful in restoring proper biomechanical balance around the joint.

Rehabilitation protocol considerations

- If a shoulder dislocation is suspected it is advisable to get guidance from a physician about the level of instability remaining in the shoulder. The shoulder should be considered highly vulnerable to movement or stretching techniques, especially those involving abduction and lateral rotation.

- Tension reduction in muscles is usually a primary goal of massage treatments. However, in a severe dislocation there may be some advantages in muscle tension around the joint as it can preserve joint stability and prevent further damage from the excess mobility.

- If there is an injury to the superior labrum along with the dislocation, any strength training activities involving the biceps brachii should be avoided until the labral damage has been addressed. Further use of the biceps brachii with strong resistance could further damage the superior labrum.

Cautions and contraindications   After a subluxation or dislocation, the body's proprioceptors strongly warn when a position or movement is coming near the position of instability. The client usually feels apprehension and/or discomfort with the motion. Be sure to watch for apprehension signs that indicate movement or positions that could jeopardize joint stability. Also use caution with range-of-motion techniques that push the humeral head against the edge of the glenoid labrum due to possible glenoid labrum damage.

Box 11.4 Case Study

Background

Sandra is a 46-year-old hair stylist with a large clientele. Two weeks ago she slipped on a wet floor in her salon and put her arm out behind her to break her fall as she fell backward. She did not break anything in the fall, but hurt her wrist in the accident as well as her shoulder. The wrist pain has since decreased, but she is having increasing discomfort in her shoulder, especially at the end of the day at work. She is also noticing that the shoulder pain is increasingly interrupting her sleep. The shoulder pain is a dull aching sensation and the pain is localized in her shoulder but also extends down her arm somewhat. This condition is making it increasingly difficult for her to perform her long days of work in the hair salon.

She saw her physician after the injury and confirmed that there were no broken bones from the accident. However, the shoulder pain was not that prominent at the time. She has not been back to see the physician again about this shoulder complaint. She is an active yoga practitioner and has tried some stretching and yoga for the shoulder problem, but this does not seem to be resolving the problem.

Questions to consider

- Sandra's shoulder pain seems to be worse now than right after her initial injury. Why might the pain be more serious now?
- Based on the mechanics of the injury and the few symptoms she has described, do you think she has injured any neurological structures in her shoulder?
- Now that she is several weeks post injury but experiencing some increasing shoulder pain do you think any thermal modalities, such as moist heat or ice would be helpful for her shoulder? Why or why not?
- If Sandra's condition turns out to involve shoulder impingement that is being aggravated by the position of her arms at work, would you want to treat this with massage?
- If the initial injury caused a supraspinatus rotator cuff tear, should this be treated with massage? If so, how often would massage treatment be helpful. If not, when would it be appropriate to begin massage treatment?
- What else can Sandra do along with massage treatment to decrease stress on this region during her daily activities?

References

1. Donatelli R. Physical Therapy of the Shoulder. 3rd ed. Philadelphia: Churchill Livingstone; 1997.
2. Pearsall AW. Adhesive Capsulitis. 7-30-2002; www.emedicine.com. Accessed January 23, 2005.
3. Malone T, McPoil T, Nitz A. Orthopedic and Sports Physical Therapy. 3rd ed. St. Louis: Mosby; 1997.
4. Neviaser RJ, Neviaser TJ. The frozen shoulder. Diagnosis and management. Clin Orthop. 1987(223):59–64.
5. Bruckner FE, Nye CJ. A prospective study of adhesive capsulitis of the shoulder ("frozen shoulder") in a high risk population. Q J Med. 1981;50(198):191–204.
6. Sandor R. Adhesive capsulitis – optimal treatment of 'frozen shoulder'. Physician Sportsmed. 2000;28(9):23–29.
7. Simons D, Travell J, Simons L. Myofascial Pain and Dysfunction: The Trigger Point Manual. Vol 1. 2nd ed. Baltimore: Williams & Wilkins; 1999.
8. Richardson J, Iglarsh ZA. Clinical Orthopaedic Physical Therapy. Philadelphia: W.B. Saunders; 1994.
9. Miller MD, Wirth MA, Rockwood CAJ. Thawing the frozen shoulder: the 'patient' patient. Orthopedics. 1996;19(10):849–853.
10. Bulgen DY, Binder AI, Hazleman BL, Dutton J, Roberts S. Frozen shoulder: prospective clinical study with an evaluation of three treatment regimens. Ann Rheum Dis. 1984;43(3):353–360.
11. Threlkeld AJ. The effects of manual therapy on connective tissue. Phys Ther. 1992;72(12):893–902.
12. Nordin M, Frankel V. Basic Biomechanics of the Musculoskeletal System. 2nd ed. Malvern: Lea & Febiger; 1989.
13. Panjabi M, White A. Biomechanics in the Musculoskeletal System. New York: Churchill Livingstone; 2001.
14. Neumann DA. Kinesiology of the Musculoskeletal System. St. Louis: Mosby; 2002.
15. Shah NN, Diamantopoulos P. Position of the humeral head and rotator cuff tear: an anatomical observation in cadavers. Acta Orthop Scand. 2004;75(6):746–749.
16. Lohr JF, Uhthoff HK. The microvascular pattern of the supraspinatus tendon. Clin Orthop. 1990(254):35–38.
17. Wolf WB. Calcific tendinitis of the shoulder. Physician Sportsmed. 1999;27(9):27–33.

18. Gotoh M, Higuchi F, Suzuki R, Yamanaka K. Progression from calcifying tendinitis to rotator cuff tear. Skeletal Radiol. 2003;32(2):86–89.

19. Porcellini G, Paladini P, Campi F, Paganelli M. Shoulder instability and related rotator cuff tears: arthroscopic findings and treatment in patients aged 40 to 60 years. Arthroscopy. 2006;22(3):270–276.

20. Neviaser RJ, Neviaser TJ, Neviaser JS. Anterior dislocation of the shoulder and rotator cuff rupture. Clin Orthop. 1993(291):103–106.

21. Fadale PD, Wiggins ME. Corticosteroid injections: their use and abuse. J Am Acad Orthop Surg. 1994;2(3):133–140.

22. Fredberg U. Local corticosteroid injection in sport – review of literature and guidelines for treatment. Scand J Med Sci Sports. 1997;7(3):131–139.

23. Goupille P, Sibilia J, Caroit M, et al. Local corticosteroid injections in the treatment of rotator cuff tendinitis (except for frozen shoulder and calcific tendinitis). Clin Exp Rheumatol. 1996;14(5):561–566.

24. Kennedy JC, Willis RB. The effects of local steroid injections on tendons: a biomechanical and microscopic correlative study. Am J Sports Med. 1976;4(1):11–21.

25. Wolin P, Tarbet J. Rotator cuff injury: addressing overhead overuse. Physician Sportsmed. 1997;25(6):263–267.

26. Fu F, Stone D. Sports Injuries: Mechanisms, Prevention, Treatment. Baltimore: Williams & Wilkins; 1994.

27. Torg J, Shephard R. Current Therapy In Sports Medicine. 3rd ed. St. Louis: Mosby; 1995.

28. Neer CS, 2nd. Impingement lesions. Clin Orthop. 1983(173):70–77.

29. McMaster WC, Roberts A, Stoddard T. A correlation between shoulder laxity and interfering pain in competitive swimmers. Am J Sports Med. 1998;26(1):83–86.

30. Ingber RS. Shoulder impingement in tennis/racquetball players treated with subscapularis myofascial treatments. Arch Phys Med Rehabil. 2000;81(5):679–682.

31. Cailliet R. Shoulder Pain. 3rd ed. Philadelphia: F.A. Davis; 1991.

32. Salzman KL, Lillegard WA, Butcher JD. Upper extremity bursitis. Am Fam Physician. 1997;56(7):1797–1806, 1811–1792.

33. Almekinders LC. Anti-inflammatory treatment of muscular injuries in sport – An update of recent studies. Sport Med. 1999;28(6):383–388.

34. Goldstein JL. Challenges in managing NSAID – associated gastrointestinal tract injury. Digestion. 2004;69(Suppl 1): 25–33.

35. Hawkey CJ. Non-steroidal anti-inflammatory drug gastropathy: causes and treatment. Scand J Gastroenterol Suppl. 1996;220:124–127.

36. Naesdal J, Brown K. NSAID-associated adverse effects and acid control aids to prevent them: a review of current treatment options. Drug Saf. 2006;29(2): 119–132.

37. Vanderwindt D, Vanderheijden G, Scholten R, Koes BW, Bouter LM. The efficacy of nonsteroidal antiinflammatory drugs (NSAIDs) for shoulder complaints – a systematic review. J Clin Epidemiol. 1995;48(5):691–704.

38. Khan KM, Cook JL, Bonar F, Harcourt P, Astrom M. Histopathology of common tendinopathies – Update and implications for clinical management. Sport Med. 1999; 27(6):393–408.

39. Pfahler M, Branner S, Refior HJ. The role of the bicipital groove in tendopathy of the long biceps tendon. J Shoulder Elbow Surg. 1999;8(5):419–424.

40. Levinsohn EM, Santelli ED. Bicipital groove dysplasia and medial dislocation of the biceps brachii tendon. Skeletal Radiol. 1991;20(6):419–423.

41. O'Donoghue DH. Subluxing biceps tendon in the athlete. Clin Orthop. 1982(164):26–29.

42. AAOS. Athletic Training and Sports Medicine. 2nd ed. Park Ridge: American Academy of Orthopaedic Surgeons; 1991.

43. Khan KM, Cook JL, Taunton JE, Bonar F. Overuse tendinosis, not tendinitis – Part 1: A new paradigm for a difficult clinical problem. Physician Sportsmed. 2000;28(5):38+.

44. Gehlsen GM, Ganion LR, Helfst R. Fibroblast responses to variation in soft tissue mobilization pressure. Med Sci Sport Exercise. 1999;31(4):531–535.

45. Davidson CJ, Ganion LR, Gehlsen GM, Verhoestra B, Roepke JE, Sevier TL. Rat tendon morphologic and functional changes resulting from soft-tissue mobilization. Med Sci Sport Exercise. 1997;29(3):313–319.

46. Weintraub W. Tendon and Ligament Healing. Berkeley: North Atlantic Books; 1999.

47. Matsen FA, 3rd, Zuckerman JD. Anterior glenohumeral instability. Clin Sports Med. 1983;2(2):319–338.

48. Wheeless C. Wheeless Textbook of Orthopaedics. World Wide Web Site. http://www.medmedia.com/med.htm. Accessed 2002.

49. Rodosky MW, Harner CD, Fu FH. The role of the long head of the biceps muscle and superior glenoid labrum in anterior stability of the shoulder. Am J Sports Med. 1994;22(1):121–130.

50. Post M, Benca P. Primary tendinitis of the long head of the biceps. Clin Orthop. 1989(246):117–125.

51. Pagnani MJ, Deng XH, Warren RF, Torzilli PA, Altchek DW. Effect of lesions of the superior portion of the glenoid labrum on glenohumeral translation. J Bone Joint Surg Am. 1995;77(7):1003–1010.

52. An YH, Friedman RJ. Multidirectional instability of the glenohumeral joint. Orthop Clin North Am. 2000; 31(2):275–285.

53. Lu Y, Markel MD, Kalscheur V, Ciullo JR, Ciullo JV. Histologic evaluation of thermal capsulorrhaphy of human shoulder joint capsule with monopolar radiofrequency energy during short- to long-term follow-up. Arthroscopy. 2008;24(2):203–209.

54. Miniaci A, Codsi MJ. Thermal capsulorrhaphy for the treatment of shoulder instability. Am J Sports Med. 2006;34(8):1356–1363.

55. Bisson LJ. Thermal capsulorrhaphy for isolated posterior instability of the glenohumeral joint without labral detachment. Am J Sports Med. 2005;33(12):1898–1904.

56. Wong KL, Williams GR. Complications of thermal capsulorrhaphy of the shoulder. J Bone Joint Surg Am. 2001;83(Suppl 2 Pt 2):151–155.

Chapter 12

Elbow, forearm, wrist and hand

The lower extremities are the limbs of motion, but the upper extremities are the limbs of activity. Whether it is occupational or recreational activity or simply going through the motions of daily living, much of each day involves using the hands. The human hand is designed for precise manipulation of objects, which means there is a fine degree of neuromuscular control. Fine motor control requires a complex interaction of numerous muscles and other soft tissues throughout the entire upper extremity.

Despite the mechanical demands on the region, the soft tissues in the distal upper extremity are not designed to handle large or repetitive force loads. As a result, soft-tissue orthopedic disorders often result from repetitive overuse injuries in the distal upper extremity. The distal upper extremity includes more peripheral nerve compression pathologies than any other area of the body. The small size of the bones, muscles, tendons, and ligaments in the wrist and hand also make them vulnerable to high force loads, such as those which occur when falling on an outstretched hand. Because orthopedic disorders often involve soft-tissue overuse, massage is an excellent treatment strategy for addressing this problem.

INJURY CONDITIONS

LATERAL EPICONDYLITIS (TENNIS ELBOW)

Description

Upper-extremity cumulative trauma disorders are increasingly problematic in Western society and account for a great percentage of all occupational injuries.[1–3] Lateral epicondylitis is one of the most common of these upper-extremity overuse problems. The condition is known as tennis elbow because of the frequency with which it affects tennis players, but the overall percentage of individuals who develop this problem are not tennis players.

Lateral epicondylitis rarely involves inflammation of the epicondyle. Like other conditions called tendinitis, lateral epicondylitis involves collagen breakdown in the tendon fibers (tendinosis) and not an actual inflammatory problem.[4,5] In order to heal the condition there must be reduced tension on the damaged tendon fibers and some reduction in hypertonicity in the associated muscles.

The primary problem in lateral epicondylitis is with the common extensor tendons of the wrist and hand. The fibers of the extensor carpi radialis brevis (ECRB) appear to be affected most. This muscle has a relatively small attachment site on the lateral epicondyle, so the force generated by the muscle is concentrated in a small, localized area. However, any of the wrist extensors could be involved in this condition.

The tendon fibers from all the wrist extensor muscles come together near the attachment site at the lateral epicondyle. There is little distinction between the separate tendons where they attach at the epicondyle.[6] Because of its anatomical location certain activities put greater loads on the ECRB than on the other extensor tendons.[7]

The majority of problems in lateral epicondylitis result from excessive concentric wrist extension or eccentric wrist flexion. Either of these actions performed repetitively can overwhelm the tendon fibers and lead to tendon degeneration. Excessive or repetitive loads on the wrist extensor muscles occur in occupations in which the hands perform a repetitive task; grocery store clerks, computer workers, and carpenters are commonly afflicted with this condition.

Chronic tension in the wrist extensor muscles (isometric contractions) can also cause fatigue and tendon degeneration. Computer use is often a cause of upper-extremity overuse problems such as lateral epicondylitis.[8] When operating the mouse tension is held in the wrist extensor muscles, which pulls on the tendons. These conditions also develop due to other complex postural, psychological, and kinetic chain relationships, not simply too much keyboard or mouse activity.[9–12]

In addition to the more obvious movements of flexion and extension, there is evidence that repetitive supination and pronation of the forearm lead to epicondylitis. Overuse occurs when the flexor and extensor muscles engage strong isometric contractions to hold implements in the hand during these motions. The constant contractions of wrist muscles can also lead to the development of myofascial trigger points in the extensor muscles. These myofascial trigger points are likely to produce symptoms similar to the pain from tendon fiber degeneration, and can be a concurrent problem.[13]

Various approaches can be used to reduce fatigue on the forearm muscles during different activities. For example, forearm support bands are routinely advocated to decrease the collagen degeneration and tendon injury of epicondylitis. Whether or not these bands actually reduce epicondylitis is still to be determined.[14,15] One study found that wearing forearm support bands actually increased the rate of fatigue in unimpaired individuals, and can contribute to the problem more than solve it.[16]

Treatment

Traditional approaches

The primary goal in treating lateral epicondylitis is to repair the damaged collagen fibers in the tendon and restore the tendon to a healthy, functioning state. Tendon repair relies on reducing or eliminating as many of the stress factors as possible that led to the tendon damage. Rest from offending activities is necessary for this repair to succeed. Rest does not mean total inactivity, but simply a reduction in activities that aggravate the problem. Ice applications are used with some success.

Traditionally ice has been used as an anti-inflammatory treatment, but it is now understood that epicondylitis is usually not an inflammatory condition. Cold treatment is still effective for its other beneficial effects, such as pain management.

Rehabilitative exercise is used to heal the damaged tissue through revascularization and collagen repair.[5] The goal of rehabilitative exercise is to improve overall strength and endurance in the muscles of the entire kinetic chain that are involved in upper-extremity activities, including muscles of the neck, shoulder, arm, and elbow regions. However, attempting strength training activities with this muscle group while the tendon fibers are still damaged can further aggravate the problem. If the problem is not sufficiently advanced, strength training is beneficial. It can condition the tendons so they are more resistant to fatigue injury. Additional physical therapy modalities such as ultrasound, phonophoresis, or electrical stimulation are commonly used in treatment as well.[17]

The pain from lateral epicondylitis can be debilitating and interfere with an individual's ability to perform daily activities. Individuals may seek the short-term pain relief offered by anti-inflammatory medications (including corticosteroid injections). While there is usually some pain relief associated with these medications, their contribution to healing of the problem is questionable. In fact, their use can be detrimental to overall tendon healing.[18–20]

If the conservative measures of bracing, strength training, and relative rest are not effective at reducing the symptoms, surgical treatment may be performed. In surgical treatment the pathologic tissue is removed. The idea is that if damaged tissue is removed, healing in the remaining tissues will allow the region to become strong again. It is suggested that care be taken so that associated structures are not significantly weakened in the surgical treatment process.[21]

New techniques with arthroscopic procedures have helped minimize additional damaged tissue, and provide for more effective surgical treatment. Physicians are experimenting with laser treatment for lateral epicondylitis and finding some success with this process, although there is a need for further research.[22–24] Despite the wide number of treatments commonly used for lateral epicondylitis, many do not have an adequate physiological rationale to support their continued use.[25]

Soft–tissue manipulation

General guidelines As in traditional approaches, rest from offending activities is a crucial part of the healing process. There are several other factors that are essential for effective soft-tissue treatment of lateral epicondylitis. Because a primary problem in this condition is excessive hypertonicity in the muscles that attach at the lateral epicondyle, reducing muscular hypertonicity is a primary goal. Massage treatment begins with compressive effleurage and general sweeping cross fiber movements to reduce tension and enhance tissue mobility. After initial muscle relaxation work, deep broadening and lengthening techniques are used on the wrist extensor muscles. Broadening techniques enhance the ability of the fibers to spread and broaden as they go into concentric contraction. Lengthening techniques enhance tissue pliability and the muscle's ability to elongate. Longitudinal stripping techniques are particularly helpful for identifying and neutralizing myofascial trigger points.

At later stages of the rehabilitation as the tendons become less sensitive, the effects of pressure and movement can be enhanced through active engagement techniques for the wrist extensors. As the rehabilitation progresses it may be beneficial to use resistance, such as rubber tubing or elastic resistance band, for recruitment of additional muscle effort.

In addition to reducing muscle tension in the wrist extensors, massage treatment addresses the primary tissue problem, which is collagen degeneration in the tendon fibers. Collagen degeneration is treated with deep friction massage, which stimulates fibroblast proliferation to help heal the damaged tendon.[26,27] Stretching of the extensor tendons is also valuable during and after soft-tissue treatment. Stretching is something the client should continue at home on a regular basis.

Suggested techniques and methods

A. Sweeping cross fiber to wrist extensors Sweeping cross fiber is helpful for reducing overall tension in the wrist extensor muscles. It can be performed in conjunction with effleurage during initial treatment of this region. Use one hand to hold the client's wrist and the other hand to perform

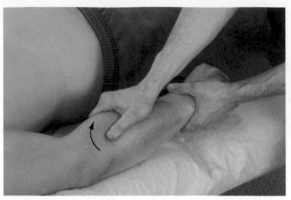

Figure 12.1 Sweeping cross fiber to wrist extensors.

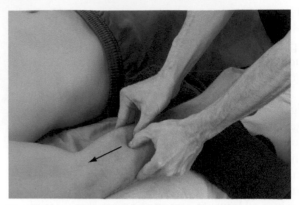

Figure 12.3 Deep stripping to extensor group.

a sweeping cross fiber technique to the wrist extensors (Fig. 12.1). Work the entire length of the forearm from the wrist to the elbow.

B. Compression broadening to wrist extensors After initial effleurage and cross fiber work, the extensor muscles can be treated at a deeper level with deep broadening techniques. The client is in a supine position with the forearm supported by the table. Perform deep compression broadening on the wrist extensor muscle group using the thenar eminence of the hand (Fig. 12.2). This is a cross fiber stroke so you can move from proximal to distal or vice versa.

C. Deep longitudinal stripping to wrist extensors Apply deep longitudinal stripping to wrist extensors to reduce tension and encouraging tissue pliability and flexibility. The client is supine on the treatment table. Use the fingers or thumb to

perform a deep longitudinal stripping technique on the wrist extensors that begins at the wrist and continues to the extensor attachment site at the lateral epicondyle (Fig. 12.3). Continue the technique in successive strips until the entire muscle group has been treated.

D. Active engagement shortening techniques At the later stages of rehabilitation the intensity of pressure can be increased with active engagement techniques. The client is supine with a towel, bolster, or other support under the wrist so full wrist flexion and extension is possible. If a wrist support is not available, this technique can be performed with the client's hand off the edge of the table. Instruct the client to move the wrist through full flexion and extension at a moderately slow pace. Perform a compression-broadening stroke during wrist extension (Fig. 12.4). Gradually work

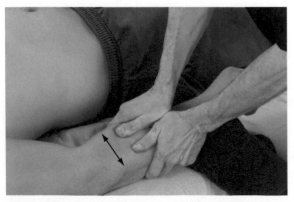

Figure 12.2 Compression broadening on wrist extensors.

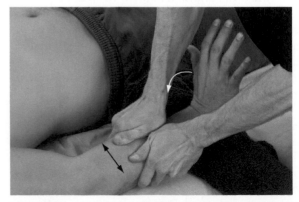

Figure 12.4 Active engagement shortening to wrist extensors.

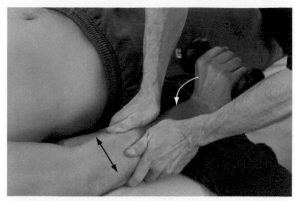

Figure 12.5 Active engagement shortening to wrist extensors with additional resistance of hand-held weight.

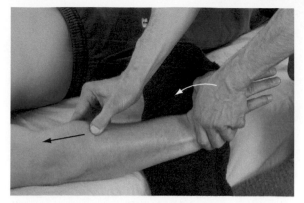

Figure 12.7 Active engagement lengthening of wrist extensors with manual resistance.

the entire length of the wrist extensor group, performing the stroke on each wrist extension. To increase the muscle recruitment and effectiveness of this technique, hand held weights or resistance bands can be used during the wrist extension (Fig. 12.5).

E. Active engagement lengthening techniques Even greater pliability and flexibility enhancement results from active engagement lengthening techniques. The client is in the same position as D above using either a support under the wrist or the hand dropped off the side of the table. Instruct the client to move the wrist through full flexion and extension at a moderately slow pace. Perform a deep longitudinal stripping technique in a distal to proximal direction during each eccentric wrist flexion movement (Fig. 12.6). Each stripping technique covers about 3–4 inches. Pause during

the wrist extension and apply another stripping technique from where the last one stopped during the next wrist flexion movement. Continue this series of stripping motions during movement until the entire muscle has been adequately covered. Hand-held weights, resistance bands or manual resistance can be used to enhance the effectiveness of this technique (Fig. 12.7).

F. Deep friction to common extensor tendons The primary function of friction techniques is to stimulate fibroblast proliferation to enhance collagen repair in the damaged tendon. The wrist is in a flexed position because keeping the tendon on stretch helps the effectiveness of this technique. Use the fingertips or thumb to perform the deep friction technique to the common wrist extensor tendons (Fig. 12.8). The deep friction technique can be performed on the tendon transversely or longitudinally.

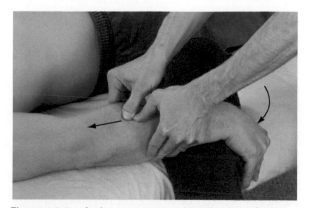

Figure 12.6 Active engagement lengthening of wrist extensors.

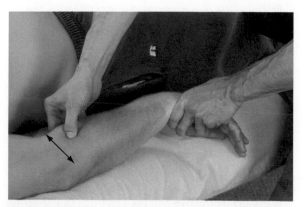

Figure 12.8 Deep friction on extensor tendons.

Rehabilitation protocol considerations

- Use appropriate assessment strategies to determine the severity of the condition. If the condition is severe, hold off on the more intense techniques such as the active engagement methods until later stages of the rehabilitation process.

- Cryotherapy is sometimes used both before and after the friction treatments to reduce discomfort.

- Stretching methods for the wrist extensors are an essential aspect of treatment. Stretching can be incorporated in the clinical session as well as by the client at home.

- Tendinosis is a slow-healing condition so encourage the client to be patient and consistent in efforts at home and in the clinic to assist in treatment.

Cautions and contraindications   Symptoms of lateral epicondylitis may be confused with those from other problems and need to be accurately clarified before initiating treatment. Compression neuropathies of the radial nerve can produce pain sensations in the same region as lateral epicondylitis. Vigorous pressure techniques such as deep friction massage could aggravate the radial nerve compression. Accurate orthopedic assessment can help clarify the condition to assure a nerve pathology is not being aggravated.

MEDIAL EPICONDYLITIS (GOLFER'S ELBOW)

Description

Just like the extensor tendons in lateral epicondylitis, the flexor tendons are susceptible to overuse pain and dysfunction at their attachment site on the medial epicondyle of the humerus. The overuse can affect any of the flexor tendons, but the flexor carpi radialis is more susceptible to damage than the others.[28]

This condition is commonly called golfer's elbow because of the frequency with which it affects those playing golf. The problem occurs from swinging the golf club and then hitting the ball at the low point of the swing. The wrist flexors are engaged in a concentric contraction to swing the club toward the ground, and then when the ball is hit there is a sudden eccentric load on the flexor group. The eccentric loading forces are exaggerated because of the golf club's length.

Medial epicondylitis, like lateral epicondylitis, rarely involves an inflammatory reaction in the tissues. Collagen degeneration in the tendon fibers from chronic tensile loads is the primary dysfunction. Medial epicondylitis develops from repetitive concentric contractions of the wrist flexor group (producing wrist flexion) or eccentric activity of these muscles as the wrist is moving in extension. This problem can arise from repetitive supination and pronation of the forearm as well.

Box 12.1   Clinical Tip

Epicondylitis is a common disorder affecting the lateral elbow region. However, because lateral epicondylitis is so common, pain in this region is sometimes mistakenly attributed to overuse of the extensor tendons when they are not the tissue at fault. A branch of the radial nerve called the posterior interosseous nerve (PIN) courses under the supinator muscle near the lateral epicondyle of the humerus. Compression of the PIN in this region, also called radial tunnel syndrome, can produce lateral elbow pain very similar to that experienced in epicondylitis. Traditional treatment for epicondylitis is usually ineffective and the condition can linger for long periods. Hence, the condition has become known as "resistant tennis elbow."

In addition to elbow pain, compression of the PIN is likely to produce weakness of all the wrist extensor muscles. Epicondylitis is more likely to be painful on resisted wrist extension while radial tunnel syndrome is more likely to indicate weakness with little increase in pain. Massage treatment for epicondylitis involves deep friction on the proximal extensor tendons. However, that treatment could exacerbate a radial tunnel syndrome so it is important to make a distinction between these different conditions so proper treatment can be devised.

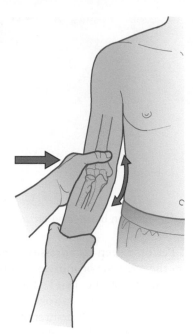

Figure 12.9 A valgus force applied to the elbow puts tensile stress on the flexor tendons.

Long periods of isometric contraction can also lead to tensile loads on the tendon fibers that cause collagen breakdown. This is especially true in occupations where the person has to grasp or hold tools or equipment in the performance of a specific job. For example, firmly holding a hammer requires strong contraction in the flexor muscles just to hold the hammer and swing it through space. Maintaining that grip when the hammer strikes a solid object is an additional load on the tendons that can lead to tendon degeneration when performed repetitively.

Medial epicondylitis also occurs from repeated throwing motions. There is a valgus force on the elbow during the throwing motion, and this force stresses the flexor tendons.[29] An illustration of valgus force on the elbow is shown in Figure 12.9. The strong valgus force on the elbow exaggerates stress on the tendons near their attachment site at the medial epicondyle.

Treatment

Traditional approaches

Conservative treatment for medial epicondylitis follows the same principles outlined above for lateral epicondylitis. A critical factor is to reduce

or eliminate activities that are causing constant or repetitive tensile loads on the tendon fibers. In most instances, conservative measures, including elbow braces, stretching, ice applications, or flexibility enhancement, are effective in treating medial epicondylitis.

Anti-inflammatory medications, whether administered orally or through corticosteroid injection, are still used to treat this condition. However, treatment with anti-inflammatory medication is questionable because the problem is not generally an inflammatory condition.[30,31] There may be short-term benefits of pain reduction with corticosteroids, but their continued use is related to long-term connective tissues damage and tendon failure.[32,33]

In some instances, conservative methods are not effective and surgery is used for treatment. Surgical treatment is similar to that used for lateral epicondylitis. Any damaged tissue will be excised and the individual is encouraged to gradually return to prior activity levels. Physical therapy and strength training during the rehabilitative phase is important to gain strength in the tissues that have been weakened by the surgical fiber disruption.

Soft-tissue manipulation

General guidelines   Soft-tissue treatment of medial epicondylitis uses the same general guidelines as treatment for lateral epicondylitis described above. The difference is that in this case attention is focused on the wrist flexors instead of the extensors. Rest from offending activities and reduction of hypertonicity in the flexor muscles are essential components of the rehabilitation process. Massage treatment begins with compressive effleurage and general sweeping cross fiber movements. Deep compression broadening to the wrist flexor muscles helps reduce hypertonicity, enhance pliability, and decrease the tensile load on the flexor tendons. In addition, deep longitudinal stripping and some of its variations are used to help encourage elongation and elasticity in the flexor muscles. These techniques are also effective for identifying and treating myofascial trigger points.

At later stages of the rehabilitation when the tendons become less sensitive, shortening and lengthening active engagement techniques are used to enhance the effects of pressure and movement. These techniques may be used earlier in the treatment program if the condition is not severe. They are also valuable as a preventive strategy when trying to keep the forearm's soft tissues resilient and prevent overuse injury.

The primary tissue dysfunction (collagen degeneration of the flexor tendons) is effectively treated with deep friction massage. The purpose of deep friction massage treatment is to stimulate collagen production in the damaged tendon tissue. Stretching of the flexor tendons is also helpful during and after the soft-tissue treatment, and should be regularly performed by the client at home.

Suggested techniques and methods

A. Sweeping cross fiber to wrist flexors This technique helps reduce tension in the wrist flexor group and prepare the muscles for deeper work. It is easily performed in conjunction with effleurage when first beginning treatment. Use one hand to hold the client's wrist and the other hand to perform a sweeping cross fiber technique to the wrist flexors (Fig. 12.10). Work the entire length of the forearm from the wrist to the elbow. Use caution with pressure applied in the sweeping thumb motion as you near the flexor attachments at the medial epicondyle. The ulnar nerve is somewhat superficial in this region and you can put adverse pressure on it.

B. Compression broadening to wrist flexors After initial effleurage and cross fiber work, the wrist flexor muscles are worked deeper in a cross fiber direction with deep broadening techniques. The client is supine with the forearm supported

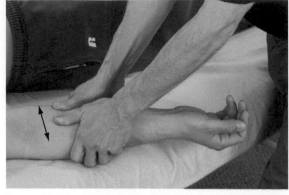

Figure 12.11   Compression broadening on wrist flexors.

by the table. Perform deep compression-broadening strokes on the wrist flexor muscle group using the thenar eminence of the hand (Fig. 12.11). Each compression-broadening stroke is a cross fiber movement so it doesn't matter if they are moving progressively toward the elbow or toward the wrist.

C. Deep longitudinal stripping to wrist flexors Tissue elasticity is enhanced and muscle tension further reduced with deep stripping techniques. The client is supine on the treatment table. Use the fingers or thumb to perform a deep longitudinal stripping technique on the wrist flexors that begins at the wrist and continues to the flexor attachment site at the medial epicondyle (Fig. 12.12). This stroke is using deep specific pressure on the extremities, so follow the venous return with this stroke and move distal to proximal with each stripping motion. Continue the technique in successive strips until the entire muscle group has been treated.

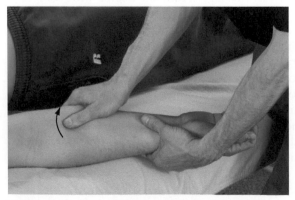

Figure 12.10   Sweeping cross fiber to wrist flexors.

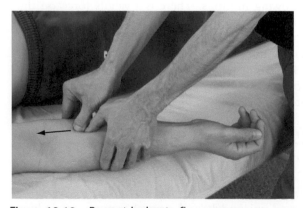

Figure 12.12   Deep stripping to flexor group.

D. Active engagement shortening techniques At the later stages of rehabilitation the intensity of pressure can be increased with active engagement techniques. The client is supine with a towel, bolster, or other support under the wrist so full wrist flexion and extension is possible. Just like for lateral epicondylitis if a wrist support is not available, the technique can be performed with the client's hand off the edge of the table. The client moves the wrist through full flexion and extension at a moderately slow pace while a compression-broadening stroke is applied to the wrist flexor muscle group (Fig. 12.13). Gradually work the entire length of the flexors, performing the stroke on each wrist flexion until the entire muscle has been treated. To increase the muscle recruitment and effectiveness of this technique, hand-held weights or resistance bands can be used during the wrist flexion in the same way it was pictured and described for lateral epicondylitis in Figure 12.5. The only difference is that the weight or resistance will be in wrist flexion instead of extension.

E. Active engagement lengthening techniques Active engagement lengthening achieves greater pliability and flexibility enhancement. The client is in the same position as D above using either a support under the wrist or the hand dropped off the side of the table. The client moves the wrist through full flexion and extension at a moderately slow pace. Perform a deep longitudinal stripping technique in a distal to proximal direction during each eccentric wrist extension movement

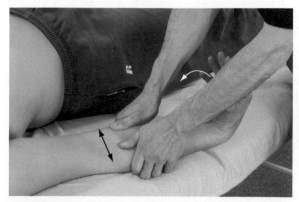

Figure 12.13 Active engagement shortening to wrist flexors.

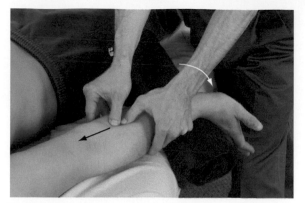

Figure 12.14 Active engagement lengthening to wrist flexors.

(Fig. 12.14). Each stripping technique covers about 3–4 inches. Pause during the wrist flexion and apply another stripping technique from where the last one stopped during the next wrist extension movement. Continue this series of stripping motions until the entire muscle has been adequately covered. Hand-held weights, resistance bands or manual resistance can be used to enhance the effectiveness of this technique just like it was described for lateral epicondylitis in Figure 12.7. The only difference is that in this technique the increased resistance is with the flexor group instead of the extensors.

F. Deep friction to common flexor tendons Friction techniques stimulate fibroblast proliferation in the tendon and enhance collagen repair in order to heal the damaged tendon. However, this is a slow physiological process, so quick or immediate results from treatment should not be expected. The wrist is in an extended position because keeping the tendon on stretch helps the effectiveness of this technique. Use the fingertips or thumb to perform the deep friction technique to the common wrist flexor tendons, transversely or longitudinally (Fig. 12.15).

Rehabilitation protocol considerations
- See the rehabilitation protocol considerations for lateral epicondylitis, which are the same for medial epicondylitis except the focus is on the wrist flexors instead of the wrist extensors.

Cautions and contraindications The ulnar nerve courses through the cubital tunnel near the medial epicondyle of the humerus (see the discussion of cubital tunnel syndrome below). Ulnar nerve

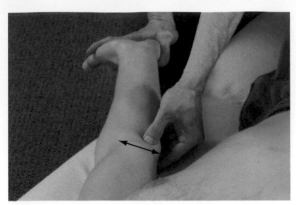

Figure 12.15 Deep friction on the common flexor tendons.

compression pathologies can produce symptoms similar to medial epicondylitis and sometimes be mistaken for this condition so proper assessment is important to distinguish these different pathologies. Use caution when performing friction techniques to the proximal flexor tendons as pressure can be accidentally applied to the nerve. The nerve is close to the skin surface in this region, so use care with cryotherapy approaches to make sure the cold application does not cause nerve damage.

CUBITAL TUNNEL SYNDROME

Description

The upper extremity is plagued by nerve compression pathologies where soft tissues compress the adjacent nerves. While carpal tunnel syndrome is a well-known, upper-extremity, nerve-compression pathology, cubital tunnel syndrome has received less attention, although it occurs with moderate frequency. The condition has been reported as the second most common peripheral compression neuropathy.[34]

The cubital tunnel is the space between two heads of the flexor carpi ulnaris muscle on the posterior side of the elbow. One head is derived from the common flexor tendon attachments at the medial epicondyle of the humerus. The other head originates on the medial aspect of the olecranon process. The two heads eventually join to form the prominent belly of the flexor carpi ulnaris. In the elbow region where the two heads are separated, the ulnar nerve travels between them and this region is the cubital tunnel (Fig. 12.16). In cubital tunnel

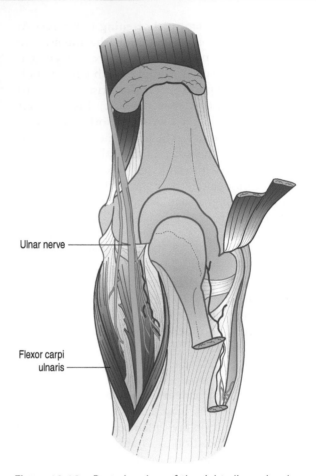

Ulnar nerve

Flexor carpi ulnaris

Figure 12.16 Posterior view of the right elbow showing the ulnar nerve entering the cubital tunnel between the two heads of the flexor carpi ulnaris.

syndrome the ulnar nerve is compressed by one or both heads of the flexor carpi ulnaris muscle.

Cubital tunnel syndrome can develop from several factors, including external forces such as leaning on the elbow for long periods, as well as repetitive motion, throwing, or prolonged elbow flexion.[35] Certain movements or positions can aggravate nerve compression in the cubital tunnel. During flexion of the elbow, the two heads of the flexor carpi ulnaris are pulled apart as the olecranon process moves slightly away from the humerus. As this occurs the tunnel becomes narrower and pressure increases on the ulnar nerve. Volume in the cubital tunnel can decrease by as much as 55% during elbow flexion.[34]

Symptoms of cubital tunnel syndrome include pain, paresthesia, or numbness in the ulnar aspect of the hand. Problems with muscle weakness in the hand can also occur because the ulnar nerve innervates a number of muscles in the hand. Atrophy or muscle wasting may be apparent on the thenar eminence of the hand from impaired nerve function. Ulnar nerve motor dysfunction causes an inability to grip and hold objects between the thumb and fingers. The adductor pollicis muscle, innervated by the ulnar nerve, is necessary for this pinch grip action of the thumb. These indicators of motor dysfunction help identify cubital tunnel syndrome. In some upper-extremity nerve compression pathologies, such as carpal tunnel syndrome, there is a greater percentage of sensory symptoms. In cubital tunnel syndrome motor symptoms are more typical.[36]

Treatment

Traditional approaches

If this condition has occurred from external pressure, such as leaning on the elbows for prolonged periods, or a direct blow to the area, the most important factor for proper rehabilitation is removal of those external forces. Nerve damage from compression can take a long time to heal, depending on the amount of compression applied and for how long (see the discussion in Chapter 2 on nerve compression injuries). In some cases a splint may be used to immobilize the elbow and wrist to keep from further aggravation of the nerve.[37] Elbow flexion at night can aggravate the problem because of increased neural compression in the cubital tunnel. Splinting the elbow at night to prevent flexion can be a valuable part of treatment.[38]

If conservative treatment is not successful, there are several surgical procedures that may be used to treat cubital tunnel syndrome. One of the most frequently used procedures is called an anterior transposition. In this procedure the ulnar nerve is repositioned so it is not compressed in the cubital tunnel. Other procedures include removing a portion of the medial epicondyle and slicing the aponeurosis that covers the tunnel to make more room for the nerve.[39]

Soft-tissue manipulation

General guidelines   Massage for cubital tunnel syndrome focuses on relieving ulnar nerve pressure by the soft tissues. The flexor carpi ulnaris is the primary problem so attention focuses on techniques designed to reduce tension in the wrist flexor group. Stretching (mobilizing) the ulnar nerve is a valuable aspect of treatment because lack of neural mobility can be a causative factor in the condition.[40]

Massage treatment should emphasize treating soft tissues throughout the entire length of the ulnar nerve in the upper extremity. A double or multiple crush nerve dysfunction could exist, so freeing the ulnar nerve along its entire path is important (see the discussion in Chapter 2 on the double or multiple nerve crush phenomenon). When addressing neural compression and tension pathologies, assume there may be more than one site of irritation. All potential sites of ulnar nerve entrapment should be addressed to give the nerve tissue the greatest chance for healthy biomechanics and function. Additional areas to focus soft-tissue treatment include the region between the anterior and middle scalene muscles, under the clavicle and pectoralis minor muscle, near the elbow, and in the wrist at the Guyon's canal.

Suggested techniques and methods

A. Sweeping cross fiber to wrist flexors Sweeping cross fiber to wrist flexors reduces tension in the wrist flexor group. Muscle tension can contribute to neural compression or restriction. Use one hand to hold the client's wrist and the other hand to perform a sweeping cross fiber technique to the wrist flexors (Fig. 12.10). Work the entire length of the forearm from the wrist to the elbow. Use caution with the amount of pressure in the sweeping thumb motion near the flexor attachments at the medial epicondyle. This is the region where the ulnar nerve is likely being compressed in the cubital tunnel.

B. Deep longitudinal stripping to flexor carpi ulnaris Tissue elasticity is enhanced and muscle tension reduced in the flexor carpi ulnaris with deep stripping techniques. Use the fingers or thumb to perform a deep longitudinal stripping technique on the flexor carpi ulnaris and other wrist flexors (Fig. 12.12). This stroke uses deep specific pressure on the extremities, so follow the venous return with this stroke and move distal to proximal with each stripping motion. Continue the technique in successive strips until the entire area has been treated. Use caution with pressure near the cubital tunnel so nerve compression is not aggravated.

C. Active engagement shortening techniques
Muscle tension in the flexor carpi ulnaris can be further reduced with active engagement techniques. The client is supine with a towel, bolster, or other support under the wrist so full wrist flexion and extension is possible. If a wrist support is not available, the technique can be performed with the client's hand off the edge of the table. The client moves the wrist through full flexion and extension at a moderately slow pace. Perform a compression broadening technique to the wrist flexor muscle group during each wrist flexion movement (Fig. 12.13). Gradually work the entire length of the flexors, performing compression broadening during each wrist flexion.

D. Active engagement lengthening techniques
Active engagement lengthening helps achieve greater pliability and flexibility enhancement. It can also encourage greater neural mobility. The client is in the same position as C above using either a support under the wrist or the hand dropped off the side of the table. The client moves the wrist through full flexion and extension at a moderately slow pace. Perform a deep longitudinal stripping technique in a distal to proximal direction during each eccentric wrist extension movement (Fig. 12.14). Each stripping technique covers about 3–4 inches. Pause during the wrist flexion and apply another stripping technique from where the last one stopped during the next wrist extension movement. Address all wrist flexors, but pay particular attention to the flexor carpi ulnaris.

E. Ulnar neural mobility If soft-tissue adhesion is binding the ulnar nerve in the cubital tunnel, neural mobility techniques help mobilize the nerve and free the adhesions restricting it. Ulnar neural mobility techniques can be performed in any position and the client can use these techniques on their own at home. Begin with the arm at the side with the elbow extended and the wrist in a neutral position. Slowly bring the extremity into a position of elbow flexion, full wrist extension and shoulder abduction to stretch the nerve and enhance mobility (Fig. 12.17). Bring the extremity only to the point where symptoms are first felt. Once that point is reached, bring the arm back into a slackened position for the nerve (toward the original starting position). Again, take the arm to the fully stretched position, stop when symptoms are felt,

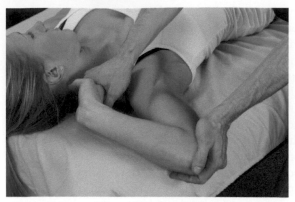

Figure 12.17   Neural stretching for ulnar nerve.

and return it to a neutral position. This cycle of neural stretch and relaxation is repeated a number of times to encourage mobility of the ulnar nerve in the cubital tunnel region. However, if neural symptoms are increased with the movements, do not continue the process.

Rehabilitation protocol consideration

- Nerves damaged by compression are slow to heal. Cubital tunnel syndrome is a chronic condition, so do not expect immediate results with treatment.

- Initial treatment should focus on reducing tension in the flexor carpi ulnaris muscle. Depending on the severity of the condition, symptoms may be too strong to initiate neural stretching procedures until later stages of rehabilitation.

- Stretching for the wrist flexor muscles should be incorporated along with soft-tissue treatment. Stretching should be encouraged at home as well.

- Some individuals find benefit with elbow braces that prevent full elbow flexion at night while asleep. This can help decrease overall compression on the ulnar nerve.

Cautions and contraindications   Use caution with massage techniques performed in this region where pressure is applied near the cubital tunnel. Additional pressure to nerve compression pathology is counterproductive and can exacerbate the condition. The space within the tunnel is reduced during elbow flexion, so be cautious with pressure applied in the cubital tunnel region when the elbow is flexed. Some people advocate ice applications to address pain sensations. However, the ulnar nerve is superficial and close to the skin in this region and thus vulnerable to nerve damage from cold applications so caution is advised.

PRONATOR TERES SYNDROME

Description

Pronator teres syndrome (PTS) is a median nerve compression pathology frequently mistaken for carpal tunnel syndrome. Carpal tunnel syndrome is a widely known nerve compression pathology. As a result, some health care providers are quick to diagnose the condition without fully exploring other possibilities. PTS produces similar symptoms and some suggest that pronator teres entrapment is under-diagnosed. This is one of the reasons for a high percentage of failed carpal tunnel syndrome surgeries.[41,42]

In PTS the pronator teres muscle is compressing the median nerve near the elbow. There are two separate heads of the pronator teres muscle (Fig. 12.18). The median nerve passes between

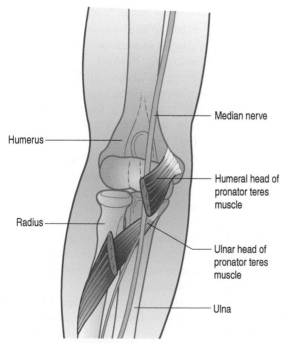

Figure 12.18   Anterior view of the right elbow showing the median nerve coursing between the two heads of the pronator teres.

the two heads of the pronator teres muscle and this is where compression occurs. Several factors can be responsible for median nerve compression in PTS. These factors include hypertonicity of the pronator teres muscle, fibrous bands within the muscle, and anatomical anomalies of the muscle. A tight pronator teres that compresses the median nerve results from repetitive motions of the elbow in flexion and/or forearm in pronation. Repetitive motions in numerous occupations, for example construction or assembly line work, create sufficient tension in the pronator teres muscle to produce nerve compression;

Muscles can also have strong fibrous bands throughout their length. These fibrous bands are tough and can compress more delicate structures like a nerve. Surgical dissections have identified fibrous bands in the pronator teres muscle and suggest these bands are frequent contributors to median nerve compression.[43]

Certain anatomical anomalies also contribute to nerve compression in PTS. In some cases, the median nerve runs deep to both heads of the pronator teres muscle. In this case, the pronator teres can compress the median nerve against the ulna. Other anatomical anomalies include nerve compression resulting from a median nerve running directly though one of the two heads of the pronator teres.[44]

Clients with pronator teres syndrome are most likely to describe mild or moderate aching in the forearm. There may also be descriptions of sharp, shooting, pains into the hand along the sensory distribution of the median nerve. Paresthesia may be present, but the paresthesia is not often as clearly limited to the hand as with carpal tunnel syndrome. Repetitive motions that involve the elbow can also aggravate the condition.

Unlike clients with carpal tunnel syndrome who may experience night pain those with pronator teres syndrome usually do not. Prolonged wrist flexion during sleep aggravates carpal tunnel syndrome because that position compresses the median nerve in the carpal tunnel. Wrist flexion does not affect the pronator teres muscle, so nerve compression by the pronator teres is not increased at night.

Another cause of median nerve compression near the pronator teres is a fibrous band from the biceps brachii muscle. This fibrous band connects the distal portion of the biceps brachii to the forearm. The fibrous band is called the lacertus fibrosus. The median nerve passes underneath the lacertus fibrosus, and can be compressed by it, especially during repetitive strong contractions of the biceps brachii. Median nerve compression by the lacertus fibrosus is easily mistaken for pronator teres syndrome, though it is treated in a similar way to PTS with more focus on the biceps brachii muscle group.

Treatment

Traditional approaches

As with all nerve compression pathologies, the primary focus of treatment is to reduce offending activities that aggravate the problem. It may not be possible to completely eliminate these activities, but they should be decreased. Splints or braces are sometimes used to alter biomechanical patterns that contribute to the problem. If conservative treatment of PTS is not successful, surgery is sometimes used. Surgical procedures focus on releasing constricting tissues such as fibrous bands within the muscle or a portion of the pronator teres muscle.[45] While surgery may be successful in relieving symptoms in some cases, it is not clear that there is a need for surgery in most cases.[36]

Soft-tissue manipulation

General guidelines The pronator teres muscle is synergistic with the wrist flexor muscles. Consequently, treatment of the wrist flexors is an important first step in addressing pronator teres dysfunction. Following general treatment of the flexor muscles in the forearm, address the pronator teres with more specific treatment. Hypertonicity of the pronator teres is a primary aspect of this condition, so techniques that are specifically designed to reduce tension in the pronator teres are particularly valuable. Specific treatment is applied through deep stripping, active engagement, as well as pin and stretch techniques.

As with other nerve compression and tension neuropathies, it is important to address additional regions along the nerve's pathway where mobility restrictions can occur. Lack of neural mobility in these regions can sensitize the median nerve and make it more prone to aggravation by pronator

teres entrapment. Additional locations of entrapment include the region between the anterior and middle scalene muscles, underneath the clavicle, underneath the pectoralis minor muscle, along the anterior aspect of the elbow, and in the wrist at the carpal tunnel. Neural stretching techniques are used to improve mobility of the median nerve as it passes through these various regions. Perform the neural stretching procedures after other soft-tissue manipulation strategies for the flexors and pronator teres. Reduced tension in these other soft-tissues enhances neural mobility.

Suggested techniques and methods

A. Deep stripping to wrist flexor group General massage applications are performed on the wrist flexor group prior to deep stripping techniques. After general applications decrease tension, more specific treatment is used on the proximal end of the wrist flexors near the pronator teres attachment. The client is supine on the treatment table. Use the fingers or thumb to perform a deep longitudinal stripping technique on the wrist flexors that begins at the wrist and continues to the flexor attachment site at the medial epicondyle (Fig. 12.12). This stroke uses deep specific pressure on the extremities, so follow the venous return with this stroke and move distal to proximal with each stripping motion. Continue the technique in successive strips until the entire muscle group has been treated.

B. Compression broadening for wrist flexors The client is supine with the forearm supported by the table. Perform compression broadening strokes on the wrist flexor muscle group using the thenar eminence of the hand (Fig. 12.11). Each compression broadening stroke is a cross fiber movement so it does not matter if the stroke moves progressively toward the elbow or toward the wrist. This technique works toward reducing tension and enhancing pliability in the wrist flexor muscles as they can contribute to developed tension in the pronator teres.

C. Active engagement lengthening to wrist flexors The client is in the same position as B above using either a support under the wrist or the hand dropped off the side of the table. The client moves the wrist through full flexion and extension at a moderately slow pace. Perform a deep longitudinal stripping technique in a distal to proximal direction during each eccentric wrist extension movement (Fig. 12.14). Each stripping technique covers about 3–4 inches. Pause during the wrist flexion. Then during the next wrist extension movement apply another stripping technique from where the last stroke stopped. Continue this series of stripping motions during movement until the entire muscle has been adequately covered. Hand-held weights, resistance bands, or manual resistance can be used to enhance the effectiveness of this technique.

D. Pin and stretch for pronator teres The pronator teres is a difficult muscle to isolate for stretching or massage treatment. The pin and stretch technique is a great way to apply more specific treatment to the pronator teres and reduce adverse compression of the median nerve. The client is in a supine position with the elbow partially flexed. Grasp the client's hand as if in a handshake position. While holding the client's hand in the handshake position, fully pronate the client's forearm, thus shortening the pronator teres muscle. Apply pressure to the pronator teres muscle with the thumb of the opposite hand (Fig. 12.19). The pronator teres can be located by first finding the gap on the anterior elbow region between the forearm flexors and extensors. Place the thumb in the gap between those two muscle groups. When the thumb is pushed medially the pronator teres is the first muscle encountered. Maintain pressure on the pronator teres while supinating the client's

forearm with the hand that is holding the client's hand. The thumb of one hand performs the pin while the thumb of the other hand performs the stretch.

E. Active engagement lengthening for pronator teres The client and practitioner are in the same starting position as in C above with one hand grasping the client's hand in the handshake position and the other thumb applying pressure to the pronator teres muscle. With the pronator teres in the shortened position, instruct the client to hold that position while attempting to supinate the client's wrist. Once an isometric contraction is established, instruct the client to slowly release the contraction. As the client slowly lets go, the client's hand turns so the forearm moves in supination. As the forearm is supinated, perform a stripping technique directly on the pronator teres muscle (Fig. 12.20).

Rehabilitation protocol considerations

- As with other nerve compression pathologies, nerve damage is slow to heal. Immediate or rapid results can occur but resolution of the condition is more likely to be a slow and gradual process.

- The symptoms of pronator teres syndrome and carpal tunnel syndrome can be identical and it can be difficult to isolate exactly where the nerve compression is occurring. In the event of apparent distal median nerve pathology it is advantageous to treat for both pronator teres and carpal tunnel syndromes as long as the symptoms are not aggravated.

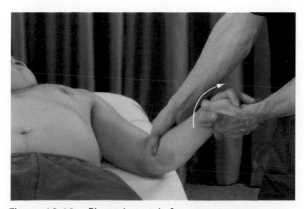

Figure 12.19 Pin and stretch for pronator teres.

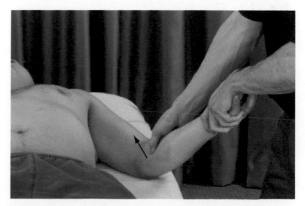

Figure 12.20 Active engagement lengthening for pronator teres.

- If the condition is severe, treatments such as the pin and stretch or active engagement lengthening for pronator teres may be too intense for the client. Reserve these techniques for later stages of the rehabilitation process or for conditions that are not severe to begin with.

- Stretching for the wrist flexor muscles should be incorporated along with soft-tissue treatment. Stretching should be encouraged at home as well.

- If symptoms are severe and soft-tissue treatment aggravates neurological sensations, decrease the pressure level and duration of treatment until a tolerable level is found for the client.

Cautions and contraindications Use caution when performing techniques directly on the pronator teres muscle because pressure might be applied very close to the region of nerve entrapment. If the client reports additional symptoms of nerve compression during the technique release pressure in that region and move to another location on the muscle that does not further compress the nerve. Pressure on hypertonic muscles can be uncomfortable and increase pain or discomfort, but is still beneficial treatment. However, additional pressure on a site of nerve compression is not helpful and should be avoided. If pressure increases radiating neurological sensations it is likely that the treatment is putting pressure on a nerve and that pressure must be ceased.

CARPAL TUNNEL SYNDROME

Description

Carpal tunnel syndrome (CTS) is the most well-defined and frequently studied upper-extremity entrapment neuropathy. As a result there is a good understanding of the various causes of this problem. Yet, because CTS has become so widely known, there is a tendency to assume CTS is the cause of symptoms, which can lead to overlooking other upper-extremity neuropathies. CTS can occur alongside another compression condition in the hand involving the ulnar nerve in the Guyon's canal (see below).

The carpal tunnel is bounded by the carpal bones and the transverse carpal ligament (TCL) (also called the flexor retinaculum). The flexor retinaculum attaches to the pisiform and hamate on the medial side and then spans the tunnel to connect with the trapezium and scaphoid on the lateral side (Fig. 12.21). Nine flexor tendons and the median nerve course through the carpal tunnel. The tendons in the tunnel include the flexor pollicis longus, four flexor digitorum superficialis tendons, and four flexor digitorum profundus tendons. The median nerve is the most superficial structure of those in the tunnel and, therefore, very likely to be compressed against the TCL.[46]

The problem of carpal tunnel syndrome is usually an intrinsic pathology. That means the nerve compression occurs from factors within the tunnel as opposed to pressure or forces applied from

---

Box 12.2   Clinical Tip

Median nerve entrapment, especially in the carpal tunnel, is one of the most common upper-extremity injuries. While the carpal tunnel is the likely site for median nerve entrapment, there are at least half a dozen potential sites of nerve entrapment between the neck and hand. In many cases, a carpal tunnel syndrome becomes more symptomatic than it normally would because there is at least one additional location of nerve compromise along the median nerve's path. Even a partial nerve entrapment can complicate the condition.

Traditional treatments for carpal tunnel syndrome often only focus attention on the carpal tunnel itself at the base of the hand. The contribution of nerve entrapments in other locations can be overlooked. An advantage of massage therapy treatment is the amount of time the practitioner spends with the client and the subsequent thoroughness of soft-tissue treatment that can be applied throughout the entire upper extremity. Extensive massage treatment along the entire path of the median nerve helps make sure any of these potential sites of nerve entrapment are properly neutralized.

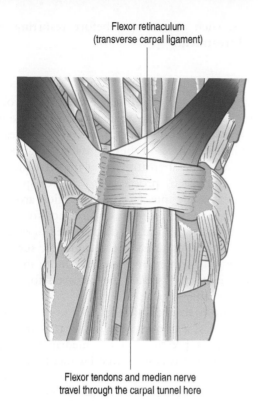

Flexor retinaculum
(transverse carpal ligament)

Flexor tendons and median nerve
travel through the carpal tunnel here

Figure 12.21   Anterior view of the left wrist showing the carpal tunnel.

outside the tunnel. One of the most common causes for tunnel compression is tenosynovitis in the flexor tendons that travel through the tunnel. The flexor tendons must bend during wrist flexion or extension. A synovial sheath encloses the tendons to reduce friction during these movements. As a result of overuse, adhesion or inflammation can develop between the tendons and their synovial sheath. This is tenosynovitis and it increases the size of the tendon sheaths due to the inflammatory reaction. The increased tendon sheath size takes up additional space in the tunnel causing compression of the median nerve.

Differences in the shape of the wrist play a role in decreasing space in the tunnel as well. Kuhlman and Hennessey present a ratio of measuring the width and height of the carpal tunnel to describe the interior shape of the tunnel.[47] Their work shows that variations in shape have a strong correlation with the likelihood for developing CTS. Cross-sections of the wrist vary in shape from square to oval. The closer a wrist cross-section

was to square, the more likely the individual would be to develop CTS. This indicates that wrist shape can be a valuable factor in assessing the presence of CTS as well.

Electrodiagnostic studies are frequently used to verify carpal tunnel syndrome, but they are not a completely reliable source of information.[48–51] In some instances, electrodiagnostic studies were not found to give any greater degree of accuracy in identifying this problem than good clinical evaluation procedures.[52] Yet, reliance on clinical tests alone also appears to lack precision, as there are significant concerns with the accuracy of commonly used clinical evaluation tests.[47,52]

Women have a greater reported incidence of CTS than men. However, it is unclear if there is a gender specific factor or if the higher occurrence is a result of greater representation of women in statistical evaluations. There are also more women in jobs that are at high risk for CTS.[53,54] These occupations generally include repetitive hand tasks, such as data entry, factory, packaging, janitorial, and cleaning jobs.

There are other factors that can lead to intrinsic compression of the median nerve in the tunnel such as fluid retention during pregnancy. Small tumors or ganglions that develop in the tunnel can also take up space. These tumor-like structures may not be painful themselves, but cause additional pressure on other structures in the tunnel such as the median nerve. An acute injury that dislocates or fractures hand bones can also create a CTS. Diabetes, arthritis, hypothyroidism, smoking, obesity, and caffeine intake have all been associated as greater risk factors for CTS.

The first and most common symptoms to appear in CTS are usually the sensory symptoms of paresthesia, numbness, and pain in the median nerve distribution of the hand. The symptoms are more often sensory than motor in CTS because the median nerve at the wrist is composed of over 90% sensory fibers and less than 10% motor fibers.[55] Symptoms are often worse at night because people bend their wrists in flexion while sleeping, and this wrist position increases compression within the tunnel. Wrist splints worn at night that keep the wrist in a neutral position can alleviate this irritation while sleeping.

If motor symptoms are present, it is usually an indication of a greater degree of pathology and nerve compression. As the condition progresses there can be a decrease in tactile sensitivity in the fingertips. Motor symptoms develop in more serious conditions and are indicated by clumsiness, loss of dexterity, and eventually a weakening of grip strength in the hand. If the condition progresses, there is a decrease in two-point discrimination ability, further sensory loss, and wasting of the muscles in the thenar aspect of the hand.

Treatment

Traditional approaches

Because CTS cases typically involve work settings, rehabilitative strategies generally focus on workplace ergonomics in an effort to reduce the aggravating occupational factors. Ergonomic interventions include wrist braces and supports, newly designed equipment, altered work schedules to mix activities, and tool redesign. There are benefits to these approaches, but no single solution is a reliable prevention strategy for work-related CTS.[56]

As with other neuropathies, reduction of offending activities is an essential aspect of the rehabilitative process. Other treatment strategies include corticosteroid injections, oral steroids, and various non-steroidal anti-inflammatory drugs. Diuretics may also be used if pressure has increased within the tunnel from fluid retention. Wrist splints are advocated, especially at night. Night splints are helpful because they do not interfere with daily activities and relief of nerve compression at night may be sufficient to adequately facilitate the healing process.

When conservative measures are unsuccessful, CTS is often treated with surgery. The primary surgical technique used to treat CTS is the release of the TCL. This procedure is performed by making an incision in the TCL in order to reduce compression of the tunnel's contents against the ligament. While this procedure can be successful, unsuccessful CTS surgery is not uncommon.[36] Because surgical outcomes for CTS are uncertain, it is valuable to fully exhaust conservative

methods, such as massage, before resorting to surgical treatment.

Soft-tissue manipulation

General guidelines   A primary part of the problem in CTS includes hypertonicity and overuse in the flexors of the wrist and hand, so CTS treatment initially focuses on these muscles. Treatment begins with general treatment on the wrist flexor muscles and then proceeds to more specific approaches on the muscles and the region around the carpal tunnel itself. Use caution not to apply adverse pressure to the median nerve, especially near the carpal tunnel. Some techniques, such as the active engagement methods are more intense for the client, and should be reserved for later stages of rehabilitation.

In addition to reducing tension on the wrist flexor muscles, a primary goal of treatment is to decrease direct pressure on the median nerve at the carpal tunnel region. While ligaments such as those that span the carpal tunnel are generally not very pliable, certain myofascial techniques have demonstrated the ability to slightly increase length in the TCL. This technique appears to be most effective when the condition is not severe.[57] There is still question about the physiology of this procedure as there are conflicting reports of how extensible and pliable the TCL actually is. Even if it is not very pliable, this technique still appears beneficial in reducing symptoms.[58]

Stretching of muscles in the forearm, especially the wrist flexors is valuable to reduce hypertonicity and overuse irritation. In addition, treat muscles and soft tissues throughout the entire upper-extremity kinetic chain, as tension in these muscles contribute to biomechanical dysfunction that eventually becomes symptomatic in the carpal tunnel.[59] In the later stages of rehabilitation neural mobilization procedures for the median nerve can also be helpful.

Suggested techniques and methods   Initial treatment of CTS focuses on the wrist flexor muscles, just as with PTS. Treatment can begin by using techniques A, B, and C listed in the previous section on PTS.

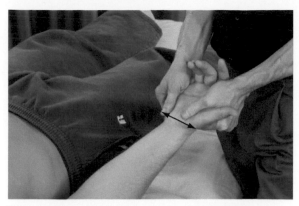

Figure 12.22 Myofascial release of transverse carpal ligament.

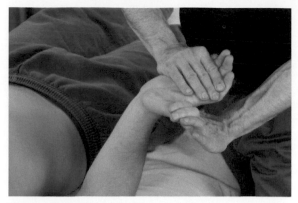

Figure 12.23 Stretching the wrist flexors and transverse carpal ligament.

A. Myofascial release of carpal tunnel This myofascial technique is used to increase length in the TCL so there is a reduction of pressure on the median nerve. The client is in a supine position with the forearm supinated so the palm is facing up. Grasp the client's hand and apply pressure in opposite directions across the base of the client's hand with the thumbs to the attachments of the TCL (Fig. 12.22). Hold this stretch position for about 20–30 seconds to enhance elongation of the TCL and flexor tendons. This technique should not increase neurological symptoms so do not continue pressure if it does. However, a short duration of symptom increase during pressure on this region should not cause adverse effects.

B. Stretching wrist flexors and transverse carpal ligament Tissue elongation for the flexor muscles and TCL is also enhanced with this myofascial procedure. Begin the technique with the client's hand in a supinated position. Pull the client's wrist into hyperextension with one hand and stretch the thumb into full extension with the other hand (Fig. 12.23). Hold this stretch position for about 20–30 seconds to enhance elongation of the TCL and flexor tendons.

C. Median nerve mobilization In the later stages of rehabilitation CTS treatment is enhanced by increasing mobilization of the median nerve so it can freely move within the tunnel. Median nerve mobilization is performed by taking the nerve to a fully stretched position, slackening the nerve somewhat, and then returning it to a stretched

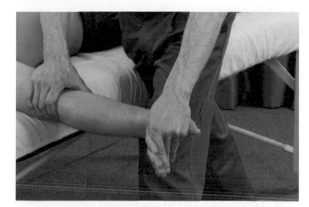

Figure 12.24 Neural stretching for median nerve.

position. The fully stretched position for the median nerve has the shoulder abducted, elbow extended, and wrist hyperextended (Fig. 12.24). Once the stretch position is reached, symptoms may recur. Do not hold the nerve in the stretched position like you would hold a muscle stretch. Immediately return the nerve to a slackened position. This stretching process is repeated multiple times to help encourage neural mobilization.

Rehabilitation protocol considerations

- As with other nerve compression pathology, nerve damage is slow to heal. Immediate or rapid results can occur but resolution of the condition is more likely to be a slow and gradual process.

- The choice of treatment techniques and approaches for this common nerve compression syndrome are highly variable. If the condition is severe and symptoms are magnified, treatment pressure, duration, and intensity must all be adjusted to the appropriate needs of the client so that aggressive work does not further exacerbate the condition.

● Techniques such as the neural mobilization procedure can aggravate nerve symptoms if performed aggressively. Use caution with these procedures and pay close attention to signs of symptom aggravation.

Cautions and contraindications Because this condition involves nerve compression, the main goal of treatment is to reduce or remove the compression on the nerve. Use caution with any technique that puts additional pressure on the carpal tunnel region. Methods such as the myofascial release technique described above may be appropriate in some cases (mild to moderate) and not appropriate in others. Appropriate clinical judgment about technique choice is essential. It is also important to evaluate the possibility of other regions of median nerve entrapment (the double or multiple crush) that can contribute to exacerbation of carpal tunnel symptoms.

DE QUERVAIN'S TENOSYNOVITIS

Description

Tenosynovitis can develop in tendons surrounded by a synovial sheath. The majority of the sheathed tendons are in the distal extremities. In tenosynovitis, repetitive overuse causes an irritation or inflammatory reaction between the tendon and its synovial sheath. The tendons of the abductor pollicis longus and extensor pollicis brevis muscles share a common synovial sheath near the styloid process of the radius. This region is known as the *anatomical snuff box* (Fig. 12.25).

The retinaculum that covers these tendons is an extension of the extensor retinaculum on the dorsal surface of the wrist. In other regions of the body, tendons course under a retinaculum without any tissue between the tendons. However, there is an anatomical variation in some individuals in which a septum or fascial wall exists between the abductor pollicis longus and extensor pollicis

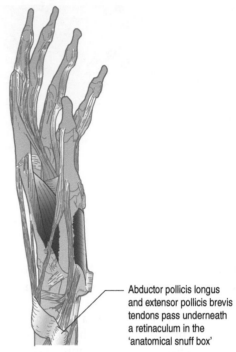

Abductor pollicis longus and extensor pollicis brevis tendons pass underneath a retinaculum in the 'anatomical snuff box'

Figure 12.25 Side view of the left wrist showing tendons of the 'anatomical snuff box.'

brevis tendons. This septum creates a smaller chamber for the extensor pollicis brevis and these individuals are more likely to develop de Quervain's tenosynovitis.[60] In a study of cadaver specimens, a septum was found in 77%, indicating that the septum is relatively common.[61]

A frequent cause of de Quervain's tenosynovitis is repetitive irritation of the tendons. The repeated friction leads to fibrous adhesion between the tendon and its synovial sheath, as well as some degree of local inflammation. This condition also develops from direct trauma, although the acute cause is not as frequent. Ordinarily, inflammation associated with de Quervain's tenosynovitis is not severe and may not be visible. Local tenderness is a more significant indicator of the underlying pathology. Tenderness is felt directly over the anatomical snuffbox when it is palpated. If the inflammation is severe, other nearby structures can be affected. The dorsal sensory branch of the radial nerve passes directly over this area. If local inflammation creates pressure on this nerve there may be paresthesia sensations in the thumb, dorsum of the hand, and index finger.[55]

Treatment

Traditional approaches

De Quervain's tenosynovitis is commonly treated with a variety of modalities, including heat, phonophoresis, and various active exercises to encourage free movement of the tendons within their sheath.[28] Cold applications may also be used to reduce local inflammatory response. If conservative treatment is not successful, corticosteroid injections are sometimes used to address the inflammation. Corticosteroids are also administered with phonophoresis or iontophoresis. There are some concerns about the effect of corticosteroids on connective tissues, so it advised that these approaches be used sparingly. If neither conservative treatment nor injection therapy yield beneficial results, surgery may be the next option. Surgical procedures focus on decompressing the tendons underneath the retinaculum. The primary problem is often the septum that exists between the abductor pollicis longus and the extensor pollicis brevis. Surgery involves cutting the septum to decompress the extensor pollicis brevis muscle.[62,63]

Soft-tissue manipulation

General guidelines Tenosynovitis develops from overuse and fatigue of the abductor pollicis longus and the extensor pollicis brevis muscles, whose tendons course underneath the retinaculum; treating the tension in these muscles is beneficial. Because they are relatively long and thin, it is most effective to treat these muscles with specific longitudinal stripping techniques. These muscles wrap around to the dorsal surface of the wrist and forearm, so the longitudinal stripping methods should focus on the distal aspect of the forearm on the dorsal surface.

Other muscles acting on the thumb can also be hypertonic from overuse, and should be treated. The extensor pollicis longus can be treated on the dorsal surface of the forearm as treatment is applied to the extensor pollicis brevis and abductor pollicis longus.

The flexor pollicis longus tendon and muscle belly are close to the anatomical snuff box, and when hypertonic can give sensations that can be confused with de Quervain's tenosynovitis. The flexor pollicis longus and eight flexor tendons lie underneath the flexor retinaculum. They can be treated with longitudinal stripping methods on the volar aspect of the distal forearm. Deep transverse friction (DTF) massage is commonly advocated for addressing tenosynovitis.[64] The pressure and transverse movement on the tendon mobilizes adhesions that have developed between the tendon and its sheath.

Prior to performing deep stripping on the thumb tendons, apply warming techniques to the area, such as effleurage or sweeping cross fiber movements. Compression broadening techniques applied to the wrist flexors and extensors is also helpful to prepare the tissues for more specific treatment.

Suggested techniques and methods

A. Deep stripping on thumb tendons Deep stripping can be used to encourage tissue lengthening after general relaxation techniques are performed on the area such as effleurage or compression broadening. Hold the client's hand or wrist in a neutral position with one hand while applying this technique with the thumb or fingers of the other hand. Apply a deep specific stripping to the tendons and muscle bellies of the abductor pollicis longus and extensor pollicis brevis (Fig. 12.26).

B. Pin and stretch on thumb tendons The primary purpose of this pin and stretch technique is to enhance mobility between the tendon and the surrounding sheath, as well as encourage

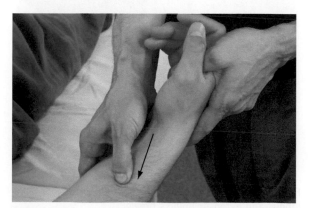

Figure 12.26 Deep stripping to abductor pollicis longus and extensor pollicis brevis.

lengthening and pliability of the affected muscles. Grasp the client's hand so that it is easy to move the hand in radial and ulnar deviation. Start with the hand in full radial deviation. While one hand holds the client's hand, apply static pressure to the abductor pollicis longus and extensor pollicis brevis muscles with the opposite thumb. While holding pressure on those muscles, pull the client's hand into ulnar deviation (Fig. 12.27). As a variation on this technique, deep stripping can be applied during the ulnar deviation instead of static compression. The deep stripping technique further enhances tissue pliability and reduction of adhesions between the tendon and synovial sheath.

C. Deep transverse friction on thumb tendons at the anatomical snuff box Adhesion between the tendons and the surrounding synovial sheath is most effectively addressed with deep transverse friction (DTF). Friction is effective in breaking up adhesions when it is performed transverse (perpendicular) to the tendon fiber direction. For best results, put the client's hand in ulnar deviation in order to keep the tendons on stretch (Fig. 12.28). Perform DTF to the affected tendons alternating the friction technique with various passive wrist movements, general effleurage, sweeping cross fiber, and other techniques to encourage greater pliability and tendon mobility. In addition to the friction

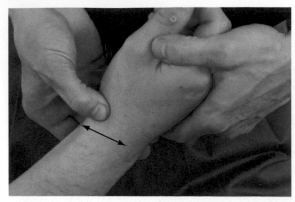

Figure 12.28   Deep transverse friction at Guyon's canal.

treatments on these tendons, encourage the client to stretch the wrist in this position on a regular basis.

Rehabilitation protocol considerations

- Reducing muscle tension in the affected muscles is an important part of addressing tendon adhesion. Make sure all forearm muscles are adequately treated in addition to the attention focused on the dysfunctional tendons.

- Friction techniques, pin and stretch, and the other techniques applied directly to the affected tendons can be uncomfortable for the client. This treatment strategy is still helpful even if it is uncomfortable. However, pain should not be unbearable. Adjust the treatment to fit the client's comfort tolerance, but explain that treatment is more effective if they can withstand tolerable discomfort.

- Ice applications are beneficial both before and after the specific stripping and friction treatments to reduce pain associated with the treatment. However, keep in mind stretching and flexibility enhancement will not be as effective immediately after the cold applications due to decreased connective tissue pliability.

Cautions and contraindications   Effective treatment of de Quervain's tenosynovitis often involves some level of discomfort for the client. Use caution when administering this treatment and pay close attention to the pain threshold of the client.

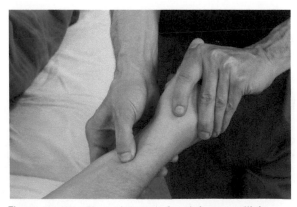

Figure 12.27   Pin and stretch for abductor pollicis longus and extensor pollicis brevis.

There are several branches of the radial nerve that are very close to the affected tendons in this region. Any sensations of paresthesia or shooting pain in the hand during treatment may indicate pressure on these nerves, and treatment should move to a different region.

Box 12.3   Clinical Tip

Few occupational injuries are as common for massage practitioners as tenosynovitis in the wrist and finger tendons. The unique hand positions used in massage and the muscular stress applied to the hands all day long put the massage practitioner's hands in a susceptible position. Tenosynovitis can be a stubborn condition that takes a long time to heal. Massage practitioners are strongly advised to take preventive measures to keep this occupational injury at bay. The techniques that are described for treating a client with this condition are easy to administer to yourself, and they are effective in prevention as well as treatment. Strength training and conditioning of the wrist, hand, and fingers is also a great way to reduce the likelihood of developing problems with overuse tenosynovitis from massage.

GUYON'S CANAL SYNDROME

Description

The ulnar nerve courses along the medial side of the forearm from the elbow to the wrist. When it reaches the wrist it enters a canal or tunnel, just like the median nerve in the carpal tunnel. This tunnel is called Guyon's canal (also called the tunnel of Guyon). The canal is the narrow space created by a division of the TCL, through which the ulnar nerve and the ulnar artery must travel (Fig. 12.28).

The space in Guyon's canal is quite narrow. However, unlike the carpal tunnel there are no tendons that pass through Guyon's canal.

Consequently, tenosynovitis causing nerve compression is not an issue for the ulnar nerve as it is for the median nerve in the carpal tunnel. Ulnar nerve compression in Guyon's canal generally results from forces outside the body pressing on the nerve as opposed to compression developing within the tunnel itself. In acute cases, the compression occurs from striking the hand. For example, banging an object or surface with the base of the palm can lead to ulnar nerve compression.

Chronic compression of the ulnar nerve at Guyon's canal is more common than acute injury. It develops in activities such as long distance cycling because of the cyclist's hand position on the handlebars and the pressure placed directly on Guyon's canal. When it occurs in cyclists, the condition is called handlebar palsy. A similar situation develops where pressure on the handle of a cane used to assist in walking creates chronic nerve compression. Guyon's canal syndrome also commonly results from occupational disorders. For example, it occurs in construction workers who hold tools in a position so that chronic pressure is placed on the nerve.

Symptoms of ulnar nerve compression in the Guyon's canal include sensory impairment or paresthesia sensations that are felt in the cutaneous distribution of the ulnar nerve which includes half of the ring finger and pinky. Pressure applied directly over Guyon's canal aggravates the sensory symptoms. Motor symptoms of weakness and/or atrophy are common for ulnar neuropathy at the wrist because the ulnar nerve supplies a number of muscles in the hand.

The ulnar nerve also supplies motor fibers to the adductor pollicis muscle of the thumb. The adductor pollicis muscle plays an important role in opposition movements of the thumb. Opposition is the combined movement of the thumb where the pad of the thumb is brought into contact with the pads of one or more of the other fingers. If there is impaired nerve function to the adductor pollicis muscle, the individual has difficulty maintaining a strong pinch grip between the thumb and fingers.

Several other factors can lead to Guyon's canal syndrome. Fractures of the carpal bones either at the time of an acute injury or sometime later during the healing process can produce nerve compression. Small fibrous tumors, cysts, or blood clots in Guyon's canal have also been identified as a cause of the condition.[65] Symptoms of ulnar nerve compression can occur along with symptoms of CTS.

Treatment

Traditional approaches

Conservative approaches are the usual treatment for Guyon's canal syndrome. Nerve compression usually results from compression on the palm so rest from aggravating activity is the first step. Reduction of offending activities is essential to allow for adequate nerve fiber healing time. Wrist splints are helpful as they can reduce additional irritation from neural tension developed during wrist extension. These are particularly useful at night to keep the hand in a neutral position to relieve pressure and encourage nerve healing. As long as compression is not severe, the nerve damage usually repairs on its own, although the rate of healing is slow. The healing rate is dependent on how long the nerve compression has existed and how severe it is. The longer the compression pathology has been present, the slower it is to heal. A nerve conduction velocity test is sometimes performed in order to identify the compression site. Surgical decompression of the nerve is sometimes performed, but not often. Since pathologies of ulnar neuropathy at the wrist likely involve external factors of compression, removal of that compression is usually sufficient to treat the problem.

Soft-tissue manipulation

Because there are no tendons traveling through Guyon's canal as there are in the carpal tunnel, there is not a significant musculotendinous contribution to this problem. External compression

of the nerve has caused the condition. For this reason, massage techniques should not put additional pressure in the Guyon's canal region. Massage may give some symptomatic relief in the region and elsewhere through the upper extremity if adverse neural tension has contributed to the nerve irritation.

Pressure on the ulnar nerve in Guyon's canal can be aggravated by adverse tension or compression on the ulnar nerve in other regions of the upper extremity. Therefore, massage treatment should focus on enhancing mobility of the nerve throughout its entire length from the brachial plexus into the hand. Particular areas to emphasize neural mobility include the thoracic outlet region and near the cubital tunnel of the elbow. While these are the most common locations of ulnar nerve entrapment, they are certainly not the only places where nerve entrapment can occur. Consult the treatment recommendations for these other conditions (thoracic outlet syndrome and cubital tunnel syndrome) to formulate a comprehensive plan for addressing these potential ulnar nerve restrictions in the upper extremity.

Suggested techniques and methods

A. Compression broadening to wrist flexors After superficial warming techniques such as effleurage and sweeping cross fiber, attention can focus on enhancing neural mobility by treating the forearm flexors. The wrist flexor muscles are worked with compression broadening techniques. The client is supine with the forearm supported by the table. Perform the strokes on the wrist flexor muscle group using the thenar eminence of the hand (Fig. 12.11). Each compression broadening stroke is a cross fiber movement so it does not matter if the strokes move progressively toward the elbow or toward the wrist.

B. Deep stripping to wrist flexor group Tissue elasticity is enhanced and muscle tension is reduced with deep stripping techniques. This technique can aid mobility of the ulnar nerve. Use the fingers or thumb to perform a deep longitudinal stripping technique on the wrist flexors that begins at the wrist and continues to the flexor attachment site at the medial epicondyle (Fig. 12.12). This stroke uses deep specific pressure on the extremities, so follow the direction of venous return and move distal to proximal with each stripping motion. Continue the technique in successive strips until the entire muscle group has been treated.

C. Myofascial release of transverse carpal ligament This technique is aimed at reducing tension in the TCL, especially in the treatment of CTS. It can also be helpful for Guyon's canal syndrome because the ulnar nerve is underneath a portion of the TCL. The client is supine with the forearm supinated so the palm is facing up. Grasp the client's hand and apply pressure in opposite directions across the base of the client's hand with the thumbs to the attachments of the TCL (Fig. 12.22). Hold this stretch position for about 20–30 seconds to enhance elongation of the TCL and flexor tendons. This technique should not increase neurological symptoms so do not continue pressure for a prolonged period if it does. However, a short duration of symptom increase during pressure on this region should not cause adverse effects.

D. Ulnar nerve mobilization Symptoms of Guyon's canal syndrome can be aggravated if there is adverse neural tension on the ulnar nerve. This technique enhances mobility throughout the length of the ulnar nerve. Begin with the client's arm at the side with the elbow extended and the wrist in a neutral position. Moving the upper extremity at a moderate pace to stretch and mobilize the ulnar nerve, bring the extremity into a position of elbow flexion, full wrist extension and shoulder abduction (Fig. 12.17). Bring the client's arm only to the point where symptoms are first felt. Once that point is reached, bring the arm back into a slackened position for

the nerve (toward the original starting position). Repeat this process of neural stretch and relaxation a number of times to encourage mobility of the ulnar nerve along its length. Emphasize the wrist extension and elbow flexion to encourage greater emphasis of mobility in the distal portion of the nerve (near Guyon's tunnel). If neural symptoms increase with the movements, do not continue the process.

Rehabilitation protocol considerations

- If the nerve compression has occurred from a direct blow to the nerve, such as hitting the hand or palm on a hard object, the canal region is likely to be tender and easily reproduce symptoms. Choose treatment techniques that do not put any additional stress on this region.

- Guyon's canal compression syndromes frequently resolve without intervention, albeit slowly, as long as the cause of external compression has been reduced or eliminated.

- Ergonomic suggestions to help reduce external nerve compression are important for those developing the condition as a result of work activities.

Cautions and contraindications Be careful about applying pressure to the anterior wrist region if the client appears to have Guyon's canal syndrome. Further compression of the nerve will not provide therapeutic benefit and will cause the condition to worsen. If irritation of the nerve is caused by a space-occupying lesion, such as a tumor or cysts, massage could be detrimental. For severe cases or when an offending activity cannot be determined, referral to another health care practitioner to rule out these causes is advised.

Box 12.4   Case Study

Background

Mia is a 37-year-old production assistant at a local news agency. She routinely works long hours and her job requires an extensive amount of work at the computer. Over the last month she has had an increased workload due to a complex story that her news organization was working on. To complete the story she had to spend several weeks traveling and doing a great deal of her work on a laptop computer, which she does not ordinarily use at the office. The laptop keyboard is much smaller than the one she is accustomed to and she had to set it on a table in her hotel room to work. She noticed that the work position felt uncomfortable and she was noticing increasing discomfort in her forearm and hand.

She describes an aching sensation on the medial side of her forearm that extends down into her hand. The pain does not appear to be localized to a single site, but is more of a generalized aching throughout the forearm. She notices that this pain is now bothering her with increasing frequency, even though she has returned to working mostly in her office once again. She has not seen a physician or other health care provider for this problem. She has had massage therapy in the past and is aware of how much it has helped her relax, so she is curious to consider if it might be helpful for this forearm and hand pain condition.

Questions to consider

- Mia's forearm pain seems to have resulted from a change in activity levels with the extensive work she was doing on a computer she was not accustomed to working on. How could this change in work environment lead to the development of her forearm pain?
- If massage treatment is deemed appropriate for her, are there other regions besides her forearm that would benefit from soft-tissue therapy?
- What kinds of things should Mia consider doing at home to help her soft-tissue treatment and prevent this kind of problem from recurring?
- If Mia has developed an overuse tendinosis in her wrist flexor muscles, would it be a good idea for her to begin a strength training and conditioning program now?
- How might muscle tightness in her upper back or neck be related to the onset of her forearm pain?
- If her forearm and hand pain appear to be caused by muscle overuse and minor nerve compression in her forearm, is massage a beneficial strategy to help her with this problem?

References

1. Melhorn JM. Cumulative trauma disorders and repetitive strain injuries. The future. Clin Orthop. 1998(351):107–126.
2. Shafer-Crane GA. Repetitive stress and strain injuries: preventive exercises for the musician. Phys Med Rehabil Clin N Am. 2006;17(4):827–842.
3. Driver DF. Occupational and physical therapy for work-related upper extremity disorders: how we can influence outcomes. Clin Occup Environ Med. 2006;5(2):471–482, xi.
4. Kraushaar BS, Nirschl RP. Tendinosis of the elbow (tennis elbow). Clinical features and findings of histological, immunohistochemical, and electron microscopy studies. J Bone Joint Surg Am. 1999;81(2):259–278.
5. Nirschl RP. Elbow tendinosis/tennis elbow. Clin Sports Med. 1992;11(4):851–870.
6. Greenbaum B, Itamura J, Vangsness CT, Tibone J, Atkinson R. Extensor carpi radialis brevis. An anatomical analysis of its origin. J Bone Joint Surg Br. 1999; 81(5):926–929.
7. Noteboom T, Cruver R, Keller J, Kellogg B, Nitz AJ. Tennis elbow: a review. J Orthop Sports Phys Ther. 1994;19(6):357–366.
8. Huysmans MA, Blatter BM, van der Beek AJ, van Mechelen W, Bongers PM. Should office workers spend fewer hours at their computer? A systematic review of the literature. Occup Environ Med. 2007;64(4):211–222.
9. Andersen JH, Harhoff M, Grimstrup S, et al. Computer mouse use predicts acute pain but not prolonged or chronic pain in the neck and shoulder. Occup Environ Med. 2008;65(2):126–131.
10. Gerr F, Monteilh CP, Marcus M. Keyboard use and musculoskeletal outcomes among computer users. J Occup Rehabil. 2006;16(3):265–277.
11. Gerr F, Marcus M, Monteilh C. Epidemiology of musculoskeletal disorders among computer users: lesson learned from the role of posture and keyboard use. J Electromyogr Kinesiol. 2004;14(1):25–31.

12. Hannan LM, Monteilh CP, Gerr F, Kleinbaum DG, Marcus M. Job strain and risk of musculoskeletal symptoms among a prospective cohort of occupational computer users. Scand J Work Environ Health. 2005;31(5):375–386.

13. Simons D, Travell J, Simons L. Myofascial Pain and Dysfunction: The Trigger Point Manual. Vol 1. 2nd ed. Baltimore: Williams & Wilkins; 1999.

14. Van De Streek MD, Van Der Schans CP, De Greef MH, Postema K. The effect of a forearm/hand splint compared with an elbow band as a treatment for lateral epicondylitis. Prosthet Orthot Int. 2004;28(2):183–189.

15. Walther M, Kirschner S, Koenig A, Barthel T, Gohlke F. Biomechanical evaluation of braces used for the treatment of epicondylitis. J Shoulder Elbow Surg. 2002;11(3):265–270.

16. Knebel PT, Avery DW, Gebhardt TL, et al. Effects of the forearm support band on wrist extensor muscle fatigue. J Orthop Sports Phys Ther. 1999;29(11):677–685.

17. Sevier TL, Wilson JK. Treating lateral epicondylitis. Sports Med. 1999;28(5):375–380.

18. Buckwalter JA. Pharmacological treatment of soft-tissue injuries. J Bone Joint Surg Amer Vol. 1995;77A(12):1902–1914.

19. Bisset L, Beller E, Jull G, Brooks P, Darnell R, Vicenzino B. Mobilisation with movement and exercise, corticosteroid injection, or wait and see for tennis elbow: randomised trial. BMJ. Nov 4 2006;333(7575):939.

20. Roberts WO. Lateral epicondylitis injection. Physician Sportsmed. 2000;28(7).

21. Organ SW, Nirschl RP, Kraushaar BS, Guidi EJ. Salvage surgery for lateral tennis elbow. Am J Sports Med. 1997;25(6):746–750.

22. Basford JR, Sheffield CG, Cieslak KR. Laser therapy: a randomized, controlled trial of the effects of low intensity Nd:YAG laser irradiation on lateral epicondylitis. Arch Phys Med Rehabil. 2000;81(11):1504–1510.

23. Stergioulas A. Effects of low-level laser and plyometric exercises in the treatment of lateral epicondylitis. Photomed Laser Surg. 2007;25(3):205–213.

24. Oken O, Kahraman Y, Ayhan F, Canpolat S, Yorgancioglu ZR, Oken OF. The short-term efficacy of laser, brace, and ultrasound treatment in lateral epicondylitis: a prospective, randomized, controlled trial. J Hand Ther. 2008;21(1):63–67; quiz 68.

25. Labelle H, Guibert R, Joncas J, Newman N, Fallaha M, Rivard CH. Lack of scientific evidence for the treatment of lateral epicondylitis of the elbow. An attempted meta-analysis. J Bone Joint Surg Br. 1992;74(5):646–651.

26. Cook JL, Khan KM, Maffulli N, Purdam C. Overuse tendinosis, not tendinitis Part 2. Applying the new approach to patellar tendinopathy. Physician Sportsmed. 2000;28(6):31+.

27. Weintraub W. Tendon and Ligament Healing. Berkeley: North Atlantic Books; 1999.

28. Malone T, McPoil T, Nitz A. Orthopedic and Sports Physical Therapy. 3rd ed. St. Louis: Mosby; 1997.

29. Chen FS, Rokito AS, Jobe FW. Medial elbow problems in the overhead-throwing athlete. J Am Acad Orthop Surg. 2001;9(2):99–113.

30. Almekinders LC, Temple JD. Etiology, diagnosis, and treatment of tendinitis – an analysis of the literature. Med Sci Sport Exercise. 1998;30(8):1183–1190.

31. Fadale PD, Wiggins ME. Corticosteroid injections: their use and abuse. J Am Acad Orthop Surg. 1994;2(3):133–140.

32. Nichols AW. Complications associated with the use of corticosteroids in the treatment of athletic injuries. Clin J Sport Med. 2005;15(5):370–375.

33. Stahl S, Kaufman T. The efficacy of an injection of steroids for medial epicondylitis – a prospective-study of 60 elbows. J Bone Joint Surg Amer Vol. 1997;79A(11):1648–1652.

34. Bozentka DJ. Cubital tunnel syndrome pathophysiology. Clin Orthop. 1998(351):90–94.

35. Aoki M, Takasaki H, Muraki T, Uchiyama E, Murakami G, Yamashita T. Strain on the ulnar nerve at the elbow and wrist during throwing motion. J Bone Joint Surg Am. 2005;87(11):2508–2514.

36. Dawson D, Hallett M, Wilbourn A. Entrapment Neuropathies. 3rd ed. Philadelphia: Lippincott–Raven; 1999.

37. Posner MA. Compressive neuropathies of the ulnar nerve at the elbow and wrist. Instr Course Lect. 2000;49:305–317.

38. Seror P. Treatment of ulnar nerve palsy at the elbow with a night splint. J Bone Joint Surg Br. 1993;75(2):322–327.

39. Mowlavi A, Andrews K, Lille S, Verhulst S, Zook EG, Milner S. The management of cubital tunnel syndrome: a meta-analysis of clinical studies. Plast Reconstr Surg. 2000;106(2):327–334.

40. Butler D. Mobilisation of the Nervous System. London: Churchill Livingstone; 1991.

41. Leahy PM. Improved treatment for carpal-tunnel and related syndromes. Chiropr Sport Med. 1995;9(1):6–9.

42. Mujadzic M, Papanicolaou G, Young H, Tsai TM. Simultaneous surgical release of ipsilateral pronator teres and carpal tunnel syndromes. Plast Reconstr Surg. 2007;119(7):2141–2147.

43. Hartz CR, Linscheid RL, Gramse RR, Daube JR. The pronator teres syndrome: compressive neuropathy of the median nerve. J Bone Joint Surg Am. 1981;63(6):885–890.

44. Tulwa N, Limb D, Brown RF. Median nerve compression within the humeral head of pronator teres. J Hand Surg [Br]. 1994;19(6):709–710.

45. Olehnik WK, Manske PR, Szerzinski J. Median nerve compression in the proximal forearm. J Hand Surg [Am]. 1994;19(1):121–126.

46. Slater R. Carpal tunnel syndrome: current concepts. Journal of Southern Orthopedic Association. 1999;8(3):203–213.

47. Kuhlman KA, Hennessey WJ. Sensitivity and specificity of carpal tunnel syndrome signs. Am J Phys Med Rehabil. 1997;76(6):451–457.

48. D'Arcy CA, McGee S. The rational clinical examination. Does this patient have carpal tunnel syndrome? JAMA. 2000;283(23):3110–3117.

49. Chan L, Turner JA, Comstock BA, et al. The relationship between electrodiagnostic findings and patient symptoms

and function in carpal tunnel syndrome. Arch Phys Med Rehabil. 2007;88(1):19–24.

50. Jarvik JG, Comstock BA, Heagerty PJ, et al. Magnetic resonance imaging compared with electrodiagnostic studies in patients with suspected carpal tunnel syndrome: predicting symptoms, function, and surgical benefit at 1 year. J Neurosurg. 2008;108(3):541–550.

51. Jordan R, Carter T, Cummins C. A systematic review of the utility of electrodiagnostic testing in carpal tunnel syndrome. Br J Gen Pract. 2002;52(481):670–673.

52. Szabo RM, Slater RR, Jr., Farver TB, Stanton DB, Sharman WK. The value of diagnostic testing in carpal tunnel syndrome. J Hand Surg [Am]. 1999;24(4): 704–714.

53. McDiarmid M, Oliver M, Ruser J, Gucer P. Male and female rate differences in carpal tunnel syndrome injuries: personal attributes or job tasks? Environ Res. 2000; 83(1):23–32.

54. Hagberg M, Morgenstern H, Kelsh M. Impact of occupations and job tasks on the prevalence of carpal tunnel syndrome. Scand J Work Environ Health. 1992; 18(6):337–345.

55. Verdon ME. Overuse syndromes of the hand and wrist. Prim Care. 1996;23(2):305–319.

56. Lincoln AE, Vernick JS, Ogaitis S, Smith GS, Mitchell CS, Agnew J. Interventions for the primary prevention of work-related carpal tunnel syndrome. Am J Prev Med. 2000;18(4 Suppl):37–50.

57. Sucher BM. Myofascial manipulative release of carpal tunnel syndrome: documentation with magnetic resonance imaging. J Am Osteopath Assoc. 1993;93(12):1273–1278.

58. Sucher BM. Myofascial release of carpal tunnel syndrome. J Am Osteopath Assoc. 1993;93(1):92–94, 100–101.

59. Donaldson CC, Nelson DV, Skubick DL, Clasby RG. Potential contributions of neck muscle dysfunctions to initiation and maintenance of carpal tunnel syndrome. Appl Psychophysiol Biofeedback. 1998;23(1):59–72.

60. Nagaoka M, Matsuzaki H, Suzuki T. Ultrasonographic examination of de Quervain's disease. J Orthop Sci. 2000; 5(2):96–99.

61. Mahakkanukrauh P, Mahakkanukrauh C. Incidence of a septum in the first dorsal compartment and its effects on therapy of de Quervain's disease. Clin Anat. 2000; 13(3):195–198.

62. Yuasa K, Kiyoshige Y. Limited surgical treatment of de Quervain's disease: decompression of only the extensor pollicis brevis subcompartment. J Hand Surg [Am]. 1998;23(5):840–843.

63. Zingas C, Failla JM, Van Holsbeeck M. Injection accuracy and clinical relief of de Quervain's tendinitis. J Hand Surg [Am]. 1998;23(1):89–96.

64. Chamberlain GL. Cyriax's friction massage: a review. J Orthop Sport Phys Therapy. 1982;4(1):16–22.

65. Sakai K, Tsutsui T, Aoi M, Sonobe H, Murakami H. Ulnar neuropathy caused by a lipoma in Guyon's canal – case report. Neurol Med Chir (Tokyo). 2000;40(6):335–338.

Index